Atlas of Oral Pathology

Current Histopathology

Consultant Editor
Professor G. Austin Gresham, TD, ScD, MD, FRC Path.
Professor of Morbid Anatomy and Histology, University of Cambridge

Volume Eight

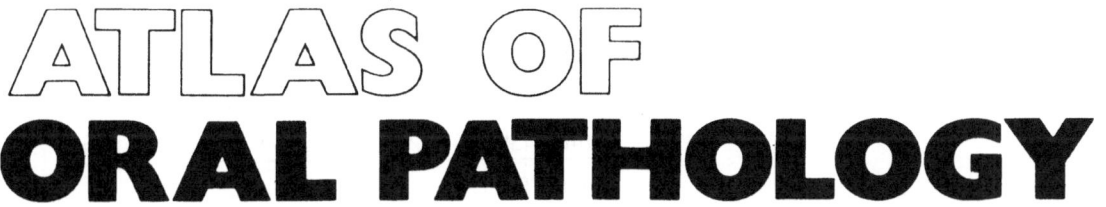

ATLAS OF ORAL PATHOLOGY

BY R. B. LUCAS

Emeritus Professor of Oral Pathology
University of London

AND J. W. EVESON

Senior Lecturer and Honorary Consultant
Department of Oral Medicine and Pathology
Guy's Hospital, London

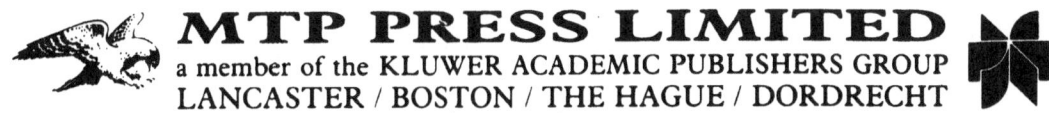

MTP PRESS LIMITED
a member of the KLUWER ACADEMIC PUBLISHERS GROUP
LANCASTER / BOSTON / THE HAGUE / DORDRECHT

Published in the UK and Europe by
MTP Press Limited
Falcon House
Queen Square
Lancaster, England

British Library Cataloguing in Publication Data

Lucas, R. B.
   Atlas of oral pathology. — (Current histopathology)
   1. Mouth—Diseases   2. Teeth—Diseases
   I. Title   II. Eveson, J. W.   III. Series
   617'.52207   RC815

Published in the USA by
MTP Press
A division of Kluwer Boston Inc.
190 Old Derby Street
Hingham, MA 02043, USA

Library of Congress Cataloging in Publication Data

Lucas, R. B. (Raleigh Barclay)
   Atlas of oral pathology.

   (Current histopathology; v. 8)
   Bibliography: p.
   Includes index.
   1. Mouth—Diseases—Atlases.   2. Histology,
Pathological—Atlases.   I. Eveson, J. W.   II. Title.
III. Series.   [DNLM: 1. Mouth diseases—Atlases.
2. Dentistry—Atlases.   W1 CU788JBA v. 8/
WU 17 L933a]
RC815.L8 1985   617'.52207   84-887
ISBN-13: 978-94-010-8959-3   e-ISBN-13: 978-94-009-5580-6
DOI: 10.1007/978-94-009-5580-6

Colour origination by Replica Photo-Litho
Reproducers Ltd, Stockport

Bound by John Sherratt and Son Limited,
Manchester

Contents

Current Histopathology Series

Consultant Editor's Note

At the present time books on morbid anatomy and histology can be divided into two broad groups: extensive textbooks often written primarily for students and monographs on research topics.

This takes no account of the fact that the vast majority of pathologists are involved in an essentially practical field of general Diagnostic Pathology providing an important service to their clinical colleagues. Many of these pathologists are expected to cover a broad range of disciplines and even those who remain solely within the field of histopathology usually have single and sole responsibility within the hospital for all this work. They may often have no chance for direct discussion on problem cases with colleagues in the same department. In the field of histopathology, no less than in other medical fields, there have been extensive and recent advances, not only in new histochemical techniques but also in the type of specimen provided by new surgical procedures.

There is a great need for the provision of appropriate information for this group. This need has been defined in the following terms:

(1) It should be aimed at the general clinical pathologist or histopathologist with existing practical training, but should also have value for the trainee pathologist.
(2) It should concentrate on the practical aspects of histopathology taking account of the new techniques which should be within the compass of the worker in a unit with reasonable facilities.
(3) New types of material, e.g. those derived from endoscopic biopsy should be covered fully.
(4) There should be an adequate number of illustrations on each subject to demonstrate the variation in appearance that is encountered.
(5) Colour illustrations should be used wherever they aid recognition.

The present concept stemmed from this definition but it was immediately realized that these aims could only be achieved within the compass of a series, of which this volume is one. Since histopathology is, by its very nature, systemized, the individual volumes deal with one system or, where this appears more appropriate, with a single organ.

Diseases of the oral tissues are dealt with in a variety of texts. There are comparatively few books that draw all aspects of oral pathology together. This book has succeeded in providing a comprehensive overview of this subject for those involved in the histopathological diagnosis of disorders of the mouth, teeth and jaws.

G. Austin Gresham
Cambridge

Preface

This *Atlas of Oral Pathology* is intended primarily as a bench companion for the general diagnostic pathologist, especially the trainee. It has not been designed to cover the subject fully and in detail, nor does it enter into the more theoretical aspects.

Since the book is essentially an atlas the text has been kept to a minimum, but in it we have tried to adopt a practical approach, with special regard to differential diagnosis. We have made some remarks about the clinical features of the various conditions dealt with, since this may help the pathologist to appreciate what is in the referring clinician's mind in an area with which the pathologist may not be particularly familiar. It is also helpful to have an idea of the clinical appearance of lesions because many oral biopsies are very small and thus the pathologist cannot obtain much assistance from the macroscopic features of specimens as they are received in the laboratory. We have therefore included a number of clinical illustrations. While these show only a few selected conditions and do not cover the full range, which would not be feasible in a work devoted essentially to histopathology, they are intended to give a general idea of the appearance and presentation of oral lesions.

In line with our endeavour to provide useful background information, we include remarks on radiographic appearances where appropriate and reproduce relevant radiographs. Every pathologist who deals with bone specimens will know the value of radiographs, and some indeed are reluctant to make a diagnosis in their absence. In addition, radiographs may give a good idea of the extent and other features of a lesion that may be represented in the first instance only by a small biopsy specimen.

While many of the illustrations have been made from sections freshly cut and stained for the purpose, others have been prepared from stained sections already in our files and since, in addition, the material comes principally from two departments, as well as from outside sources, there is appreciable variation in the final appearances of specimens stained ostensibly by the same methods. We preferred to let this variation remain, as more truly representative of day-to-day conditions in various laboratories, rather than to strive for uniformity.

Finally, while we are well aware that histopathology is best, and perhaps only, learnt by precept and personal instruction from an expert, this must be a counsel of perfection that can hardly be attainable in every field for every pathologist. We hope, therefore, that this book may be of some help to those who might not otherwise be able to obtain more adequate counsel.

Acknowledgements

We are very grateful to the numerous colleagues, in our own institutions and elsewhere, who have provided us with material. In particular, we thank Mr C. D. Allen (Figure 4.6), Professor H. J. J. Blackwood (Figures 6.39, 6.40, 6.41, 6.42), Mr R. C. Bret Day (Figure 6.30), Professor R. A. Cawson (Figures 1.24, 2.1, 2.3, 2.4, 2.20, 6.22), Professor N. F. C. Gowing (Figure 11.35), Professor I. R. H. Kramer (Figures 2.2, 2.14, 2.15), Mr P. Longhurst (Figure 2.13), Dr D. A. Luke (Figure 1.16), Dr D. G. MacDonald (Figure 11.20), Professor J. J. Pindborg (Figures 11.6, 11.7) and Professor A. C. Thackray (Figures 5.3, 5.4, 7.1, 7.2, 7.17, 7.30, 8.14, 8.38, 8.63).

Our grateful thanks are also due to Miss P. Archer for the line drawing, Figure 1.1, to Mr A. Woodman for low power photomicrography and to Mrs A. Batchelor and Miss L. Van Laere for secretarial help and typing the manuscript.

Structure and Development of the Teeth and Related Tissues

1

The Teeth

Structure

The fully developed tooth consists of the three calcified tissues, dentine, enamel and cementum, and the connective tissue pulp (Figures 1.1 and 1.2). The dentine, cementum and pulp are of mesodermal origin. The enamel is of epithelial origin[1-5].

Dentine, which constitutes the bulk of the tooth, is very similar physically and chemically to bone, but whereas bone contains osteocytes in lacunae, dentine contains cell processes but no cell bodies. The processes, which are those of the odontoblasts, lie in tubules some 2 to 3 μm wide that pass through the dentine from the pulp to the dentine-enamel junction (Figures 1.3 and 1.4). As in bone, there is sufficient organic matrix (20%) in dentine to maintain its general structure after routine decalcification. Dentine first calcifies as globules or calcospherites which eventually fuse to form a homogeneous material (Figure 1.4). In some cases calcification is incomplete and the calcospherites remain unfused and thus separated by uncalcified organic matrix. This is termed interglobular dentine.

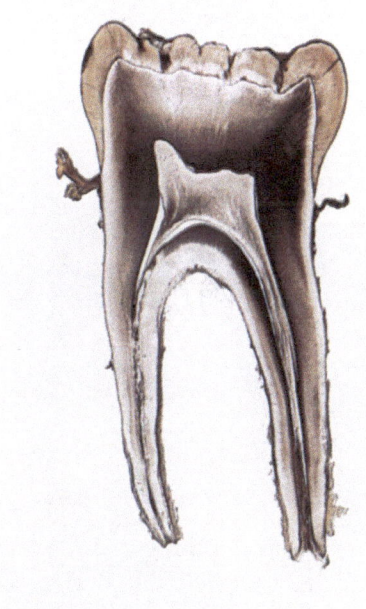

Figure 1.2 Ground section of a molar tooth. The greater part of the tooth consists of dentine. This is covered by enamel at the crown and by cementum over the roots. The gingiva is attached to the tooth at the junction of the enamel and the cementum, and its remnants can be seen in this section. The central cavity is the pulp chamber. In multirooted teeth, as here, it divides into a root canal for each root. × 3·2

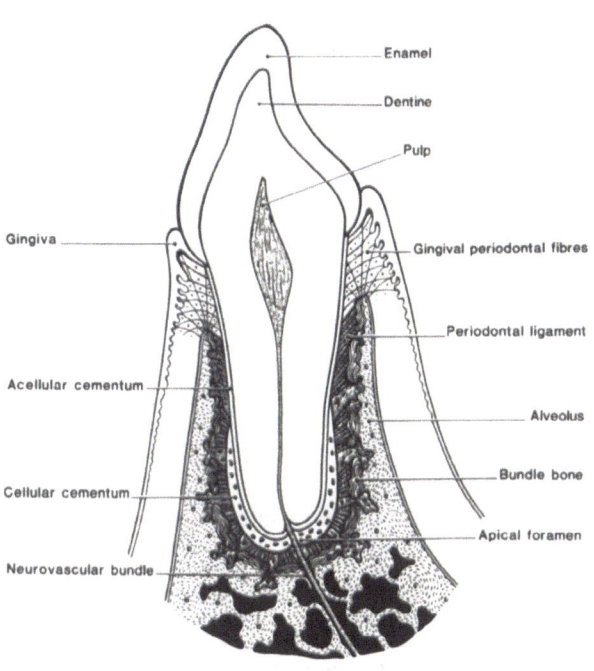

Enamel

Dentine

Pulp

Gingiva

Gingival periodontal fibres

Periodontal ligament

Acellular cementum

Alveolus

Bundle bone

Cellular cementum

Apical foramen

Neurovascular bundle

Figure 1.1 A tooth *in situ*, in the mandible

Figure 1.3 Transverse section of dentine, showing the dentinal tubules. H & E × 400

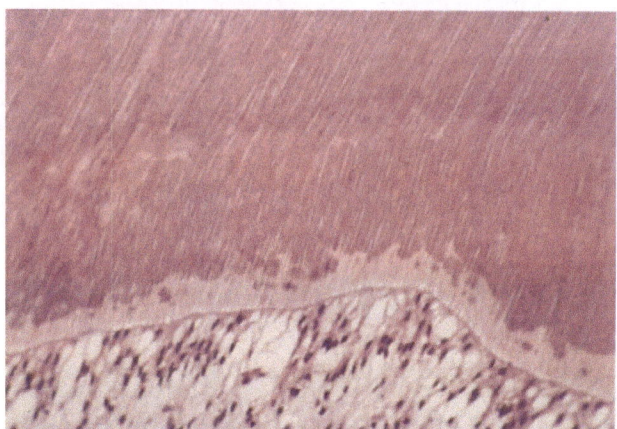

Figure 1.4 Longitudinal section showing, from below upwards, pulp with odontoblasts, the narrow zone of predentine with small calcospherites and mature dentine with tubules.   H & E × 200

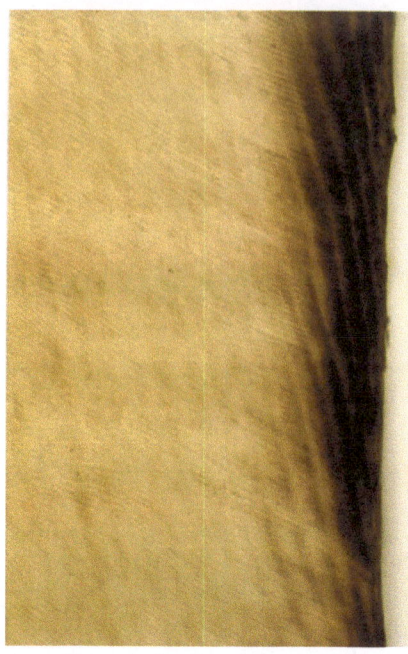

Figure 1.6 Ground section of enamel. Higher magnification to show the rod structure. The oblique striations are incremental lines, resulting from the successional deposition of layers of enamel matrix during development.   × 400

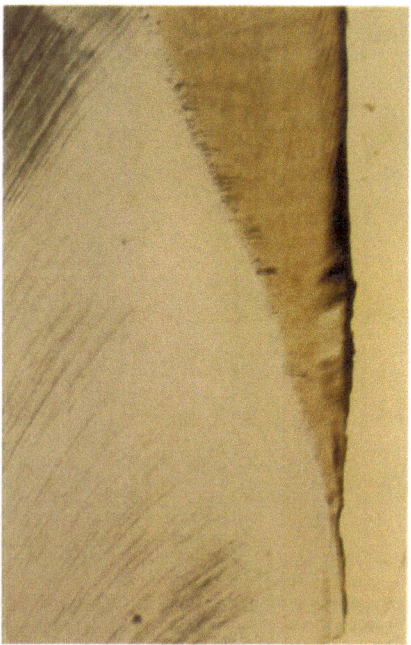

Figure 1.5 Longitudinal ground section showing enamel, dentine and the enamel–cementum junction. The rod structure of the enamel can be seen, the rods running the full thickness of the enamel from the enamel–dentine junction to the surface.   × 40

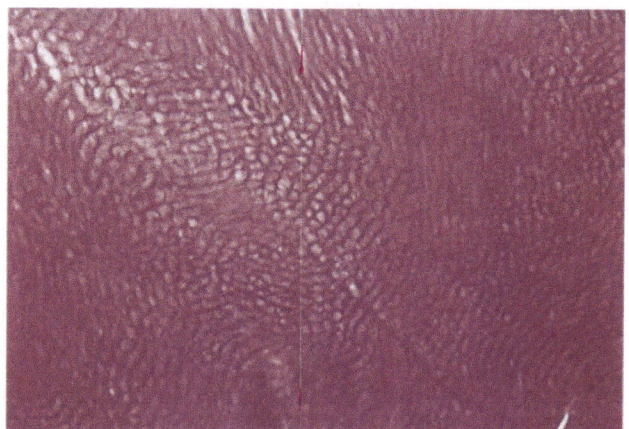

Figure 1.7 Decalcified section of immature enamel, showing the organic enamel matrix and the roughly hexagonal appearance of enamel rods in cross-section. H & E × 400

Enamel covers the dentine of that portion of the tooth that is visible in the mouth (the crown). Since over 97% of mature enamel consists of mineral, it is almost completely lost on decalcification and therefore requires ground sections or other special procedures for its study (Figures 1.5 and 1.6). However, since organic matrix forms a greater proportion of developing enamel it can often be observed in decalcified sections of immature teeth, where it can be seen to consist of roughly hexagonal rods or prisms about 4 µm in diameter (Figure 1.7).

Cementum is a bone-like tissue that covers the root of the tooth. The first formed cementum is acellular and covers the whole root surface. Cellular or secondary cementum usually covers the apical third of the root and has lacunae containing cementocytes (Figure 1.8). Cementocytes are similar to osteocytes but their cell processes tend to be orientated in one direction, towards the periodontal liga-

ment, rather than equally around the cell body as in osteocytes (Figures 1.8 and 1.9).

The pulp, which consists of connective tissue rich in blood vessels and nerves, contains the odontoblasts, arranged in a layer over its surface. The odontoblasts are columnar cells with oval nuclei and long cytoplasmic processes that lie in the dentinal tubules as they traverse the full thickness of the dentine. It is usual to see a relatively cell-free zone in the pulp immediately deep to the layer of odontoblasts (Figures 1.10 and 1.11). The central cavity in the tooth that contains the pulp is the pulp chamber. The cavity becomes much narrower in the root of the tooth, where it is termed the root canal. At the extremity or apex of the root is the apical foramen, through which the blood vessels, lymphatics and nerves gain access to the pulp (Figure 1.12).

The periodontal ligament (periodontal membrane) is

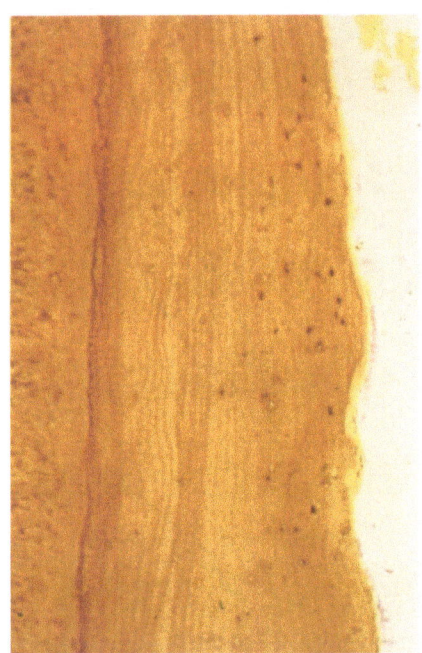

Figure 1.8 Longitudinal section showing dentine, acellular cementum and cellular cementum containing cementocytes. Prominent incremental lines are present in both the cellular and the acellular cementum.   Picrothionin × 100

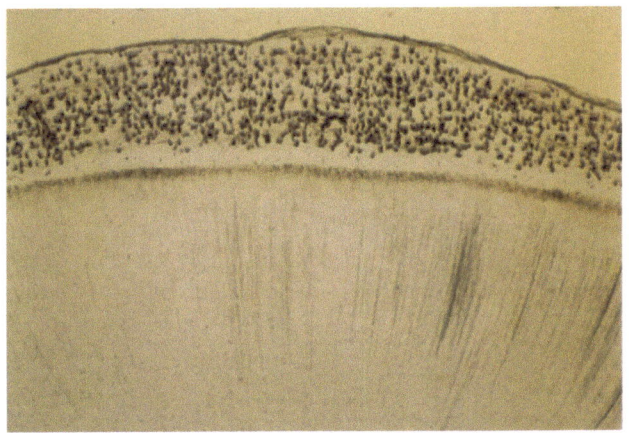

Figure 1.9 Transverse ground section showing cellular cementum and dentinal tubules.   × 40

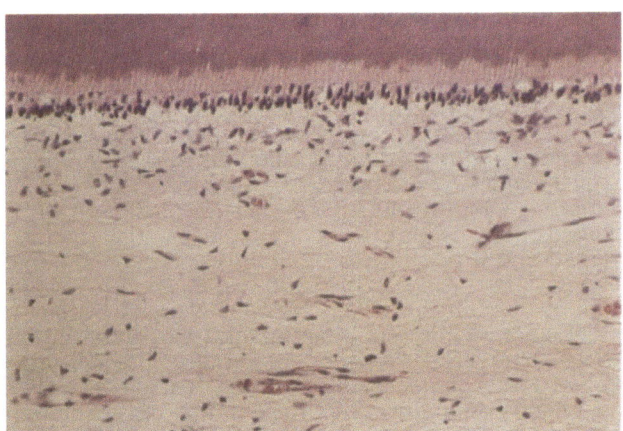

Figure 1.10 Dental pulp. The connective tissue pulp supports the odontoblasts, which are seen as a single layer of cells apposed to the predentine.   H & E × 200

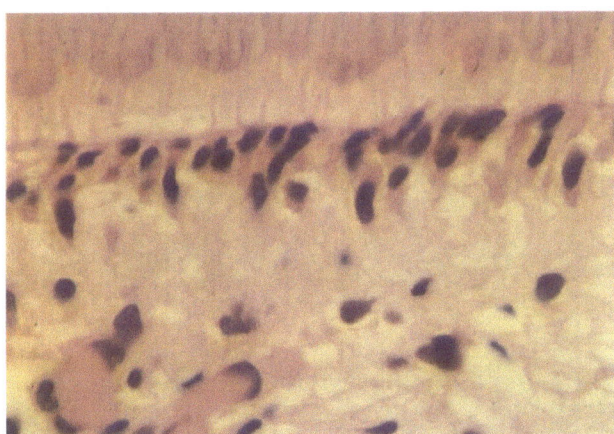

Figure 1.11 Higher magnification of the pulpodentinal junction, showing dentinal tubules, predentine and the odontoblasts. The cell-free zone is also seen. H & E × 1000

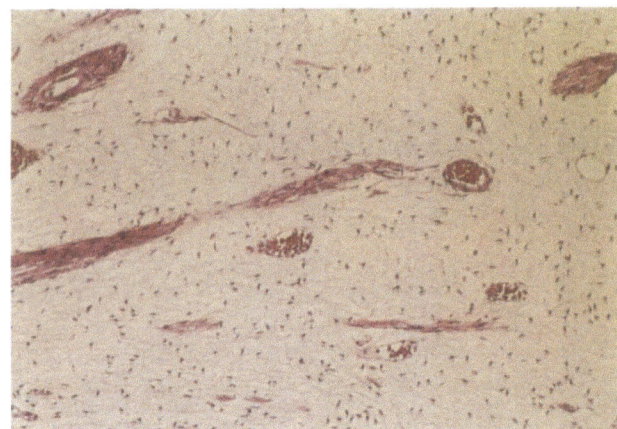

Figure 1.12 Dental pulp, showing neurovascular bundles.   H & E × 100

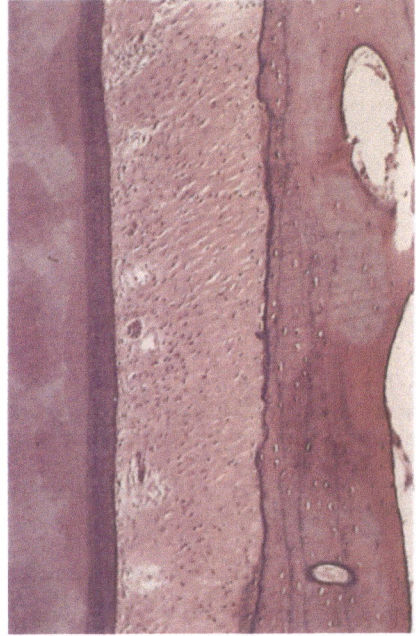

Figure 1.13 Periodontal ligament. The fibres are inserted into acellular cementum (left) and coarse bundle bone of the alveolus (right). Small residues of odontogenic epithelium (cell rests of Malassez) are present in the periodontal ligament. H & E × 100

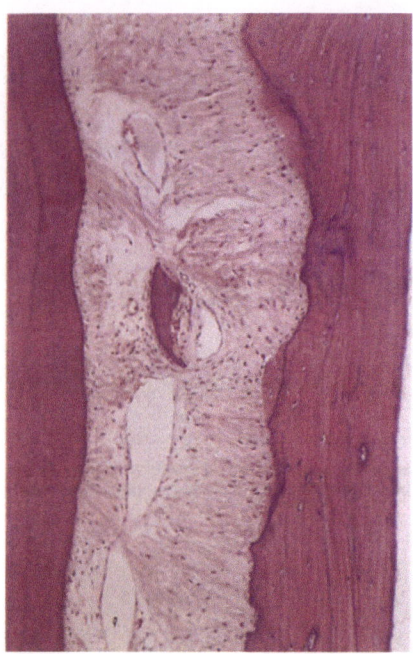

Figure 1.14 Periodontal ligament with a detached fragment of cementum (cemental spur), the result of trauma to the tooth.   H & E × 100

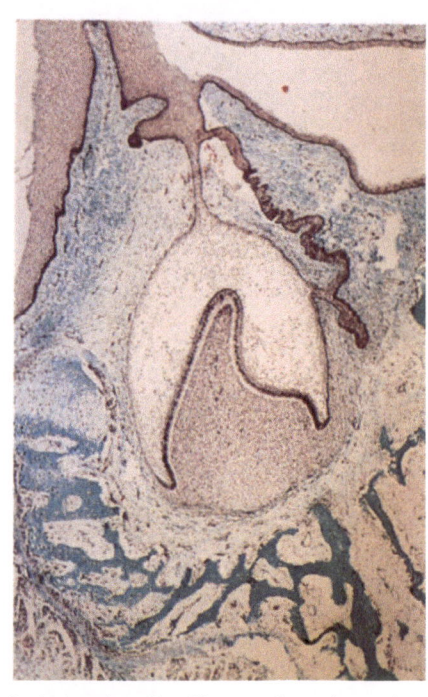

Figure 1.16 Sagittal section of jaw. The enamel organ has reached the bell stage. The lamina which gives rise to the permanent tooth is clearly visible. Trichrome × 40

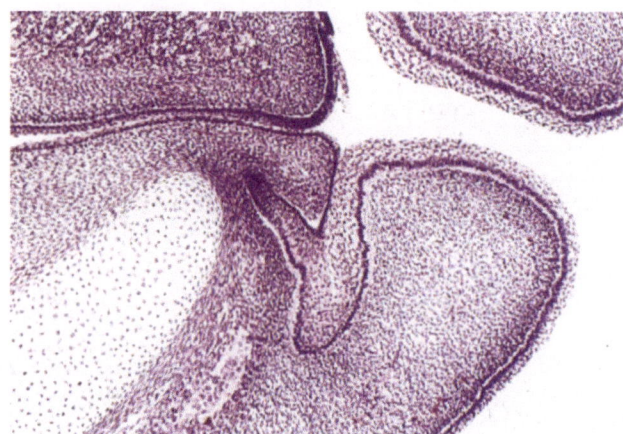

Figure 1.15 Sagittal section of developing mandible showing the early cap stage of the enamel organ.   H & E × 100

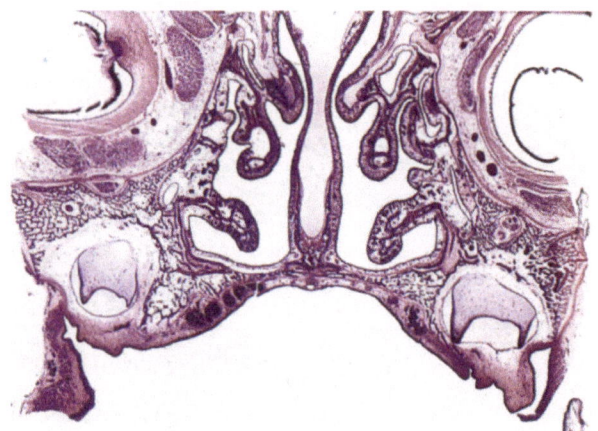

Figure 1.17 Coronal section through the embryonic maxilla and nasal cavities. A tooth germ is seen on each side.   H & E × 3

constituted by the connective tissue fibres that attach the tooth to the socket (alveolus). Inserted into the cementum of the tooth, they run from there to be attached to the alveolar bone of the socket wall (Figure 1.13). In addition to these fibres, which form a kind of shock-absorbing suspensory ligament for the tooth, other fibres run across the alveolar crest to join adjacent teeth and also pass into the gingiva, which they help to keep firmly attached to the tooth surface. Occasionally, trauma to a tooth may result in a fragment of cementum being broken off, to lie free in the periodontal ligament (Figure 1.14).

Development

Dental development begins during the sixth week of embryonic life with the formation of an ectodermal ridge from the oral epithelium of each maxillary and mandibular process. This ridge grows into the underlying mesoderm, where it subsequently divides into an outer and an inner process. The outer process marks off the lips and cheeks from the gums. The inner process or dental lamina gives rise to the teeth. Discrete swellings appear in the dental lamina to form the early enamel organs of the deciduous teeth. Each enamel organ assumes a cap-like shape and the underlying mesoderm proliferates to form the dental papilla, which will ultimately become the dental pulp (Figure 1.15). Continued epithelial proliferation in the enamel organ results in its becoming bell- rather than cap-shaped and it now encloses much of the dental papilla (Figure 1.16). The successional or permanent teeth arise as buds of epithelium from the enamel organ close to its attachment to the dental lamina and they pass through similar stages. The permanent molar teeth, however, have no deciduous predecessors and arise from the dental lamina, which continues to proliferate backwards behind the deciduous molars as an epithelial process with no direct attachment to the overlying epithelium. When the dental lamina breaks down in due course, each tooth germ lies

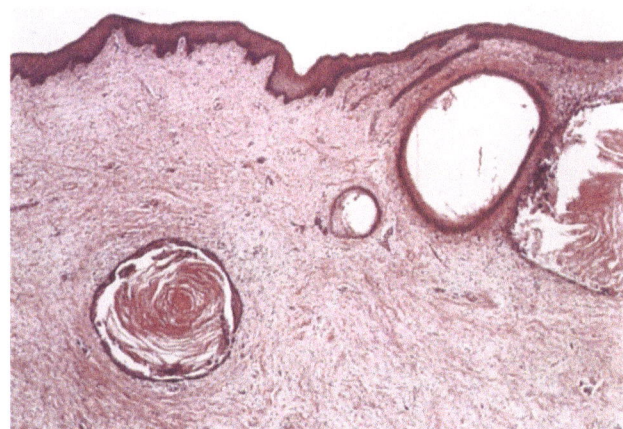

Figure 1.18 Cell rests of Serres, some of which have undergone cystic change. H & E × 40

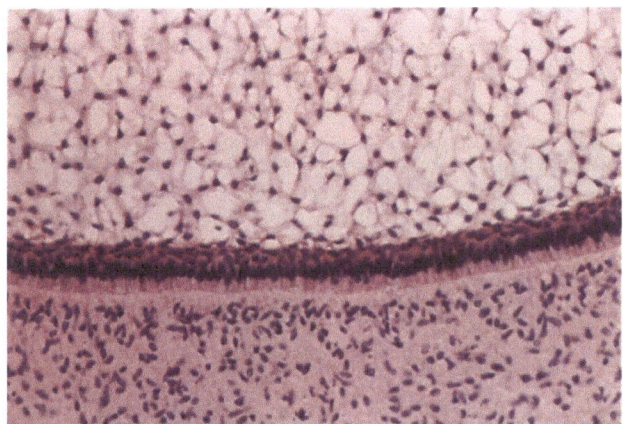

Figure 1.19 Enamel organ showing, from above down, stellate reticulum, stratum intermedium, the layer of ameloblasts with nuclei polarized away from the basement membrane, and the dental papilla.   H & E × 400

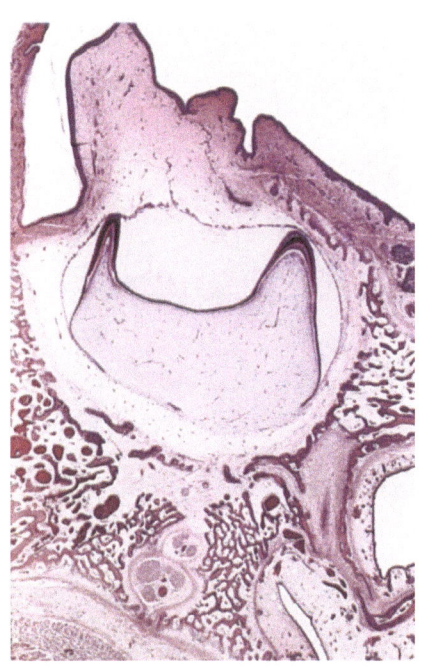

Figure 1.20 Enamel organ showing early enamel and dentine formation in the cusp tips.   H & E × 12·5

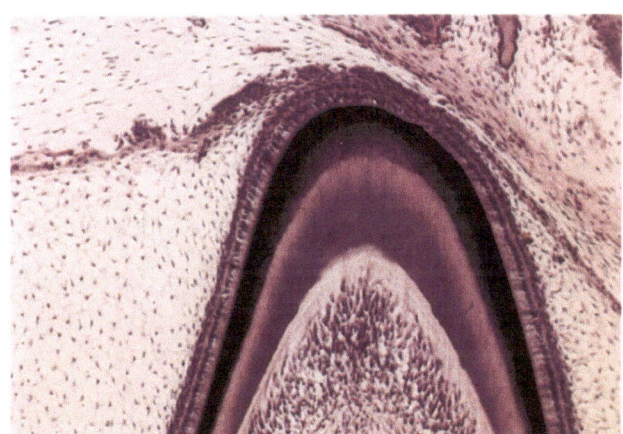

Figure 1.21 Enamel organ. Higher magnification to show early enamel and dentine formation.   H & E × 100

free in the jaws (Figure 1.17). Small groups of dental lamina cells may persist, as the cell rests of Serres. These rests appear to be important in the pathogenesis of some odontogenic cysts and tumours (Figure 1.18).

The cells of the outer layer of the enamel organ are low and columnar and are separated from the surrounding mesenchyme by a basement membrane. As the enamel organ enters the cap stage the epithelial cells in contact with the dental papilla become taller and are called the internal enamel epithelium to distinguish them from the rest of the outer layer cells, which constitute the external enamel epithelium. Later, the cells in the interior of the enamel organ become separated from one another by intercellular fluid accumulation but remain in contact by delicate processes and form the stellate reticulum. In the late bell stage a further layer of flattened cells some 2–3 cells thick forms between the internal enamel epithelium and the stellate reticulum. This is the stratum intermedium (Figure 1.19). The area where the internal and external enamel epithelium

meet is the cervical loop. This is a zone of active growth which eventually forms the root sheath of Hertwig.

Meanwhile, odontoblasts differentiate from the cells of the dental papilla adjacent to the internal enamel epithelium under the inductive influence of the epithelial cells. The odontoblasts lay down dentine between the two layers of cells as an organic matrix which later calcifies. The most recently formed dentine is always uncalcified and is termed predentine. Processes from the odontoblasts become enclosed in tubules in the forming dentine.

At the same time, the cells of the internal enamel epithelium become elongated and the nuclei become polarized away from the basement membrane. Once dentine formation starts these cells shorten slightly and become ameloblasts which lay down enamel, first as an organic matrix and then as hydroxyapatite crystals arranged in a prismatic manner (Figures 1.20, 1.21 and 1.6). When enamel formation is complete the stellate reticulum is greatly

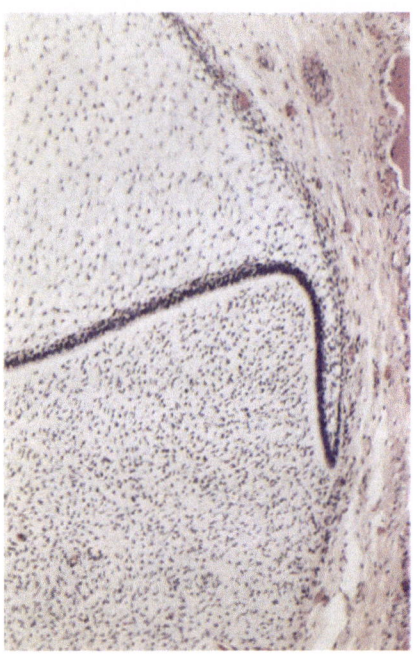

Figure 1.22 Cervical loop, where the inner and outer enamel epithelium fuse to form Hertwig's sheath which maps out the form of the root.   H & E × 100

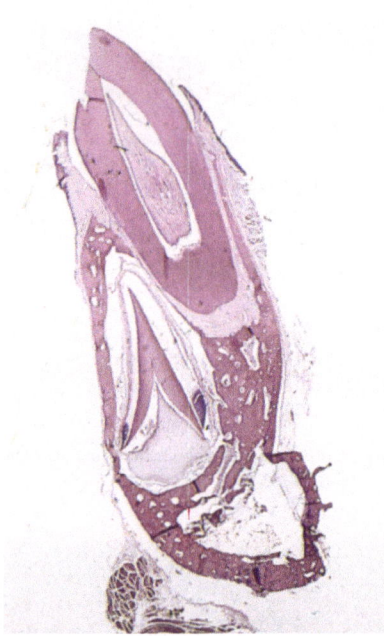

Figure 1.24 Sagittal section through the mandible, showing an erupted deciduous tooth and the unerupted permanent successor in its follicle.   H & E × 4·5

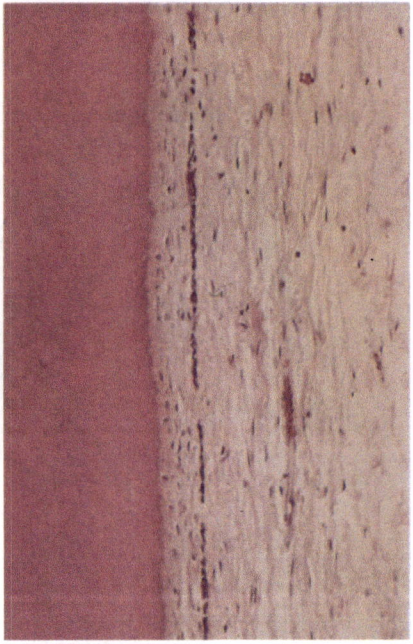

Figure 1.23 Hertwig's sheath breaking down to form the cell rests of Malassez, before the start of cementum formation.   H & E × 200

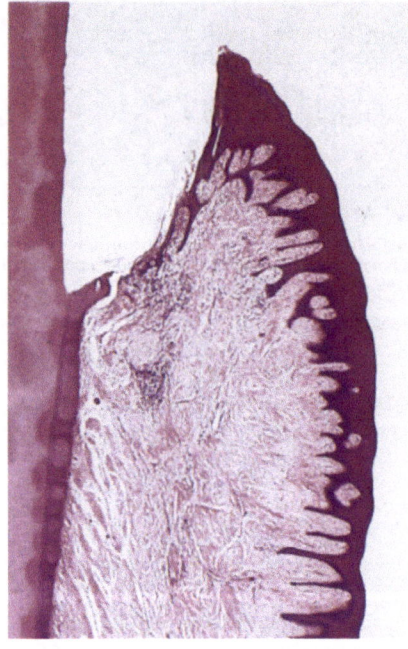

Figure 1.25 Gingiva. There is mild chronic inflammatory infiltration of the corium subjacent to the base of the sulcular epithelium H & E × 40.

reduced in size and the internal and external enamel epithelium fuse to form the reduced enamel epithelium.

The internal and external enamel epithelium fuse at the cervical loop to form the root sheath of Hertwig which maps out the root area of the tooth (Figure 1.22). Dentine is deposited by the odontoblasts to form the tooth root, but no enamel is formed in this region. When root formation is complete the root sheath degenerates, but remnants persist as interconnected cords and small islands of cells around the root – the cell rests of Malassez (Figure 1.23). As the root sheath breaks down, the dentine of the root

comes into contact with the surrounding connective tissue, from which mesenchymal cells differentiate into cementoblasts. These cells deposit cementum on the root surface.

From an early stage in development the tooth germ becomes surrounded by a condensation of mesoderm which eventually forms a fibrous sac or follicle within which the tooth develops. This is the dental follicle (Figure 1.24). The follicle around the root portion of the tooth finally becomes the periodontal ligament.

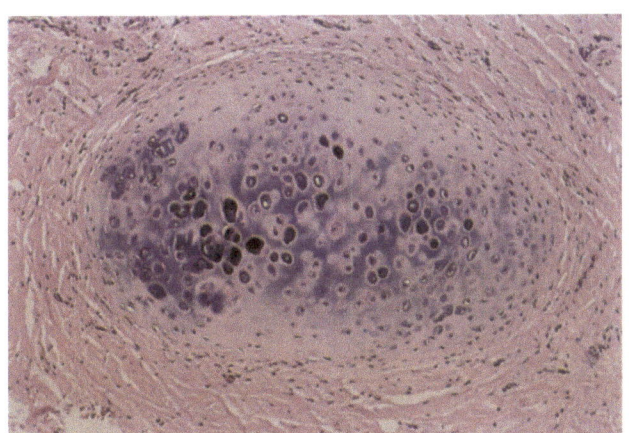

Figure 1.26 Ectopic cartilage in a gingivectomy specimen from the palatal gingiva between the upper central incisor teeth.   H & E × 100

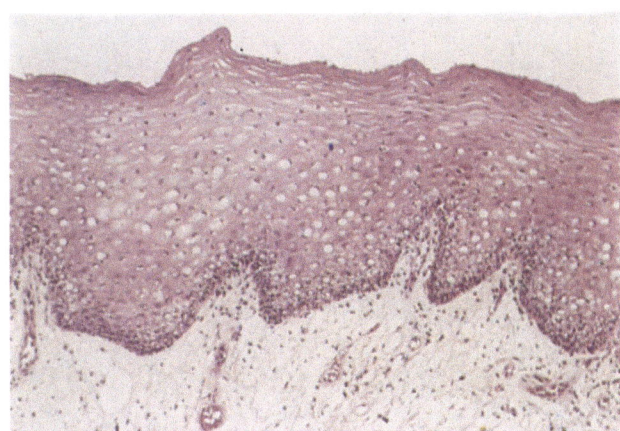

Figure 1.28   Buccal mucosa. The epithelium is thick and nonkeratinized.   H & E × 100

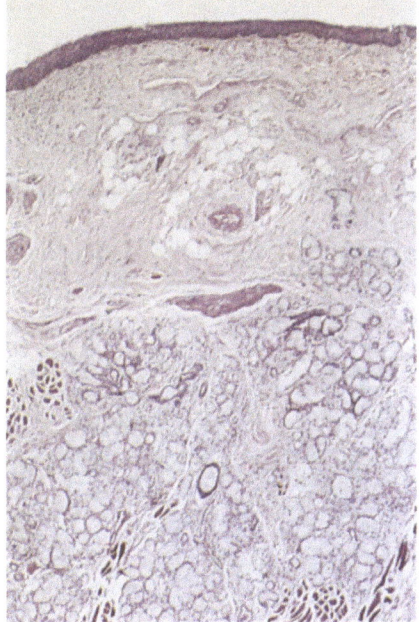

Figure 1.27   Soft palate. There are many mucous salivary glands in the submucosa.   H & E × 40

The Soft Tissues

Gingiva

The mucous membrane related to the neck of the tooth and the adjacent alveolar bone is the gingiva or gum. The gingiva is continuous with the alveolar mucosa that covers the rest of the alveolar bone. Except for a small marginal area, healthy gingiva is firmly attached to the neck of the tooth and the adjacent bone. Between the marginal or free gingiva and the tooth is the gingival crevice or sulcus which, in the absence of adequate cleansing, is a stagnation area where plaque tends to accumulate. The epithelium of the sulcus (sulcular epithelium) is continuous at the bottom of the gingival crevice with the epithelium

that is attached to the tooth surface (epithelial attachment). The epithelium of the marginal gingiva is usually keratinized, but parakeratosis is not uncommon. The sulcular epithelium is nonkeratinized. The epithelial ridges are long and slender, and mild chronic inflammatory infiltration of the gingival corium close to the gingival sulcus is usually present, even in clinically normal gingivae (Figure 1.25). The alveolar mucosa, which is nonkeratinized, has few small rete ridges and is not firmly attached to the underlying bone.

Hard Palate

The epithelium of the palate shows orthokeratosis and has numerous long rete ridges. Towards the midline of the palate and also towards the gingiva the mucosa is firmly adherent to the periosteum, forming a mucoperiosteum. In other areas, particularly towards the soft palate, there are many mucous glands in the submucosa. Behind the upper central incisor teeth it is not uncommon to see small cartilaginous residues in biopsy specimens (Figure 1.26). These may be cartilage sequestered from the nasal septum or from the paraseptal cartilages during development. The palatine papilla, which is situated in the midline just behind the incisor teeth, contains many nerve endings and may also contain the blind endings of the nasopalatine ducts, which are lined by columnar epithelium containing goblet cells.

Soft Palate

The oral surface of the soft palate is covered by nonkeratinized stratified squamous epithelium and has numerous minor mucous salivary glands in the submucosa (Figure 1.27). The nasal surface is covered by columnar ciliated epithelium.

Cheeks

The nonkeratinized buccal mucosa is thick and the cells are frequently distended with glycogen (Figure 1.28). Along the line of mucosa adjacent to where the cheek teeth meet there is frequently mild parakeratosis and there may be keratosis if the patient indulges in cheek-sucking or biting. The cheeks are a common place to see ectopic sebaceous glands (Figure 1.29). These appear clinically as small yellowish granules (Fordyce granules)[6].

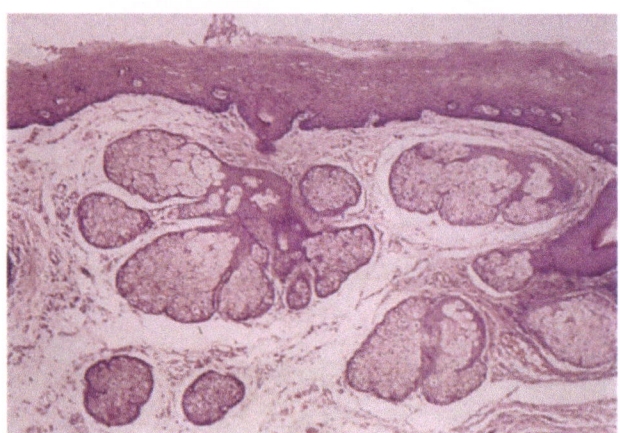

Figure 1.29 Fordyce granules. These sebaceous glands are common in the oral mucosa of adults, especially the buccal mucosa and lips.   H & E × 40

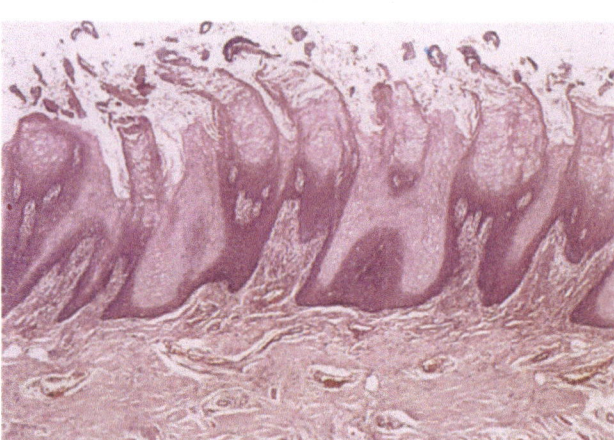

Figure 1.31 Dorsal tongue mucosa showing filiform papillae and colonies of bacteria in the superficial keratin layers and on the surface.   H & E × 40

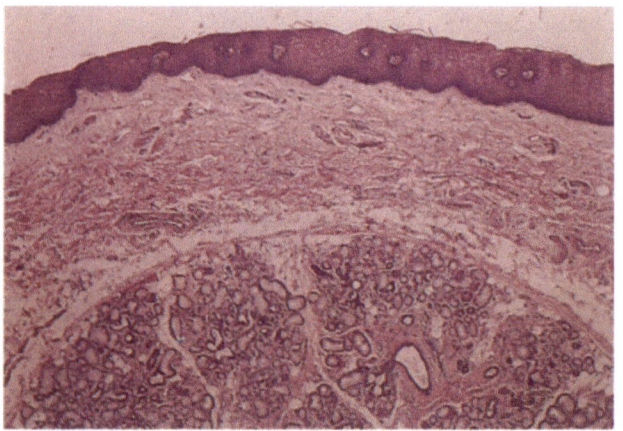

Figure 1.30 Lip mucosa. The epithelium of the oral portion of the lip is relatively thin, with short and blunt rete processes. Seromucinous minor salivary glands are plentiful.   H & E × 40

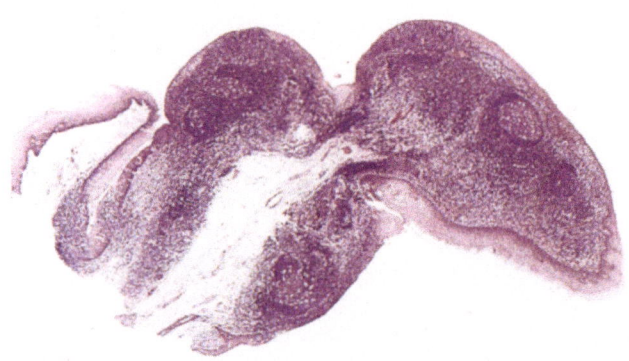

Figure 1.32 Foliate papilla, showing lymphoid aggregates with germinal centres.   H & E × 18

Lips

The vermilion borders are keratinized and have numerous long rete ridges. Although hair follicles and sweat glands are absent, there may be many sebaceous glands. The epithelium of the oral portion of the lip is nonkeratinized. The rete ridges are short and blunt and minor salivary glands are present in the submucosa (Figure 1.30).

Tongue and Floor of Mouth

The ventral lingual mucosa and the floor of the mouth are covered by thin nonkeratinized epithelium. The dorsum of the tongue is covered by papillae, with a rather variable arrangement. The filiform papillae are the most numerous and are conical with a central connective tissue core covered by keratinized stratified squamous epithelium (Figure 1.31). The fungiform papillae are much less numerous and consist of rounded elevations covered by thinly keratinized or nonkeratinized epithelium. The vallate papillae, 10 to 12 in number, are situated mainly in the posterior third of the tongue in relation to the V-shaped sulcus terminalis. Each vallate papilla is delimited by a deep circular groove and the epithelium forming the inner wall of this groove contains numerous taste buds. Small serous glands open into the bottom of each groove. Several leaf-like papillae are present on the lateral margin of the tongue at the junction of the anterior two-thirds and the posterior third. The cores of these foliate papillae contain lymphoid tissue (Figure 1.32). They not infrequently become irritated and inflamed, when they cause considerable discomfort[7].

References

1. Berkovitz, B. K., Holland, G. R. and Moxham, B. J. (1978). *A Colour Atlas and Textbook of Oral Anatomy*. (London : Wolfe Medical Publications Ltd)

2. Scott, J. H. and Symons, N. B. B. (1982). *Introduction to Dental Anatomy*. 9th Edn. (Edinburgh, London, Melbourne, New York: Churchill Livingstone)

3. Squier, C. A., Johnson, N. W. and Hopps, R. M. (1976). *Human Oral Mucosa. Development, Structure and Function*. (Oxford, London, Edinburgh, Melbourne: Blackwell Scientific Publications)

4. Ten Cate, A. R. (1980). *Oral Histology. Development, Structure and Function*. (St Louis, Toronto, London: C. V. Mosby Company)

5. Bhaskar, S. N. (1980). *Orban's Oral Histology and Embryology*. 9th Edn. (St Louis, Toronto, London: C. V. Mosby Company)

6. Miles, A. E. W. (1958). Sebaceous glands in the lip and cheek mucosa of man. *Brit. Dent. J.*, **105**, 235

7. Simpson, H. E. (1964). Lymphocyte hyperplasia in foliate papillitis. *Oral Surg.*, **22**, 209

Developmental and Acquired Abnormalities of the Teeth

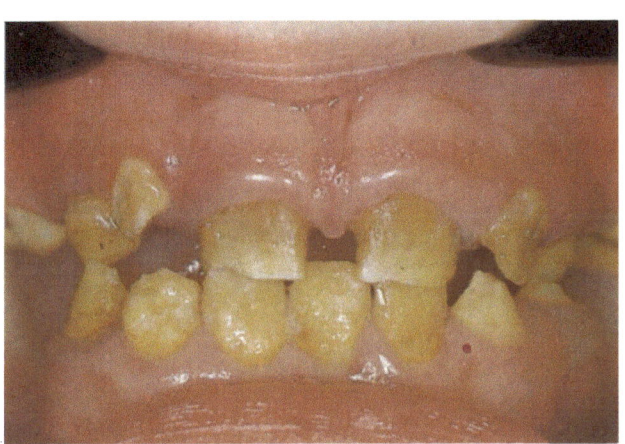

2

Figure 2.1 Amelogenesis imperfecta. The enamel is hypoplastic and pitted but normally calcified in this example of hereditary enamel hypoplasia

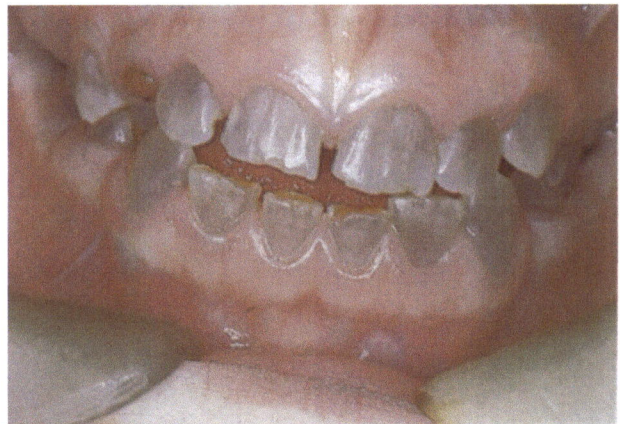

Figure 2.3 Dentinogenesis imperfecta. The teeth have a purplish colour and are distinctly opalescent. These teeth will soon wear to a similar state to those in Figure 2.4

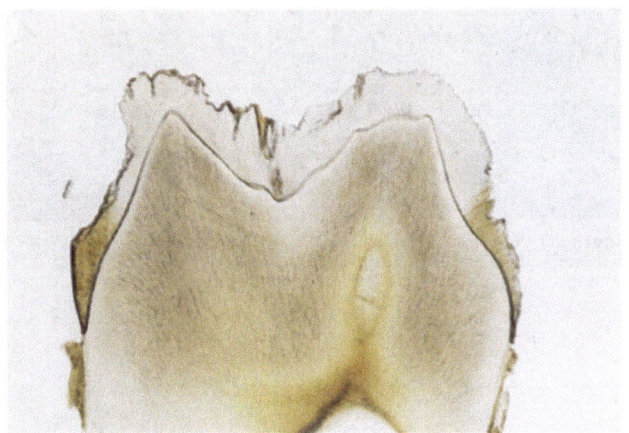

Figure 2.2 Amelogenesis imperfecta. Ground section of molar tooth showing irregular enamel hypoplasia. ×9

Developmental Abnormalities

Local disease or trauma, or systemic disease or other general factors, may affect developing teeth, interfering with the formation of enamel or dentine or both[1]. When the affected teeth erupt a variety of defects in structure may be seen. The following are among those most likely to be encountered by the pathologist.

Amelogenesis Imperfecta

This is an inherited disorder, usually involving all the teeth, which has two common clinical presentations[2]. In *hereditary enamel hypoplasia* the enamel is normally calcified but deficient in quantity (Figures 2.1 and 2.2). It is thin and in some cases the surface is pitted and the teeth wear very rapidly under normal masticatory stress. In *hereditary enamel hypomineralization* the enamel is formed in normal quantities but is poorly mineralized. The soft enamel becomes stained, quickly chips off the underlying dentine and easily wears away.

Dentinogenesis Imperfecta
(hereditary opalescent dentine)

This condition, which is usually inherited as an autosomal dominant trait, can appear alone or in combination with osteogenesis imperfecta[3]. It tends to affect all teeth in both dentitions. The enamel is normal in form but the tooth crown has a brownish or purplish opalescent appearance (Figure 2.3). The crown is bulbous and the roots are

There are a large number of developmental and acquired abnormalities of dental tissues that are mainly of specialist interest. Many of these abnormalities can only be studied in undecalcified ground sections and by other techniques that are not routinely undertaken in most general pathology laboratories. The following brief account is therefore limited to the more common disorders, and a few less common but particularly distinctive lesions.

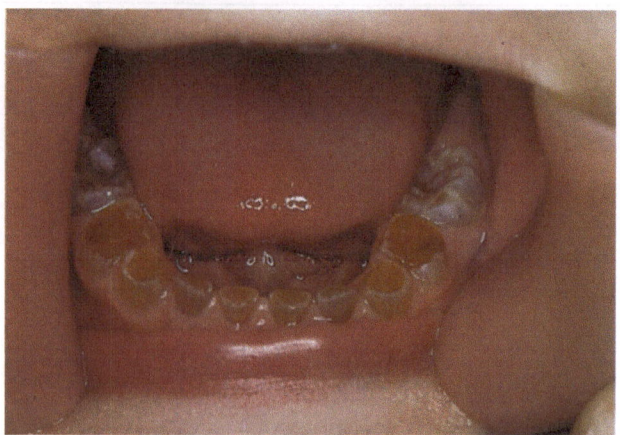

Figure 2.4 Dentinogenesis imperfecta. The enamel has chipped off to expose the softer dentine, which has rapidly worn down

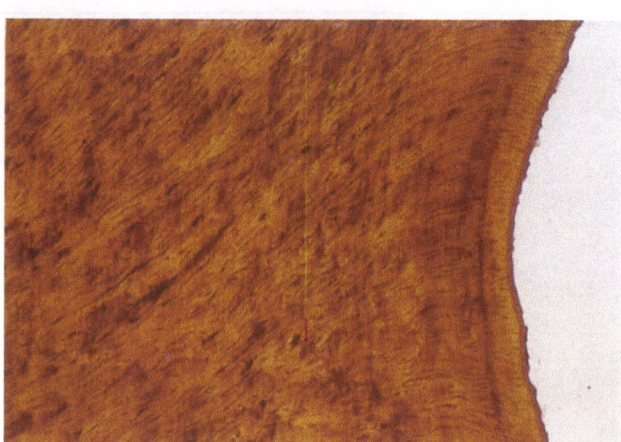

Figure 2.6 Dentinogenesis imperfecta. The first formed or mantle dentine is normal. The remainder of the dentine shows reduced numbers of irregular dentinal tubules and cellular inclusions.   Picrothionin × 100

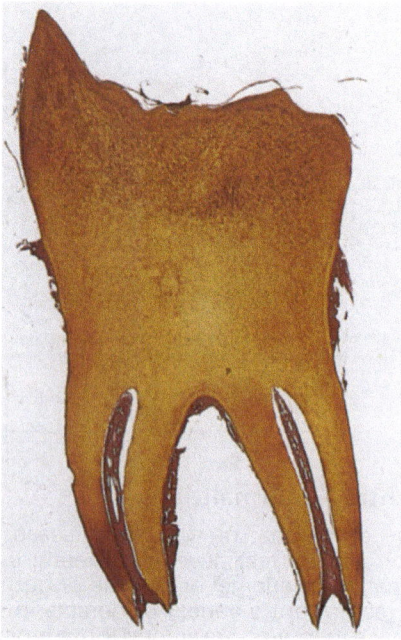

Figure 2.5 Dentinogenesis imperfecta. The roots are short and the pulp chamber has been obliterated by continued irregular dentine formation.   Picrothionin × 5

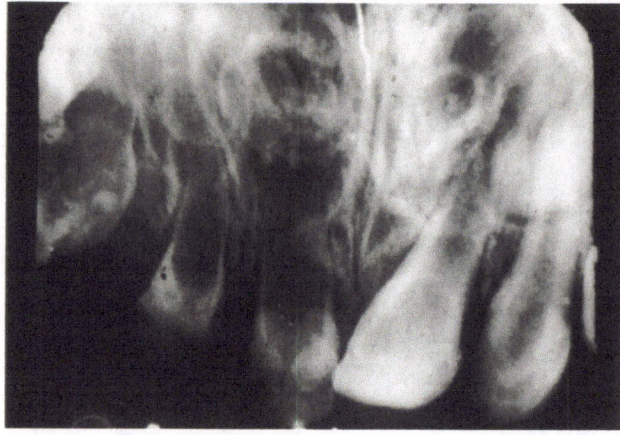

Figure 2.7 Regional odontodysplasia. The radiograph shows the ghost-like appearance of the unerupted teeth. Both enamel and dentine are very thin

short. The union between enamel and dentine is defective and the enamel chips away to expose the softer dentine, which rapidly wears down (Figure 2.4).

Microscopy shows that the earliest formed dentine is normal but the deeper layers have fewer tubules which are often obliterated by continuous dentine deposition (Figures 2.5 and 2.6). The enamel is normal but the usual scalloping of the enamel-dentine junction is said to be absent.

Regional Odontodysplasia

In this uncommon but distinctive anomaly there is localized arrest in tooth development[4,5]. The condition affects one or several adjacent teeth, most commonly in the anterior maxillary region and usually unilaterally. Both the deciduous and permanent dentitions can be affected. Radiography shows hypoplastic, partly mineralized teeth (hence the alternative name of ghost teeth). The crowns characteristically have a somewhat crumpled appearance (Figure 2.7).

Microscopically, the enamel is thin and irregular with the cells of the reduced enamel epithelium adherent to the enamel and showing irregular calcification (Figure 2.8). Focal collections of odontogenic epithelium, frequently calcified, can be seen scattered throughout the follicle (Figure 2.9). The coronal dentine is severely disorganized and poorly mineralized with large areas of interglobular dentine. Zones of amorphous, collagen-free dentine in the coronal area are a particularly characteristic feature (Figure 2.10). The root dentine has a more nearly normal

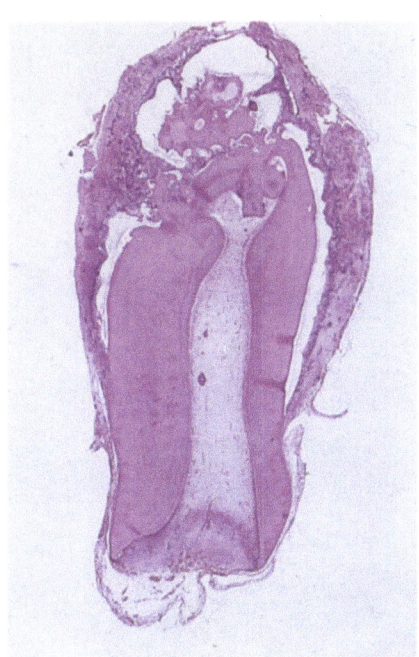

Figure 2.8 Regional odontodysplasia. A low power view showing the calcified reduced enamel epithelium externally, the irregular space left by the decalcification of enamel and the grossly irregular dentine. H & E × 7·5

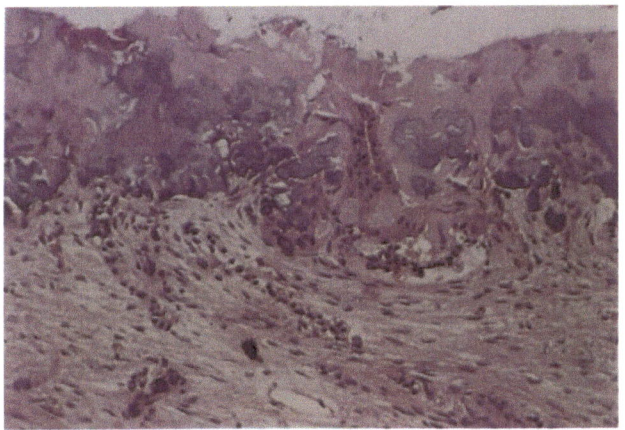

Figure 2.9 Regional odontodysplasia. There is calcification of the reduced enamel epithelium and odontogenic epithelial rests are present in the follicle. H & E × 400

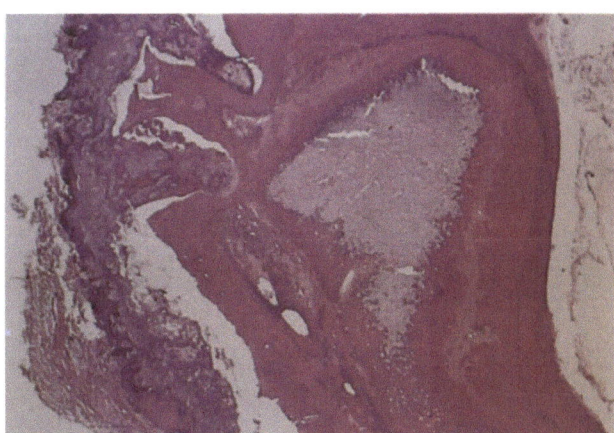

Figure 2.10 Regional odontodysplasia. The dentine is severely disorganized. It contains characteristic pale-staining collagen-free areas. H & E × 200

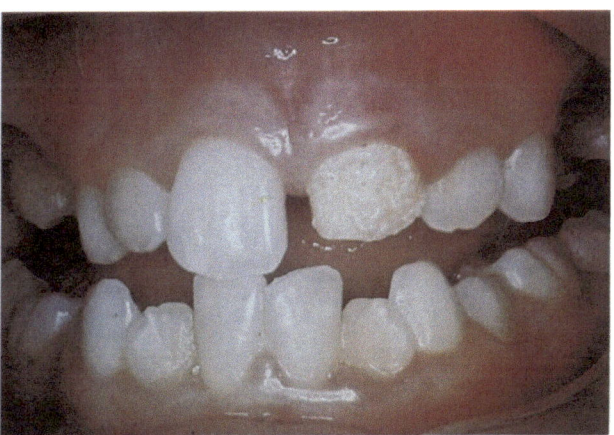

Figure 2.11 Hypoplastic tooth. The upper central incisor is hypoplastic due to damage before eruption from infection around the root of the deciduous predecessor

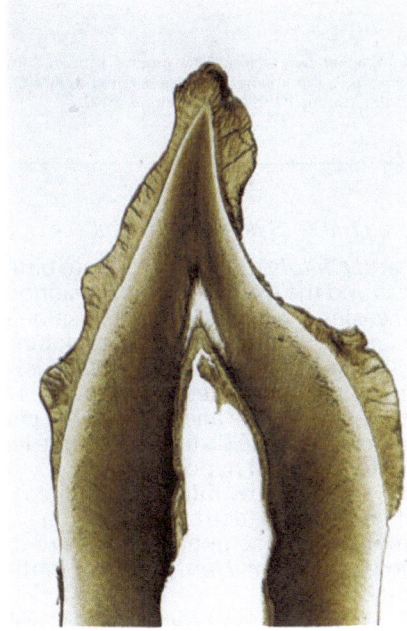

Figure 2.12 Hypoplastic tooth. Ground section showing gross enamel hypoplasia and interglobular dentine. × 7·5

structure, although areas of interglobular dentine may be present. The pulp may show degenerative changes or it may be necrotic.

Hypoplasia Due to Local Infection or Trauma

Infection in the periapical area of a deciduous tooth, or trauma to the tooth, can damage the underlying permanent successor. When this tooth eventually erupts and appears in the mouth, it may show abnormalities in size and shape and the enamel may be pitted (Figures 2.11 and 2.12). The pits in the enamel are often filled by deposition of cementum on to the enamel surface before the tooth has erupted. There is defective mineralization in the dentine and there may be wide areas of interglobular dentine similar to those seen in renal rickets.

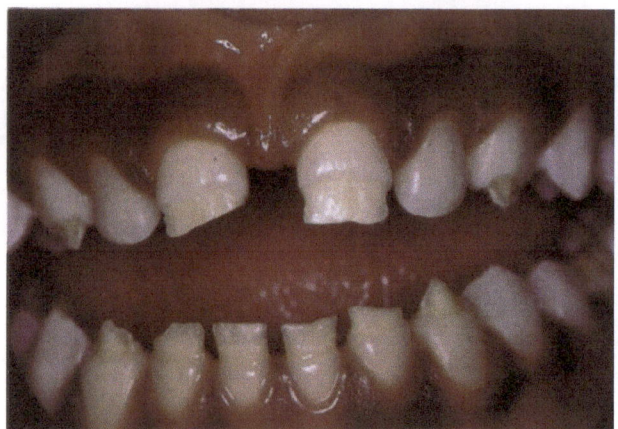

Figure 2.13 Enamel hypoplasia. The teeth show linear hypoplasia caused by severe illness in early childhood

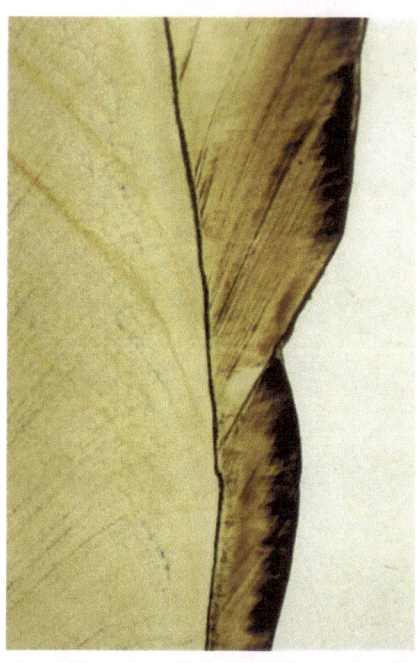

Figure 2.15 Enamel hypoplasia. Higher magnification from Figure 2.14 shows the hypoplastic groove in the enamel and interglobular dentine. The tetracycline bands in the dentine are clearly visible. × 40

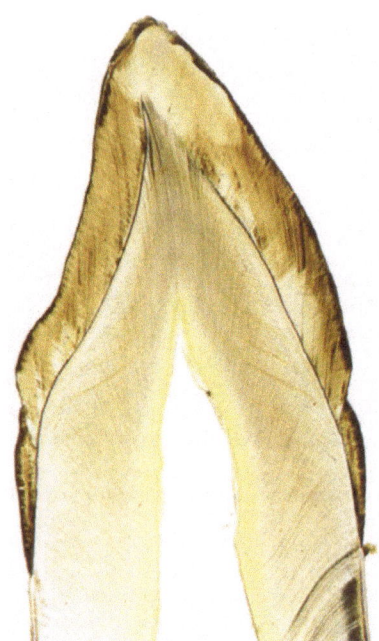

Figure 2.14 Enamel hypoplasia. This ground section shows the horizontal hypoplastic groove in the enamel that has resulted from a childhood infection. There are also tetracycline bands in the dentine. × 9

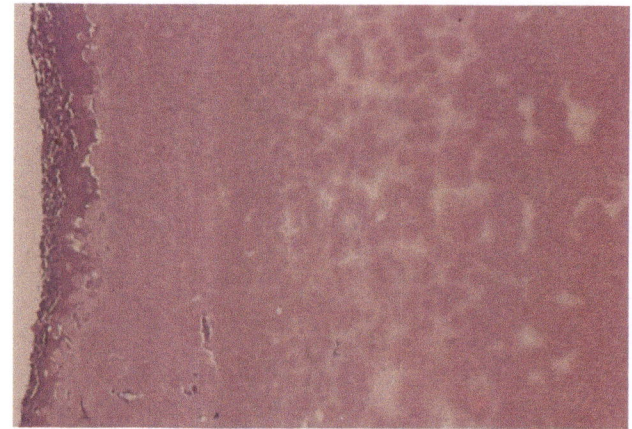

Figure 2.16 Rickets. Decalcified section showing extensive areas of interglobular dentine. × 100

Hypoplasia Due to Systemic Factors

Perinatal and Childhood Illness. Severe birth injury, neonatal illness and the exanthematous childhood fevers (especially measles nowadays) may cause defective matrix formation in the teeth that are developing during the period of the illness. This is usually manifest as hypoplastic pits or grooves in the teeth (Figures 2.13–2.15). It is possible to determine the age at which the patient suffered from the illness from the distribution of the lesions (hence the term chronological hypoplasia).

Prenatal syphilis, now rare, can produce characteristic abnormalities in the teeth (Hutchinson's incisors and Moon's molars). These abnormalities are thought to be due to the presence of *Trep. pallidum* in the developing tooth germs.

Rickets. In Western countries rickets is usually secondary to renal disease and, apart from its more serious effects on the skeleton, there are characteristic changes in the

teeth[6]. The enamel may be hypoplastic, showing a series of pits and grooves on its surface. The dentine is poorly mineralized and shows extensive areas of interglobular dentine formation and a widened zone of predentine (Figures 2.16 and 2.17).

Tetracycline Staining. Tetracycline is incorporated into calcifying tissues of the fetus and the young child, being deposited as a yellowish pigment along the incremental lines of developing dentine and enamel[7]. The staining is permanent and darkens with time so that involved teeth become greyish brown and relatively opaque (Figure 2.18). In sections, the tetracycline fluoresces as bright yellow in ultraviolet light (Figure 2.19).

Dental Fluorosis. Although fluoride in the drinking water in concentrations of one part per million protects the teeth from caries, higher concentrations may damage the enamel, the effects tending to be proportional to the concentration[8]. If the concentration is between 2 and 6 ppm

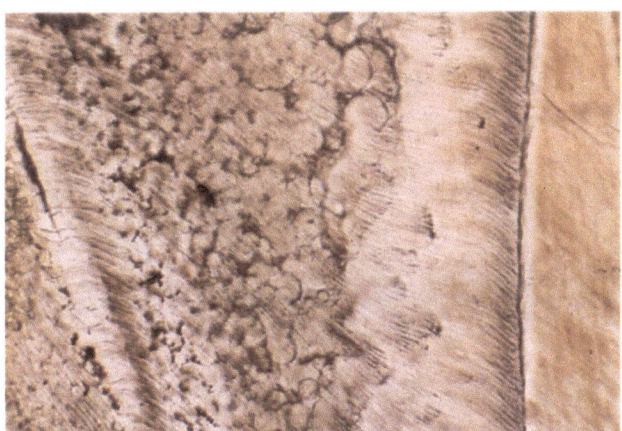

Figure 2.17 Rickets. Ground section showing extensive areas of interglobular dentine. The enamel is normal. ×100

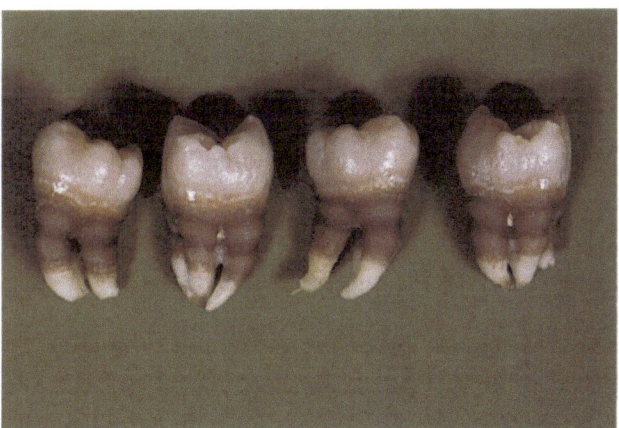

Figure 2.18 Tetracycline staining. There are linear deposits of staining in the roots of these third molar teeth from a patient who had been treated with tetracycline for acne between the ages of 11 and 13 years

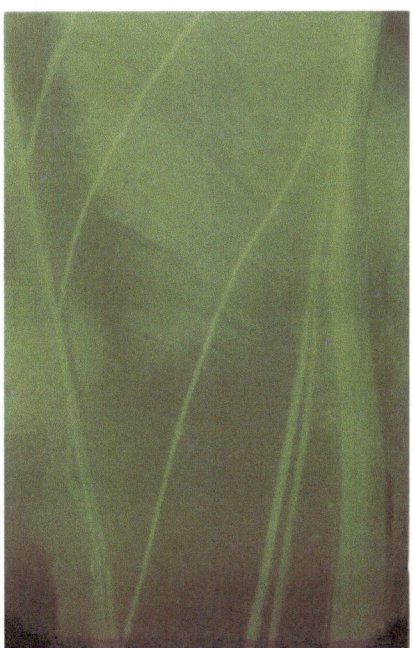

Figure 2.19 Tetracycline staining. Ground section of tooth viewed under ultraviolet light shows intensely fluorescent bands in the dentine. ×40

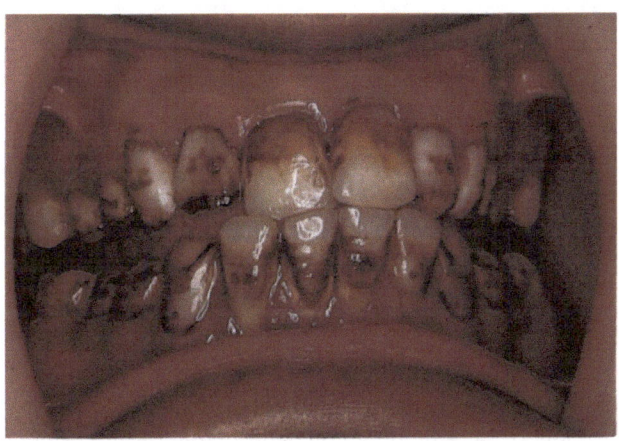

Figure 2.20 Dental fluorosis. The teeth show severe mottling of the enamel with brown staining

matrix formation is unaffected but the enamel shows areas of defective mineralization, appearing as irregular mottling. With higher concentrations of fluoride the enamel is hypoplastic, showing pitting and staining (Figure 2.20). In addition, it is brittle and can chip away from the tooth, especially on the incisal edges.

Acquired Abnormalities of the Teeth

The most important acquired abnormality of the teeth is dental caries, which is considered in Chapter 3. Regressive and degenerative changes in the pulp and the effects of injury on developing and formed teeth are described here.

Regressive and Degenerative Changes in the Pulp

A number of regressive or degenerative changes have been described in the dental pulp[9]. These are usually seen as coincidental features and most are of limited, if any, clinical significance. Indeed, it is likely that some of the changes so described are fixation artifacts due to the slow penetration of fixatives through the narrow apical foramen.

Oedema appears as droplets of fluid between the odontoblasts, pushing them apart and producing a characteristic wheatsheaf appearance (Figure 2.21).

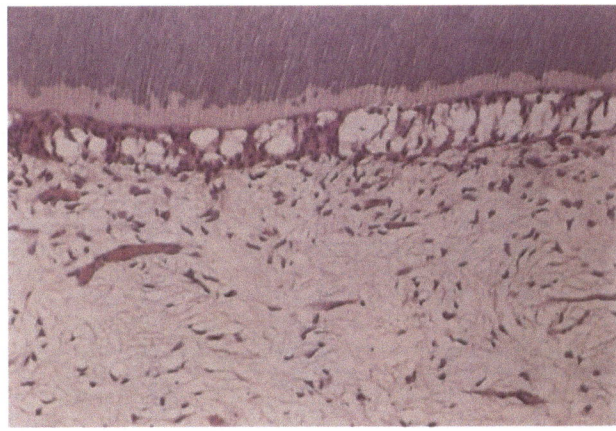

Figure 2.21 Oedema of the pulp causing separation of the odontoblasts. H & E ×200

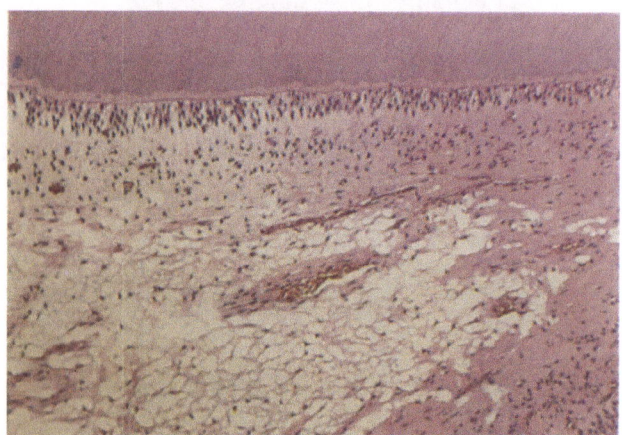

Figure 2.22   Fatty change and fibrosis of the pulp.   H & E × 100

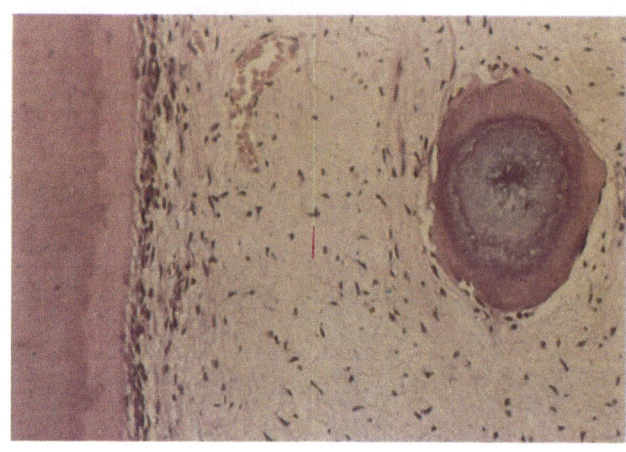

Figure 2.24   Concentrically laminated true pulp stone.   H & E × 200

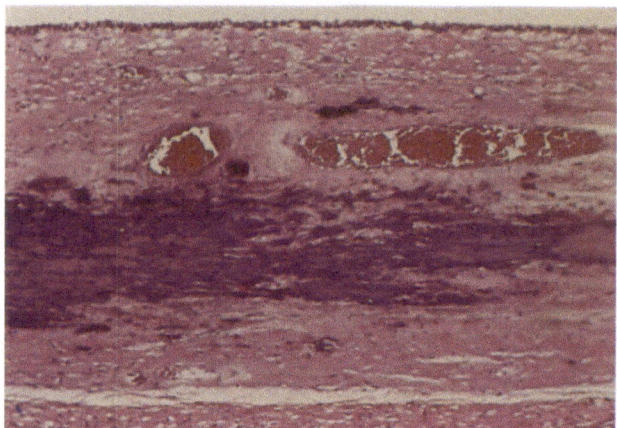

Figure 2.23   Pulpal fibrosis and amorphous calcium deposits in the root canal.
H & E × 100

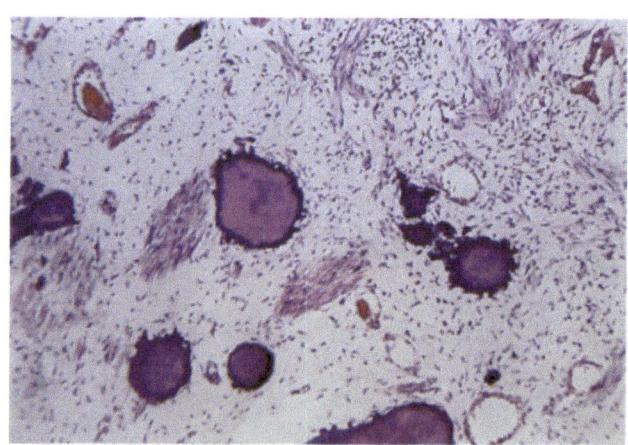

Figure 2.25   Relatively structureless pulp stones and small amorphous calcifications.   H & E × 100

Fatty change is uncommonly present in ageing teeth as droplets of fat which can be demonstrated with conventional fat stains. It is probably the result of progressive ischaemia related to the narrowing of the apical foramen that takes place with increasing age (Figure 2.22).

Fibrosis. The pulp of young teeth has a fine connective tissue which matures only to the reticulin stage. As the tooth ages a large part of the pulp is replaced by collagenous fibrous tissue and becomes less cellular (Figure 2.22).

Pulpal calcification. Dystrophic calcification in the pulp is extremely common. Diffuse calcification appears as granules of densely haematoxyphilic material, especially in the root canals (Figure 2.23). Focal areas of calcification (pulp stones) may be seen lying either free within the pulp or attached to the dentine of the pulp wall (Figures 2.24 and 2.25). They are usually concentrically lamellated and may contain dentinal tubules (true pulp stones) or they may be relatively structureless (false pulp stones). Pulp stones can be large enough to be detected radiographically, but, despite popular misconception, do not cause any symptoms.

Idiopathic internal resorption. In this uncommon condition of unknown aetiology there is chronic inflammation of the pulp with granulation tissue formation. Osteoclasts cause focal resorption of the dentine and there may be

areas of repair with atubular dentine or cementum. Sometimes the process extends throughout the coronal dentine and enamel and results in exposure of the pulp (Figures 2.26 and 2.27).

Injuries to the Teeth[1]

Acute Injuries

Physical injury to developing teeth is not uncommon and usually results from a blow to the overlying deciduous tooth. If the injury involves the crown of an early tooth germ enamel and dentine formation are impaired, producing hypoplastic defects in the tooth as described previously. At a later stage in development the crown may be temporarily displaced without serious damage, or root formation may continue at an angle to the displaced crown, resulting in a bent or dilacerated tooth which frequently fails to erupt (Figure 2.28).

A blow to an erupted tooth may cause displacement or fracture. If the degree of displacement is minimal there may be haemorrhage into the pulp. Often, however, the periapical vessels are severed and the pulp undergoes infarction. The necrotic pulp is frequently invaded by bacteria, which leads to inflammation in the periapical

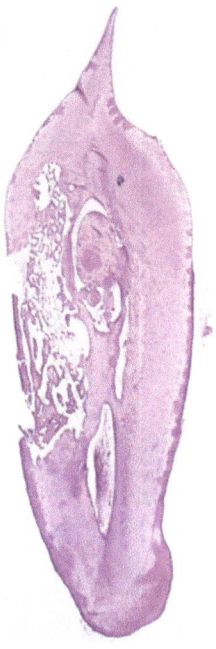

Figure 2.26 Idiopathic internal resorption. There has been severe resorption of the dentine and perforation of the enamel near the cervical margin, with consequent exposure of the pulp.   H & E × 4·5

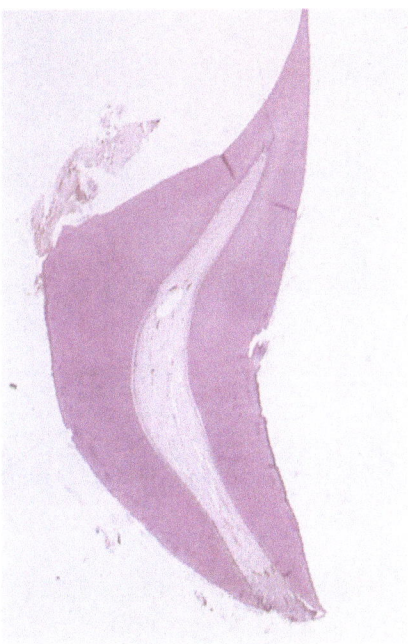

Figure 2.28 Dilaceration. Injury to the tooth germ has caused the root to develop at an angle to the crown.   H & E × 4

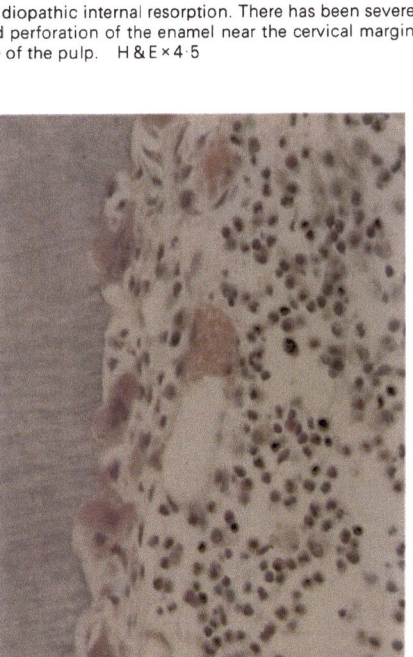

Figure 2.27 Idiopathic internal resorption, showing the inflamed pulp and resorption of dentine by osteoclast-like giant cells.   H & E × 400

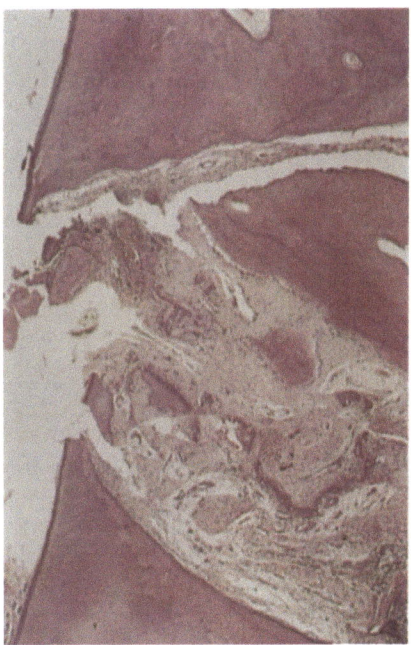

Figure 2.29 Root fracture. Irregular cementum has been deposited over the fractured root surfaces and there has been fibrous union.   H & E × 40

tissues and may result in the formation of a periapical granuloma (see Chapter 3).

If the crown of a tooth is fractured but a sufficient thickness of dentine remains around the pulp the latter responds by transient inflammation followed by the deposition of an irregular type of secondary or reparative dentine. This seals off any open dentinal tubules. If the fracture involves the pulp there is usually severe inflammation and pulpal necrosis rapidly follows.

Root fractures may be followed by repair if the line of the fracture is not exposed to the oral fluids. At the time of injury there is haemorrhage around the root fragments and this haematoma later organizes. There is osteoclastic resorption of the exposed root surfaces and irregular cementum is deposited over the fractured surfaces. It is uncommon for complete hard tissue union of the root fragments to ensue. The typical end result is fibrous union (Figure 2.29).

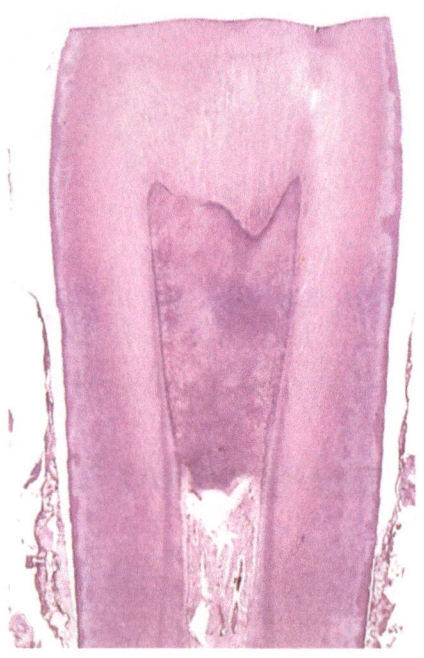

Figure 2.30 Attrition. Irregular reparative dentine has been deposited in response to the low grade injury of attrition.   H & E × 12

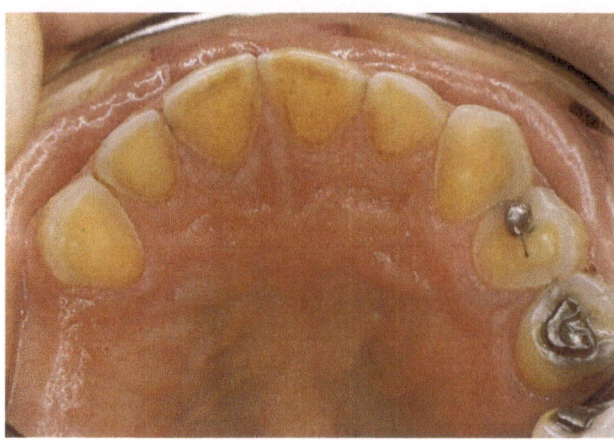

Figure 2.32 Erosion. Habitual vomiting has caused loss of enamel on the palatal aspect of the upper anterior teeth and the yellowish colour of the dentine is now visible

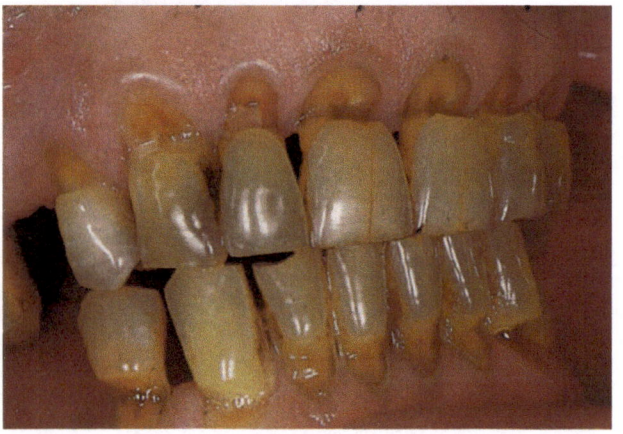

Figure 2.31 Toothbrush abrasion. Deep grooves have been worn into the teeth by excessive and incorrect toothbrushing

Chronic Injuries

The teeth are subjected to wear and damage by a variety of physical and chemical agents.

Attrition is the wearing away of tooth substance due to tooth-to-tooth contact and is most conspicuous on the occlusal and incisal surfaces of the teeth. It is most severe in people living on a coarse, gritty diet or in patients with abnormal teeth, e.g. dentinogenesis imperfecta (Figure 2.4). Severe attrition is also seen in persons who habitually grind their teeth, especially at night. Wear facets develop in the enamel and later the underlying dentine becomes exposed and often stained. On the pulpal aspect variable amounts of secondary (reparative) dentine form and this helps to compensate for the loss of tooth substance (Figure 2.30).

Abrasion is pathological wear of tooth substance caused by foreign bodies. Incorrect and excessive toothbrushing and chewing on a pipe stem are the most common causes (Figure 2.31). The microscopical changes are similar to those of attrition.

Erosion is loss of tooth tissue due to the action of chemical substances and not mediated by bacterial action (as is caries). It may be seen in workers in the battery and pickling industries, in habitual vomiting and in those who consume excessive amounts of acidic drinks, fruits or medicines (Figure 2.32). There is progressive superficial loss of enamel (without the softening typical of caries). This is followed by reparative dentine formation.

References

1. Pindborg, J. J. (1970). *Pathology of the Dental Hard Tissues.* (Copenhagen : Munksgaard)

2. Sedano, H. O., Sauk, J. J. and Gorlin, R. J. (1977). *Oral Manifestations of Inherited Disorders.* (Boston, London : Butterworth)

3. Sunderland, E. P. and Smith, C. J. (1980). The teeth in osteogenesis and dentinogenesis imperfecta. *Brit. Dent. J.,* **149**, 287

4. Gibbard, P. D., Lee, K. W. and Winter, G. B. (1973). Odontodysplasia. *Brit. Dent. J.,* **135**, 525

5. Gardner, D. G. and Sapp, J. (1977). Ultrastructural, electron-probe, and microhardness studies of the controversial amorphous areas in the dentine of regional odontodysplasia. *Oral Surg.,* **44**, 549

6. Cohen, S. and Becker, G. L. (1976). Origin, diagnosis, and treatment of the dental manifestations of vitamin-D resistant rickets: review of the literature and report of a case. *J. Am. Dent. Ass.,* **92**, 120

7. Ulvestad, H., Lökken, P. and Mjörud, F. (1978). Discoloration of permanent front teeth in 3,157 Norwegian children due to tetracyclines and other factors. *Scand. J. Dent. Res.,* **86**, 147

8. Murray, J. J. (1973). A history of water fluoridation. *Brit. Dent. J.,* **134**, 247, 299, 347

9. Seltzer, S. and Bender, I. B. (1975). *The Dental Pulp.* 2nd Edn. (Philadelphia, Toronto : J. B. Lippincott Company)

3

Dental Caries and its Sequelae

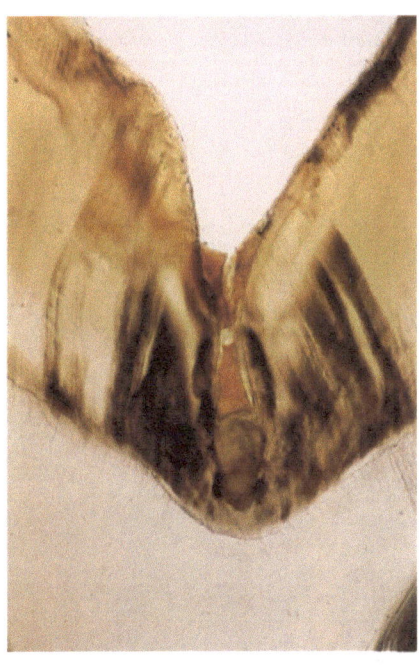

Figure 3.1 Ground section of tooth showing early dental caries. The lesion appears as an arc-shaped area of demineralization in the enamel. The translucent zone at the periphery of the lesion is the earliest detectable change. ×40

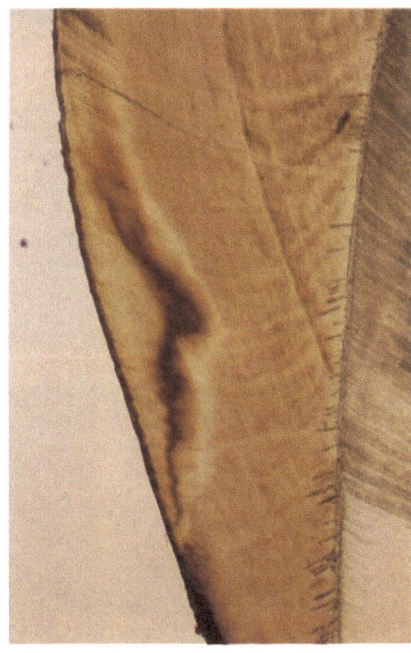

Figure 3.2 Ground section showing a flask-shaped fissure filled with organic debris. Caries begins in the walls of the fissure rather than the base and produces lesions identical to that shown in Figure 3.1. ×40

Dental caries is a bacterial disease characterized by demineralization and dissolution of the dental hard tissues[1]. It arises in the crown of the tooth, or the root if this has become exposed to oral fluids, and usually starts in areas of stagnation such as the deep grooves and pits that are normally present in the occlusal surfaces of the molars and premolars and around the areas of contact of adjacent teeth (the interproximal surfaces). It is at these sites that dental or bacterial plaque accumulates.

Dental plaque, the sticky film that forms on the surface of the teeth in the absence of adequate cleaning, consists of micro-organisms in a matrix of polysaccharides and protein. The matrix is derived partly from bacterial metabolism and partly from saliva. The exact composition of plaque varies according to whether it is situated above or below the gingival margin and it is now regarded as the principle etiological factor in both caries and periodontal disease. Initially, plaque consists mainly of streptococci, especially *Strep. mutans*, but as it matures filamentous organisms become much more numerous and often seem to form the bulk of the organisms seen in histological sections. Other less conspicuous organisms in plaque include lactobacilli, actinomyces and gram negative anaerobes. Plaque micro-organisms metabolize carbohydrates in the diet, particularly sucrose, and form lactic acid which can cause demineralization of dental hard tissues. The extracellular polysaccharides produced by plaque organisms such as *Strep. mutans* appear to be of considerable importance in the pathogenesis of caries, not only by contributing to the bulk and adhesiveness of the plaque, but also by retaining close to the tooth surface the acid produced by bacterial metabolism and by inhibiting the diffusion of salivary buffers.

The earliest macroscopic indication of dental caries is a white spot or opacity in the enamel of a tooth in a stagnation area such as a pit or fissure or below an interstitial contact point. A ground section of the tooth at this stage shows an arc-shaped area of demineralization extending from the enamel surface towards the enamel-dentine junction (Figures 3.1 and 3.2). The process spreads rapidly

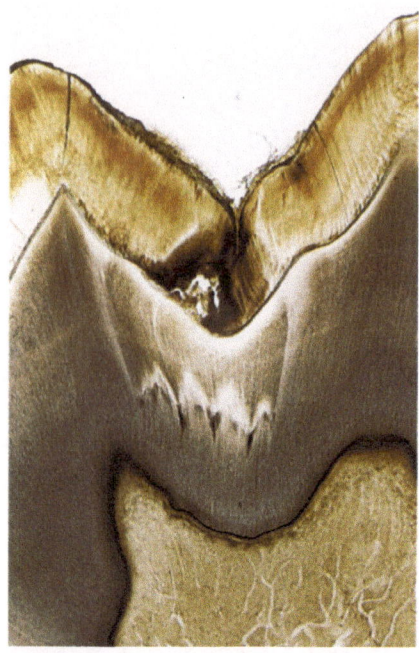

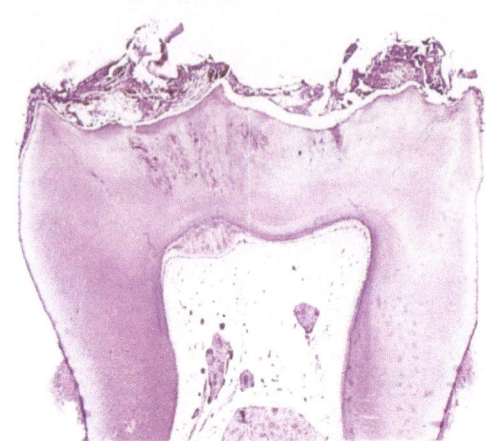

Figure 3.5 This decalcified section shows remnants of the organic matrix of enamel and food debris on the surface of the dentine. Organisms have penetrated deeply into the dentinal tubules and below this area of caries there has been reparative dentine formation.   H & E × 7·5

Figure 3.3 When caries reaches the enamel–dentine junction the process spreads rapidly in a lateral direction and involves a relatively larger area of the underlying dentine.   × 25

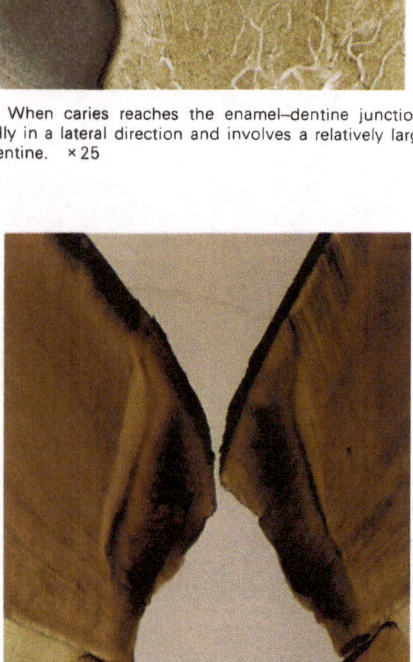

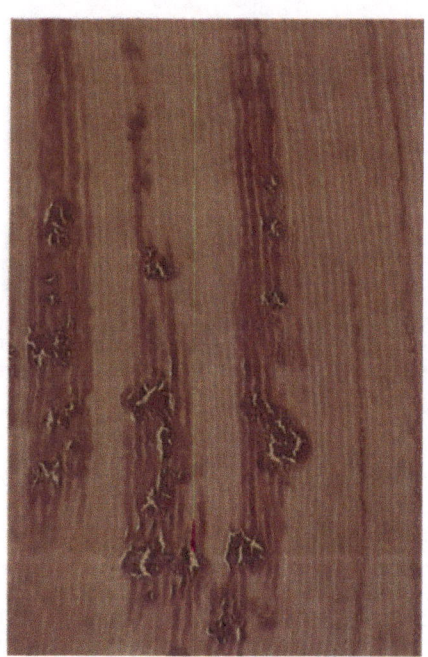

Figure 3.4 The weakened enamel eventually fractures and this allows the ingress of bacteria to the dentine.   × 40

Figure 3.6 The dentinal tubules are filled with large numbers of organisms. Foci where the dentine has softened and the tubules are distended are seen. H & E × 200

and in a lateral direction once it reaches the junction and a relatively large area of enamel thus becomes undermined (Figure 3.3). This causes the weakened enamel to fracture and bacteria can then invade the underlying, and now exposed, dentinal tubules (Figure 3.4). So-called pioneer organisms invade the tubules and can often be seen at a considerable distance from the main carious lesion (Figure

3.5). The tubules then become packed with micro-organisms, which may be cocci, bacilli or filamentous types, and eventually they become grossly distended and liquefaction foci form (Figures 3.6 and 3.7). A particularly characteristic feature of advanced dentine caries is the formation of transverse clefts (Figure 3.8).

Unlike enamel, which is an essentially inert substance,

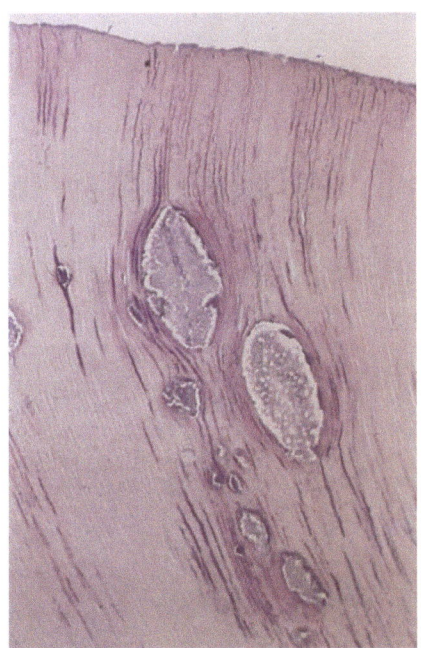

Figure 3.7 Caries of dentine showing liquefaction foci.   H & E × 100

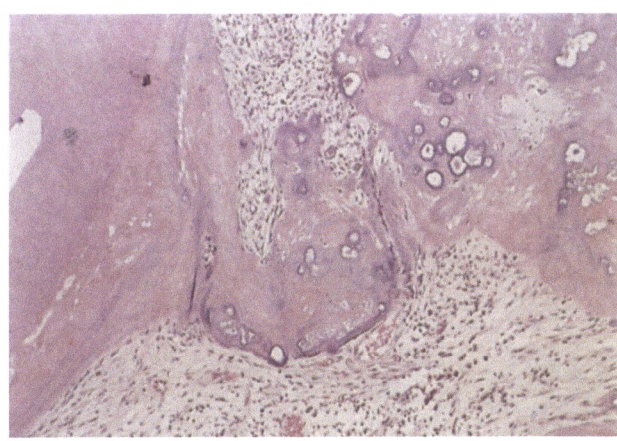

Figure 3.9 Irregular reparative dentine formation and pulpal inflammation
H & E × 100

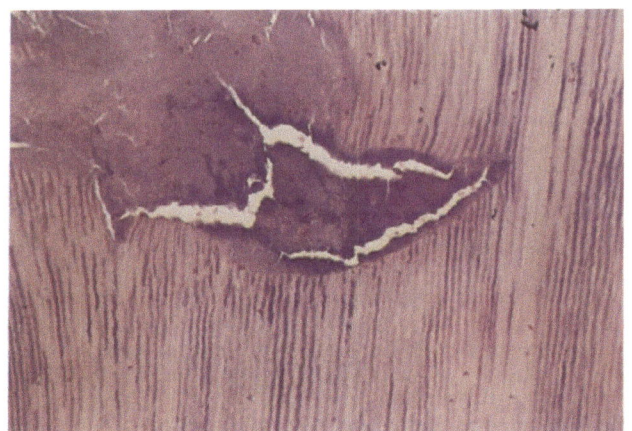

Figure 3.8 Caries of dentine showing transverse clefts.   H & E × 200

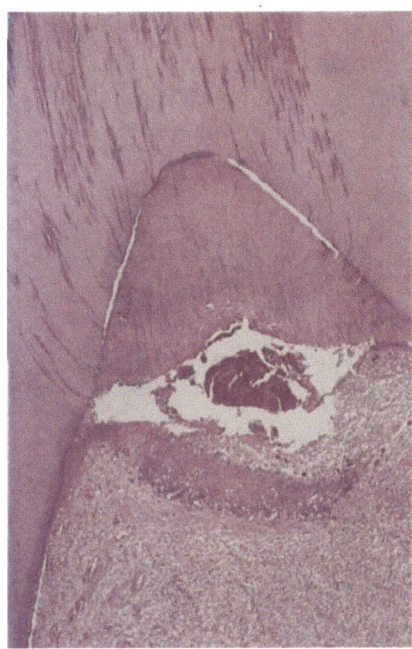

Figure 3.10 Advanced caries. Organisms are penetrating the barrier of reparative dentine and causing pulpal inflammation.   H & E × 40

the dentine is capable of undergoing a vital reaction to the carious process, mediated by the odontoblasts and other cells in the pulp. At the periphery of the lesion there is calcification within the dentinal tubules to form a translucent zone which can be seen only in ground sections. If the irritation to the odontoblast process is sufficiently severe, the odontoblast dies and the affected area of dentine is then termed a dead tract. An acellular, hyaline, calcified barrier seals off the pulpal end of the tubules and an irregular type of secondary dentine (reparative dentine) is formed by surviving odontoblasts or by odontoblasts which form from adjacent undifferentiated mesenchymal cells (Figure 3.9). In advanced caries this protective barrier is eventually breached and organisms then have direct access to the pulp (Figure 3.10).

Pulpitis[2,3]

Pulpitis is the commonest cause of toothache and accounts for the majority of teeth extracted in young people. It is usually a consequence of dental caries but may be the result of physical or chemical injury. Pulpitis frequently leads to pulpal necrosis and infection can spread through the apical foramen to involve the periapical and adjacent hard and soft tissues.

The main clinical manifestation of pulpitis is pain, often exacerbated by changes in temperature. Pulpitis is usually described as acute or chronic, according to the severity and duration of the symptoms, but there is often a distinct lack of correlation between the clinical features and the histological appearances.

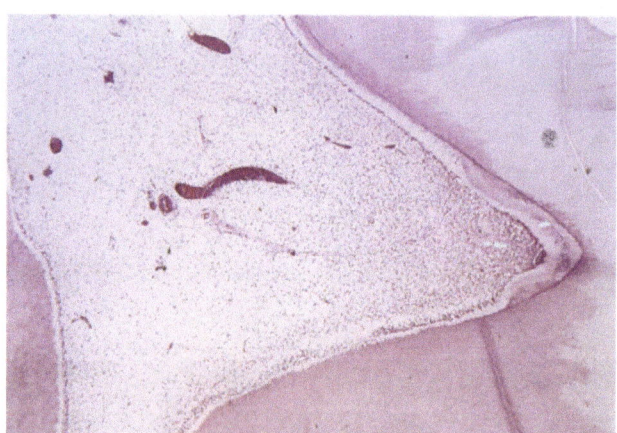

Figure 3.11 Early acute pulpitis. There is hyperaemia and early neutrophil accumulation in the pulp horn.   H & E × 40

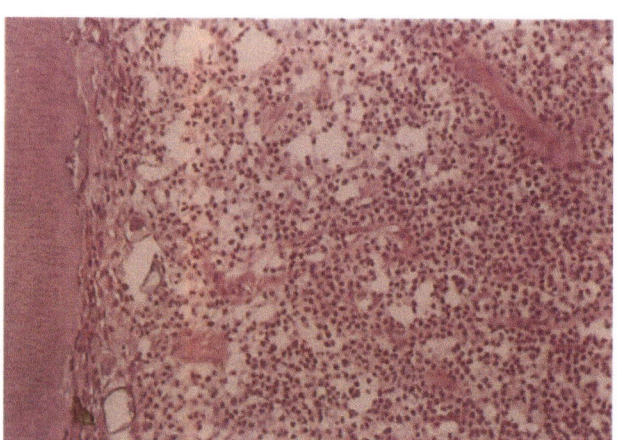

Figure 3.12 Late acute pulpitis. The odontoblast layer has been destroyed and the pulp chamber is filled with neutrophils and macrophages. Impairment of the pulpal blood supply usually leads to necrosis of the pulp.   H & E × 200

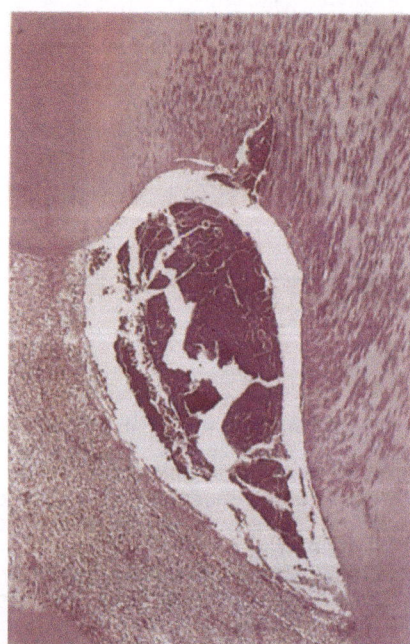

Figure 3.13 Acute pulpitis with abscess formation. Occasionally fibrosis at the periphery of an abscess walls off the lesion, at least temporarily.   H & E × 40

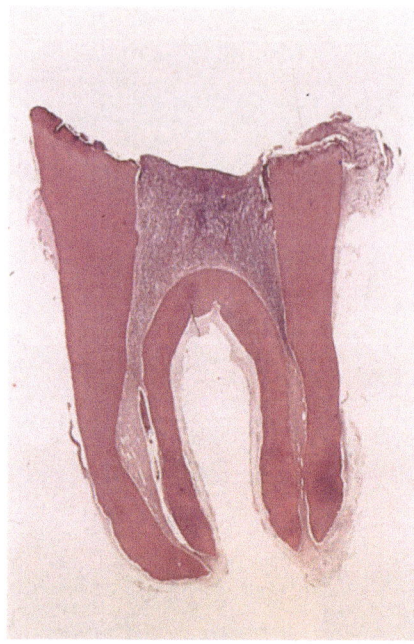

Figure 3.14 Chronic open pulpitis. The pulp chamber is filled with chronically inflamed granulation tissue.   H & E × 6·5

Acute Pulpitis

The micro-organisms that have reached the pulp from the carious dentine elicit an acute inflammatory reaction (Figure 3.11). In the early stages the inflammation is confined to the area of pulp underlying the zone of carious dentine and a localized pulp abscess may form, but the process usually extends within a short period to involve the entire pulp. The inflammatory congestion and oedema cannot easily be accommodated within the rigid walls of the pulp chamber, and the consequent increase in pressure leads to impairment of the pulpal circulation (Figures 3.12 and 3.13). In addition, the vessels passing through the relatively narrow apical foramen are also compressed and this further compromises the blood supply, leading to rapid pulpal necrosis.

Chronic Pulpitis

Although a frequent outcome of pulpitis is pulp death, on occasion a pulp abscess may remain localized and become surrounded by chronic inflammatory cells and granulation tissue. There may be attempts at repair at the periphery. In other cases there is slow progression of the chronic inflammation throughout the pulp with mild hyperaemia and infiltration of lymphocytes and plasma cells. The pulp may show fibrosis and areas of dystrophic calcification.

Chronic Hyperplastic Pulpitis (pulp polyp)

In large carious cavities there may be exposure of a wide area of pulp. By this stage the pulp is usually necrotic but occasionally it survives, and may even become hyperplastic (Figure 3.14). Chronic open pulpitis of this type is

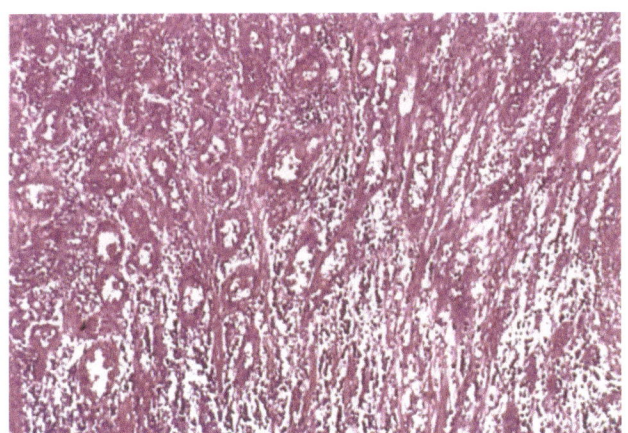

Figure 3.15 Chronic open pulpitis. Higher magnification showing severely inflamed granulation tissue.   H & E × 100

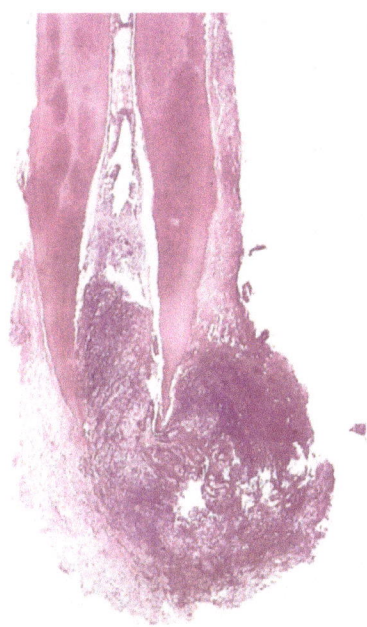

Figure 3.17 Periapical granuloma. There is pulpal necrosis and a dense mass of chronic inflammatory cells around the root of the tooth. The granuloma is permeated by epithelium derived from the cell rests of Malassez: H & E × 14

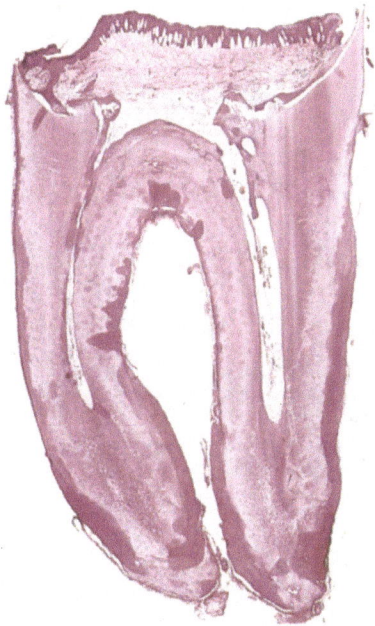

Figure 3.16 Pulp polyp. There is chronic hyperplastic pulpitis and the inflamed fibrous and granulation tissue is covered by stratified squamous epithelium. H & E × 6

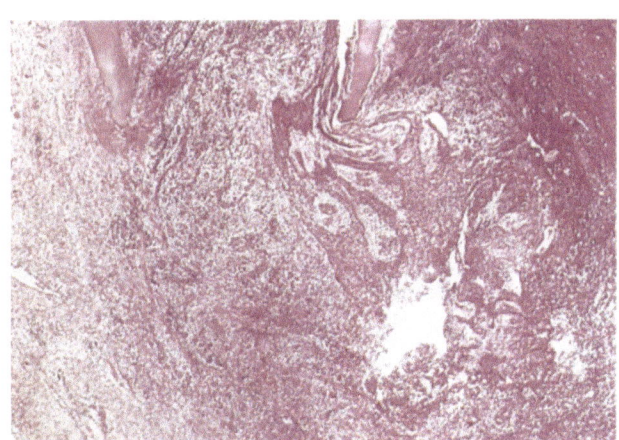

Figure 3.18 Higher magnification, showing cell rests of Malassez proliferating in a heavily inflamed periapical granuloma.   H & E × 40

most often seen in the teeth of children where the apices are not fully formed and the pulp therefore has a good blood supply. The hyperplastic pulp tissue bulges into the carious cavity as a red or pink nodule or polyp. Microscopically, the pulp chamber is seen to be filled with granulation tissue which is often severely inflamed (Figure 3.15). When this tissue has proliferated sufficiently to protrude into the carious cavity the surface may become epithelialized, presumably as a result of implantation of epithelial cells desquamated from the oral mucosa (Figure 3.16). The polyp is then covered by stratified squamous epithelium and the underlying pulpal inflammation tends to subside. This is followed by fibroblastic proliferation and collagenization.

Periapical Granuloma/Abscess
(periapical periodontitis)[3]

Following the death of the pulp inflammatory changes extend by way of the root canal and the apical foramen to the tissues surrounding the root of the tooth. A mass of granulation tissue forms, usually in relation to the apical foramen but occasionally on the lateral aspect of the tooth when a lateral or accessory root canal has been involved (Figures 3.17 and 3.18). The lesion is often symptomless, but it may be painful, especially when biting or chewing or when the affected tooth is gently percussed. Radiographs show a periapical radiolucency, sometimes with resorption of part of the involved root. The radiolucent area may

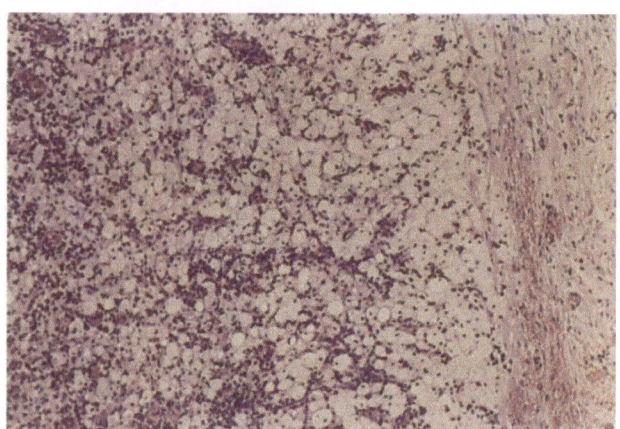

Figure 3.19 Periapical granuloma with numerous foamy macrophages. H & E × 100

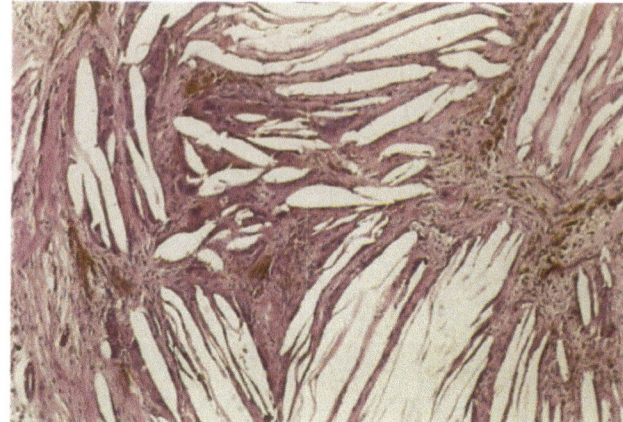

Figure 3.21 Periapical granuloma with cholesterol clefts and related multi-nucleated giant cells and foci of haemosiderin deposition. H & E × 100

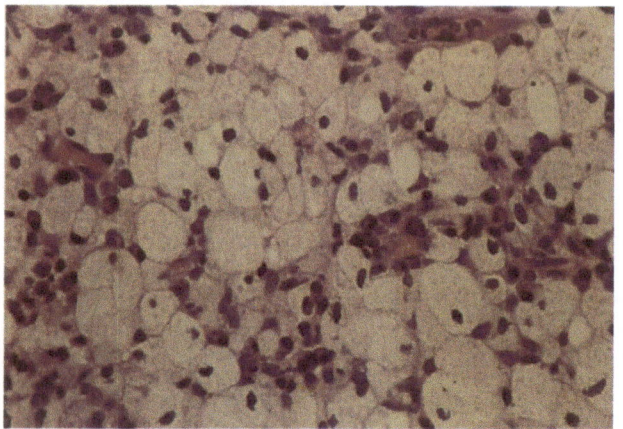

Figure 3.20 Higher magnification to show foamy macrophages. H & E × 400

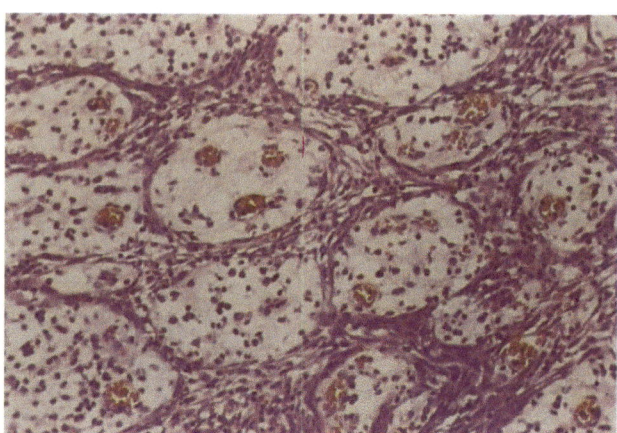

Figure 3.22 Intercellular oedema and neutrophil infiltration of odontogenic epithelium in a periapical granuloma. H & E × 200

be surrounded by a thin osteosclerotic rim or there may be a more diffuse periphery. Lesions of this type are frequently removed together with a portion of the apex of the affected tooth (apicectomy) and sent for microscopical examination.

The histological appearances depend on the stage of the lesion. Initially there is hyperaemia, oedema and intense neutrophil infiltration. As the lesion matures there is progressive infiltration of lymphocytes and plasma cells, and resorption of the surrounding bone. Vascular granulation tissue is formed and there is fibroblastic proliferation and collagenization. Large foamy macrophages, sometimes in considerable numbers, are common and in older lesions cholesterol clefts and associated multinucleated giant cells are frequently present (Figures 3.19–3.21). An important feature of apical granulomas is the presence of epithelium, derived from previously quiescent cell rests in the adjacent periodontal ligament (the cell rests of Malassez, remnants of the epithelial root sheath). The irritation causes these cells to proliferate and extend into the mass of granulation tissue as thin sheets and strands. There is often severe intercellular oedema and extensive infiltration

of the epithelium by neutrophils (Figure 3.22). There may be small areas of breakdown in the epithelium and these represent the beginning of cyst formation. When there is an acute exacerbation neutrophils continue to migrate into the area, with suppuration and abscess formation. The pus tends to track through the surrounding bone, usually on the buccal aspect, and discharges through a sinus over the apex of the involved tooth.

An infected root canal can be reamed out, cleaned and filled with inert material. Occasionally substantial quantities of such material may be inadvertently forced through the apex and be seen in a subsequent apicectomy specimen. Similarly, during the operation for apicectomy the end of the root canal is filled, usually with silver amalgam. Portions of this amalgam may be accidentally dropped into the bony cavity and later be seen microscopically in a specimen submitted as a 'failed apicectomy' (Figure 3.23).

Colonies of filamentous micro-organisms are occasionally seen in periapical granulomas (Figure 3.24). It is not generally possible reliably to identify these organisms as actinomyces, but their presence in this situation is usually of no clinical significance.

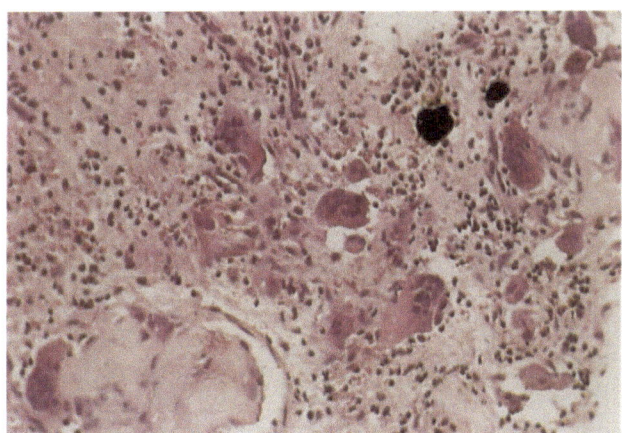

Figure 3.23 Periapical granuloma. Black fragments of silver amalgam and foreign body giant cells in a lesion removed after a failed apicectomy.   H & E × 200

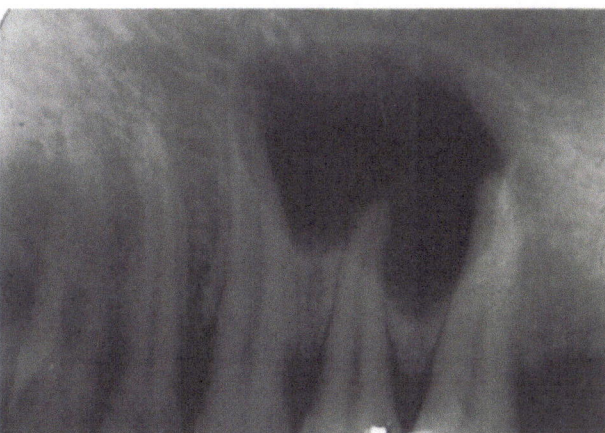

Figure 3.25 Periapical radiograph of a large radicular cyst. The lesion appears as a well defined area of radiolucency at the apex of the affected tooth

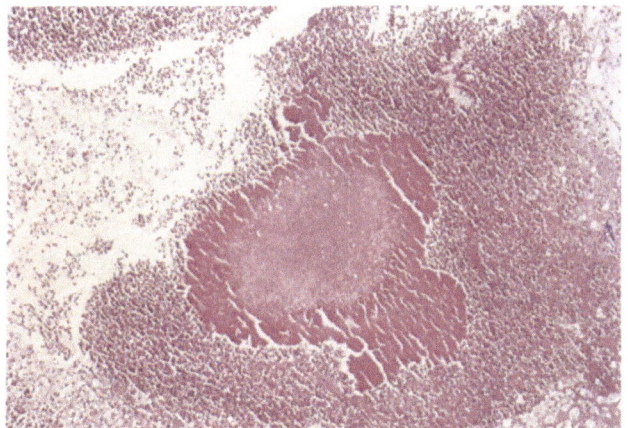

Figure 3.24 Colony of filamentous bacteria in a periapical granuloma. H & E × 100

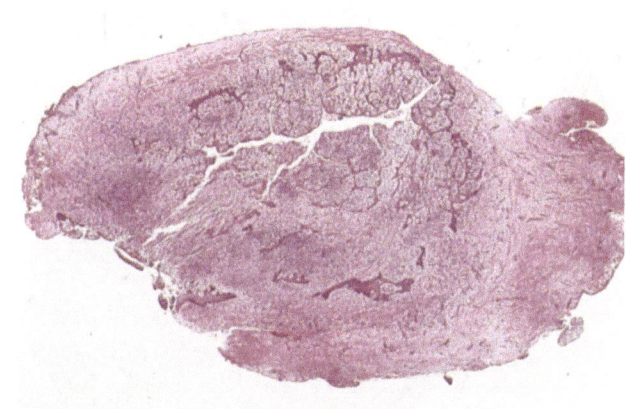

Figure 3.26 Low power view of an inflamed periapical granuloma which is extensively infiltrated by odontogenic epithelium and shows early cyst formation. × 6

Radicular Cyst
(Apical cyst, periapical cyst, dental cyst)[4]

Cysts lined by epithelium derived from the cell rests of Malassez in the periodontal ligament are the commonest cysts of the jaws[5]. Most are associated with the apex of a tooth or less commonly with a lateral root canal. The pulp of the associated tooth is invariably necrotic and this has been followed by the formation of a periapical granuloma in which the cyst arises, as described above.

The radiographic features are similar to those of a periapical granuloma, but cysts are usually larger and have a better defined periphery (Figure 3.25). A radicular cyst may remain after extraction of the related tooth, when it is termed a *residual cyst*.

Early in its formation a periapical cyst is lined by hyperplastic stratified squamous epithelium which in some areas forms an incomplete lining, while elsewhere it penetrates extensively the underlying chronically inflamed fibrous wall (Figures 3.26 and 3.27). There is often gross intercellular oedema in the epithelium and the fluid spaces frequently contain neutrophils. Dilated capillaries are

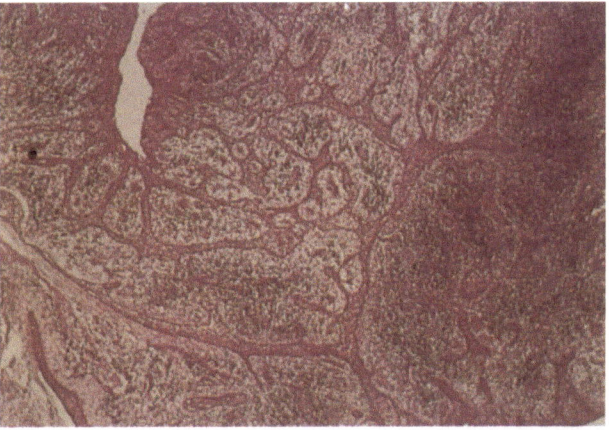

Figure 3.27 Higher magnification of proliferating odontogenic epithelium in the wall of an early radicular cyst.   H & E × 40

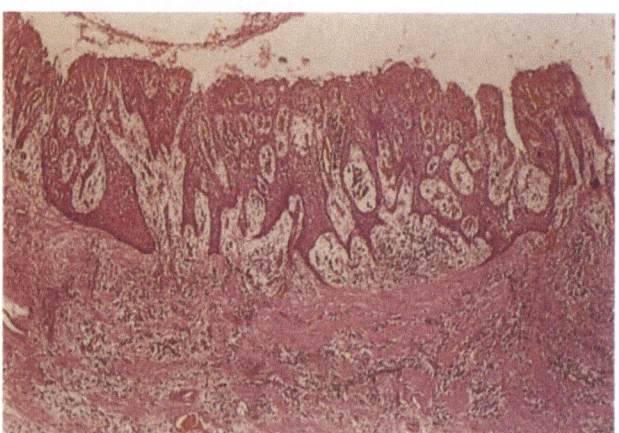

Figure 3.28 Epithelial lining of an early radicular cyst. The prominent superficial blood vessels are typical.   H & E × 40

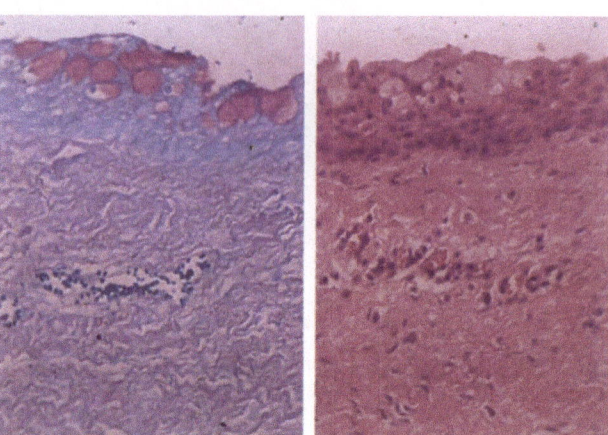

Figure 3.31 Mucous metaplasia in the epithelium of a radicular cyst. Right H & E. Left Mucicarmine.   × 100

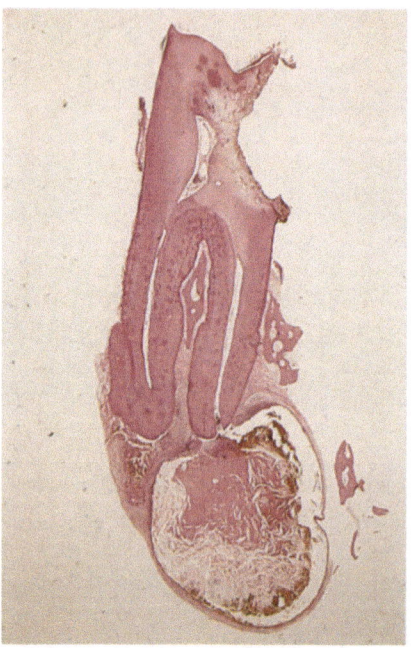

Figure 3.29 Radicular cyst. A mature cyst is attached to a root of a grossly carious tooth. The cyst is lined by attenuated epithelium and contains amorphous material in which cholesterol clefts are seen.   × 3

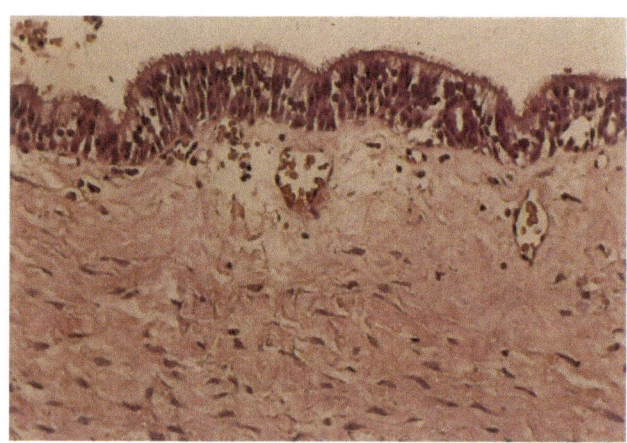

Figure 3.32 Ciliated epithelium in a radicular cyst.   H & E × 200

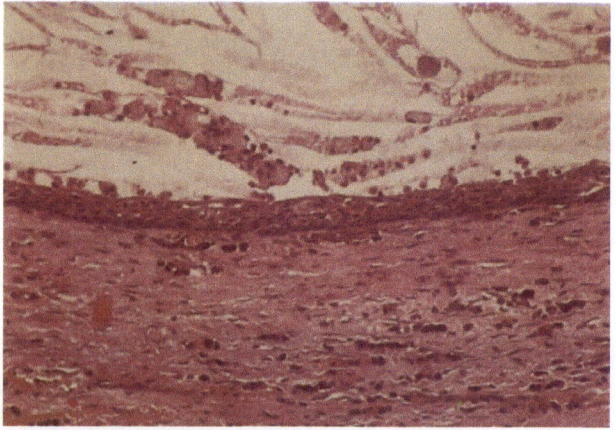

Figure 3.30 Radicular cyst. Higher magnification to show the lining of a mature cyst.   H & E × 200

present in the fibrous cyst wall adjacent to the cyst lining (Figure 3.28). Foamy macrophages are often seen, sometimes in large numbers, both within the wall of the cyst and in the cyst cavity. The cyst wall tends to become less inflamed and more fibrous towards the periphery of the lesion and the collagen bundles appear to be arranged concentrically around the cyst.

As the cyst matures it becomes less inflamed and the epithelial lining becomes thinner and more regular (Figures 3.29 and 3.30). Cholesterol clefts and associated giant cells may be seen in thickened nodules in the walls of long-standing lesions and sometimes the epithelial lining breaks down so that large amounts of cholesterol leak into the lumen of the cyst. Occasionally foci of multinucleated giant cells can be seen in the wall, apparently unrelated to cholesterol deposition or foreign material.

The lining may contain mucous cells or it may consist of respiratory-type epithelium, even in mandibular cysts (Figures 3.31 and 3.32). Characteristic hyaline bodies are seen in the epithelium in about 10% of cases. These

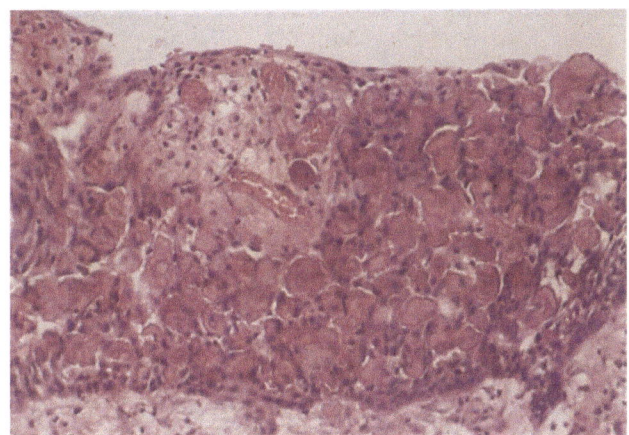

Figure 3.33 Hyaline bodies. In this cyst lining there are many eosinophilic structures, some of which are concentrically laminated.   H & E × 100

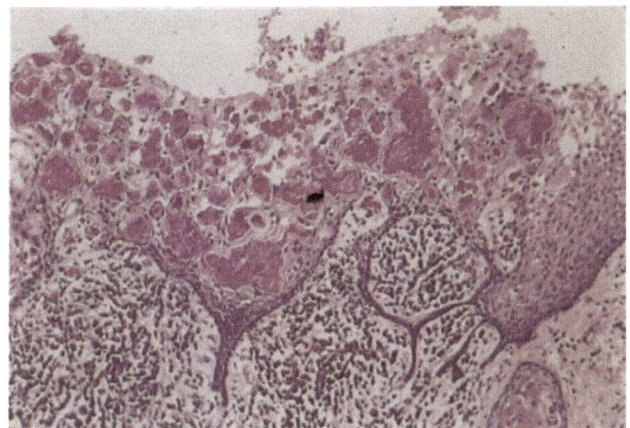

Figure 3.34 Hyaline bodies. In this specimen many of the hyaline bodies are of the granular variety.   H & E × 100

structures are eosinophilic and are straight or curved. They are concentrically laminated or, less frequently, somewhat granular in appearance (Figures 3.33 and 3.34). Their exact nature is not known.

References

1. Silverstone, L. M., Johnstone, N. W., Hardie, J. M. and Williams, R. A. D. (1981). *Dental Caries: Aetiology, Pathology and Prevention*. (London, Basingstoke: The MacMillan Press Limited)
2. Seltzer, S. and Bender, I. B. (1975). *The Dental Pulp*. 2nd Edn. (Philadelphia, Toronto: J. B. Lippincott Company)
3. Shafer, W. G., Hine, M. K. and Levy, B. M. (1983). *A Textbook of Oral Pathology*. 4th Edn. (Philadelphia: W. B. Saunders Company)
4. Shear, M. (1983). *Cysts of the Oral Region*. 2nd Edn. (Bristol: Wright PSG)
5. Tencate, A. R. (1972). The epithelial cell rests of Malassez and the genesis of the dental cyst. *Oral Surg.*, **34**, 956

The Gingivae and Periodontium

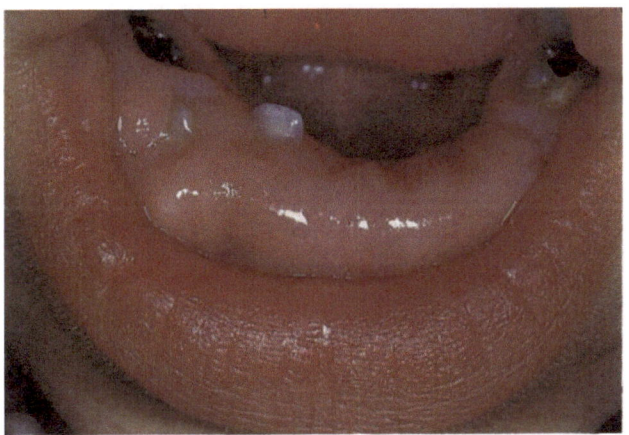

Figure 4.1 Idiopathic gingival fibromatosis. There is gross gingival hyperplasia and the teeth are nearly covered by pale firm gingivae.

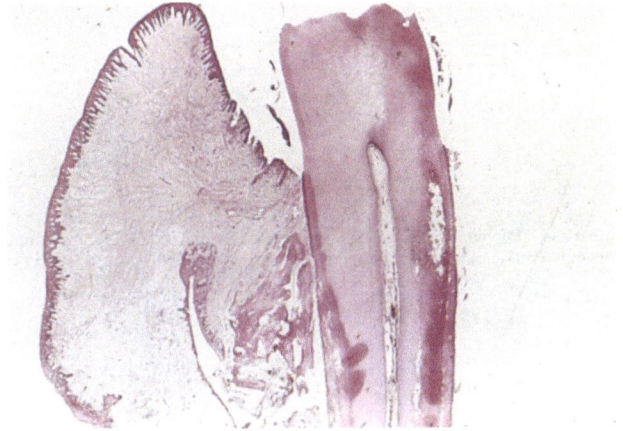

Figure 4.2 Idiopathic gingival fibromatosis. This *in situ* specimen shows gross gingival enlargement. H & E × 4·5

HYPERPLASIA

Gingival Fibromatosis

Idiopathic Fibromatosis

This uncommon condition is characterized by extensive and often severe gingival hyperplasia. Gingival enlargement may precede or follow tooth eruption and teeth in the affected areas are sometimes completely covered by firm, pale gingiva (Figure 4.1). Occasionally there is a familial history and the condition may be associated with hypertrichosis, coarse, thickened tissues and other abnormalities[1,2]. Microscopy shows coarse bundles of sparsely cellular collagen, often with areas of myxomatous change (Figures 4.2 and 4.3). Inflammatory infiltration is usually minimal. The covering epithelium shows mild acanthosis, and mild keratosis may also be seen.

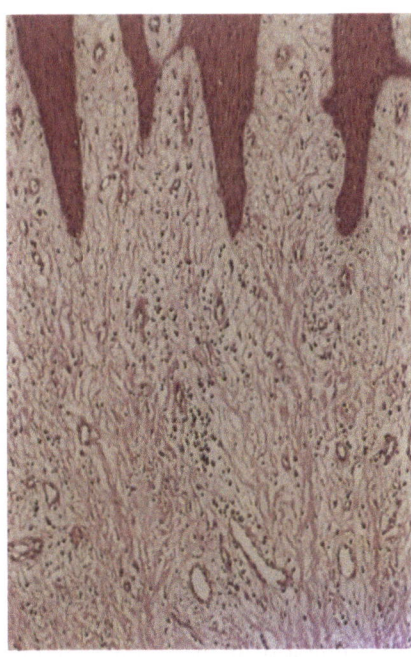

Figure 4.3 Idiopathic gingival fibromatosis. Higher magnification showing sparsely cellular fibrous tissue and patchy chronic inflammatory cell infiltration. H & E × 100

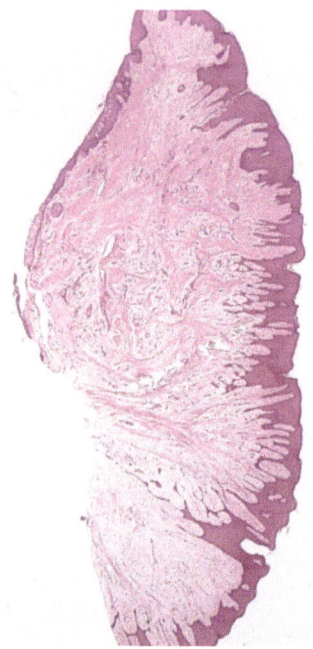

Figure 4.4 Phenytoin-induced gingival hyperplasia. There is a conspicuous increase in fibrous tissue and hyperplasia of the overlying epithelium. H & E × 12·5

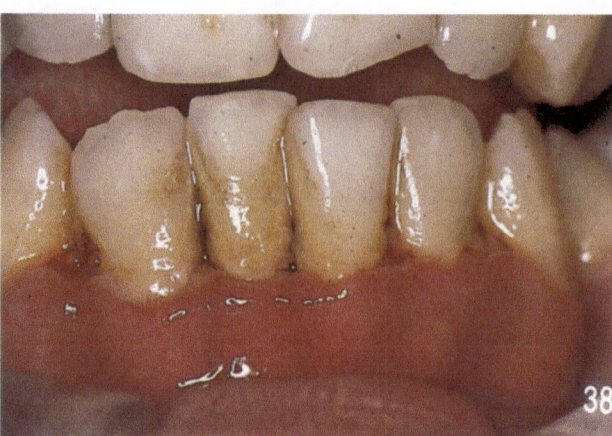

Figure 4.6 Vincent's disease. There are deposits of plaque and calculus on the teeth and the normally pyramidal interdental papillae have been destroyed, leaving crater-shaped ulcers covered by yellowish slough

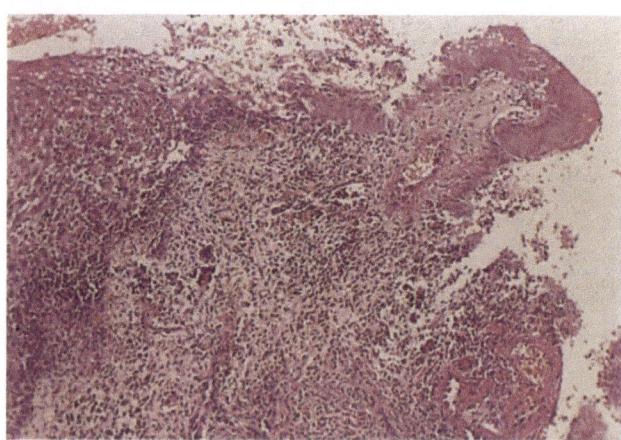

Figure 4.7 Vincent's disease. In this biopsy specimen there is severe intercellular oedema and neutrophil infiltration of the epithelium and corium. The ulcerated area is covered by a fibrinous exudate which contains numerous micro-organisms. H & E × 100

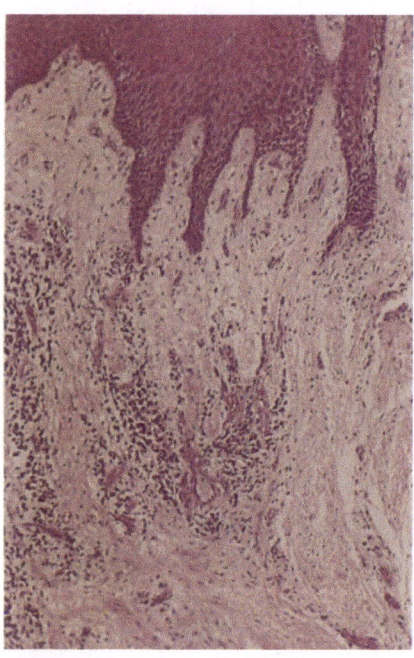

Figure 4.5 Phenytoin-induced gingival hyperplasia. Higher magnification showing fibroblastic proliferation and chronic inflammatory cell infiltration. H & E × 100

Gingival fibromatosis of either variety is usually treated by surgical excision (gingivectomy) but recurrence is very common.

Inflammatory Diseases

Chronic inflammation of the gingiva and periodontium is extremely common and is the major cause of tooth loss in older individuals. Acute inflammatory lesions are much less common and, apart from Vincent's infection, lack specific characteristics.

Acute Necrotizing Ulcerative Gingivitis
(Vincent's disease)

Vincent's disease is characterized by necrosis and destruction of the interdental papillae and marginal gingivae (Figure 4.6). Sometimes the lesions spread from the gingivae to involve adjacent cheek mucosa and this is particularly likely when the disease affects the soft tissue around the

Phenytoin-induced Gingival Hyperplasia

Gingival enlargement is common in patients taking the anti-epileptic drug phenytoin (Epanutin, Dilantin)[3]. The gingival overgrowth tends to be most severe in the interdental region, where the hyperplastic gingiva is pale and firm, with accentuation of the normal stippled pattern. Microscopically there is usually more fibroblastic activity than in the idiopathic lesion and chronic inflammatory infiltration may be pronounced (Figures 4.4 and 4.5).

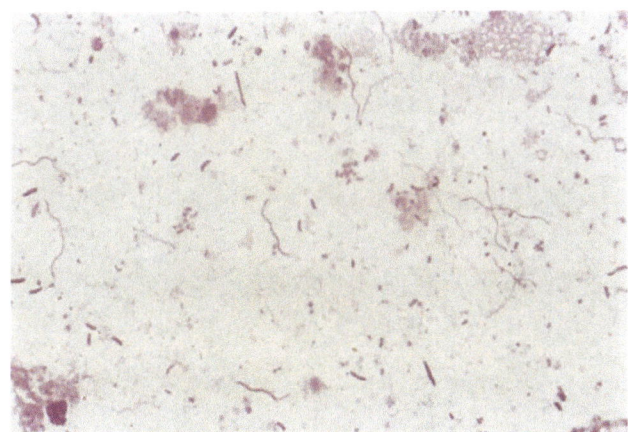

Figure 4.8 Vincent's disease. Smear from gingival exudate showing *Borrelia vincenti* and *Fusobacteria nucleatum*. Fuchsin × 1000

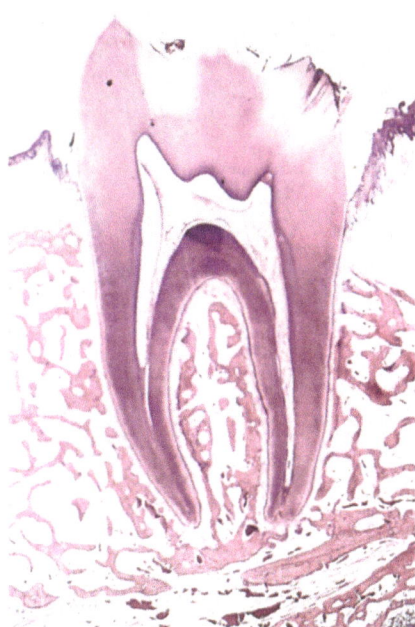

Figure 4.9 Molar tooth, *in situ* in the mandible, with early chronic marginal gingivitis. Detail is minimal at this magnification, but it can be seen that there has been no significant apical migration of the epithelial attachment. H & E × 4·5

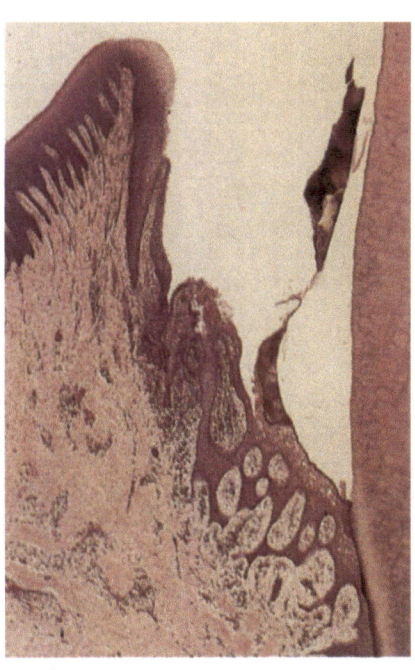

Figure 4.10 Higher magnification showing early chronic marginal gingivitis. There is proliferation and ulceration of the crevicular epithelium and chronic inflammatory infiltration of the subjacent corium. H & E × 40

crown of a partially erupted lower wisdom tooth. The lesions cause pain and bleeding and are associated with bad taste and often severe halitosis. There may be mild constitutional symptoms and occasionally regional lymphadenopathy.

It is very uncommon to receive a biopsy specimen from a patient with active disease (Figure 4.7), but clinicians often take scrapings from the base of an ulcer. Microscopy then shows numerous neutrophils, fibrin and debris and suitable staining demonstrates the characteristic Vincent's organisms (*Borrelia vincenti* and *Fusobacterium nucleatum*) (Figure 4.8). These organisms are also associated with cancrum oris (noma), in which there is massive destruction of the facial tissues. This is seen mainly in children in underdeveloped countries. It is probable that a combination of factors, including gross malnutrition and concomitant systemic infections like measles or malaria, predispose to cancrum oris in these individuals.

Acute Non-specific Gingivitis

This is seen as bright red, oedematous swelling of the gingivae in patients with febrile infections such as acute herpetic stomatitis and streptococcal pharyngitis. The gingival lesions are usually painless and in most cases represent an acute exacerbation of a pre-existing chronic gingivitis. It is very rare for such lesions to be biopsied, when microscopy shows nonspecific acute inflammation only.

Chronic Marginal Gingivitis

Chronic inflammation of the gingivae, of variable degree, is extremely common and represents the response of the gingival tissues to accumulation of dental plaque around the necks of the teeth. When the deposits of plaque are persistent and longstanding there may be more severe inflammation which can spread to involve the underlying periodontal tissues and eventually the supporting bone.

Chronic marginal gingivitis is characterized microscopically by hyperaemia, oedema and chronic inflammatory cell infiltration (Figure 4.9). The crevicular epithelium may be ulcerated and is often hyperplastic with thin, irregular prolongations into the underlying corium (Figure 4.10).

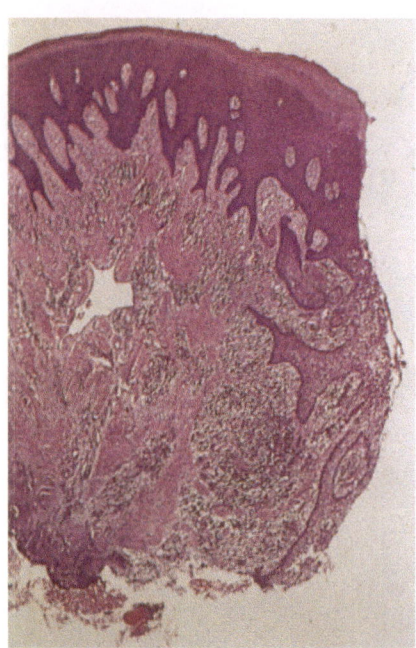

Figure 4.11   Chronic marginal gingivitis. Gingivectomy specimen, showing proliferation of the crevicular epithelium and inflammation of the underlying corium. H & E × 40

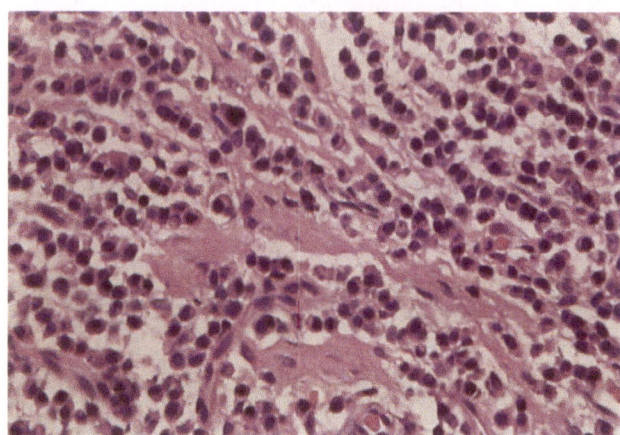

Figure 4.13   Chronic marginal gingivitis. Many lymphocytes and plasma cells are present in the deeper corium.   H & E × 400

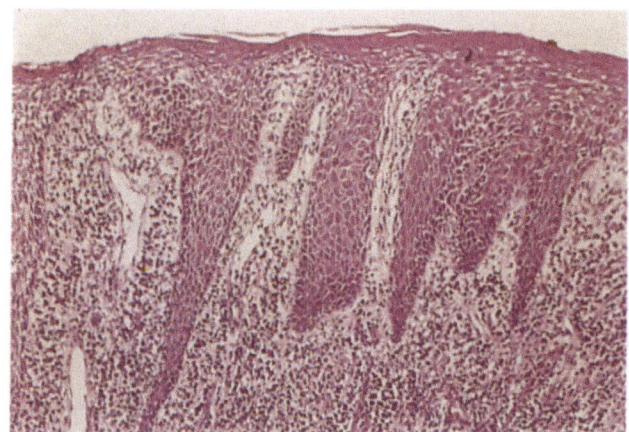

Figure 4.14   Plasma cell gingivitis. There is psoriasiform hyperplasia of the epithelium and dense plasma cell infiltration of the corium.   H & E × 100

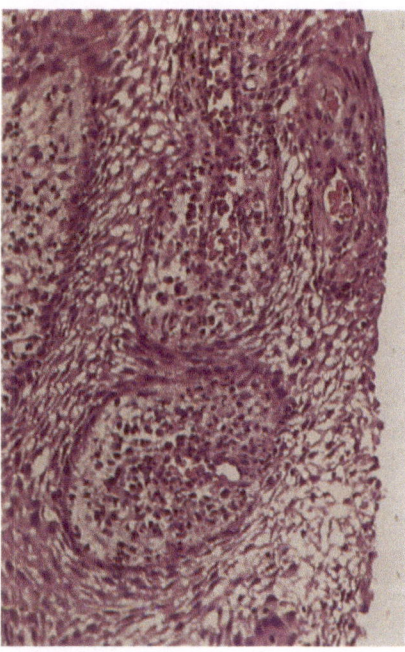

Figure 4.12   Chronic marginal gingivitis. Higher magnification showing the oedematous crevicular epithelium and inflammatory infiltration of the underlying corium.   H & E × 200

Much intercellular oedema and infiltration of the intercellular spaces by neutrophils is seen, especially in the presence of gross plaque or calculus deposits (Figures 4.11 and 4.12). Large numbers of lymphocytes and plasma cells may be present (Figure 4.13) and dense aggregates of extracellular immunoglobulin are frequently seen. Russell bodies are often conspicuous.

There is variable loss of collagen in areas of severe inflammation, but in the peripheral parts of the lesion, especially in young individuals, there may be extensive formation of new fibrous tissue.

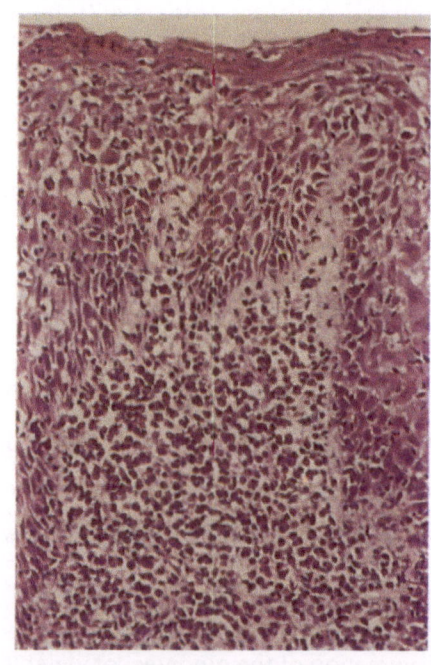

Figure 4.15   Plasma cell gingivitis. Higher magnification showing neutrophils in the superficial epithelium and dense plasma cell infiltration of the corium. H & E × 200

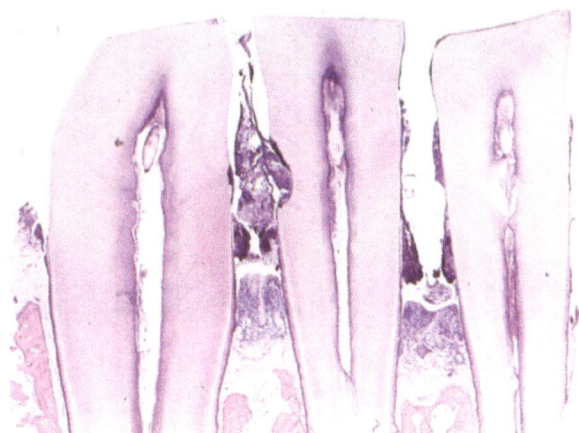

Figure 4.16 Chronic periodontitis. There is gingival recession and chronic periodontitis. There is also cervical caries of the middle tooth and there are gross deposits of plaque and calculus. All the teeth show attrition.   H & E × 5

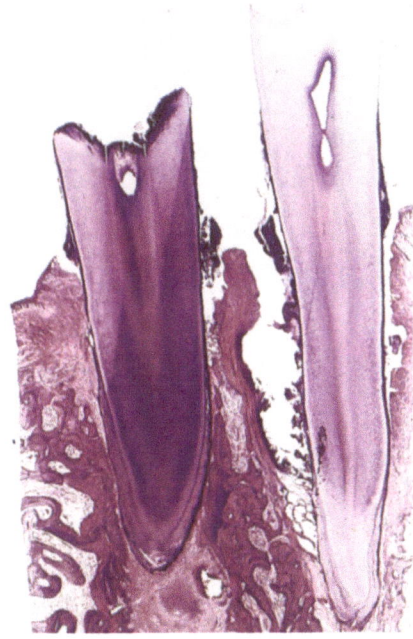

Figure 4.18 Advanced chronic periodontitis with extensive bone loss and loss of attachment of periodontal ligament to the tooth with consequent formation of deep pockets. There are gross deposits of calculus and plaque above and within the pockets.   H & E × 4

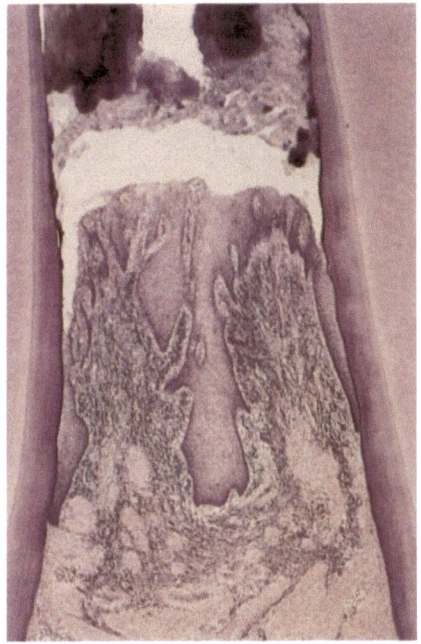

Figure 4.17 Chronic periodontitis. Higher magnification showing migration of the epithelial attachment down the cementum and dense chronic inflammatory infiltration of the corium.   H & E × 40

Plasma Cell Gingivitis

In chronic periodontal disease the presence of many plasma cells can on occasion lead to difficulty in distinguishing this common condition from other plasma-cell lesions of the gingiva. These include extramedullary plasmacytoma (page 145) and an uncommon lesion termed plasma cell gingivitis[4]. In this condition the affected mucosa is bright red and the lesion may spread from the gingival margin on to the alveolar mucosa. The lesions are not associated with blisters or ulcers and are not related to plaque accumulation. Microscopy shows psoriasiform epithelial hyperplasia with spongiosis and infiltration of the epithelium by inflammatory cells, mainly neutrophils (Figure 4.14). There is dense, mainly plasma cell infiltration of the corium (Figure 4.15). The lesion needs to be distinguished microscopically from candidosis, geographic stomatitis, intraoral psoriasis and extramedullary plasmacytoma. Although initially the disease was thought to be an allergic reaction the etiology is essentially unknown.

Chronic Periodontitis[5,6,7]

Long-standing chronic gingivitis slowly progresses to involve the underlying periodontal tissues with eventual loosening and sometimes exfoliation of the teeth (Figures 4.16 and 4.17). The essential feature of chronic periodontal disease is the destruction of the periodontal ligament and supporting alveolar bone. This results in the formation of pockets between the tooth and the supporting soft tissues in which bacterial and organic debris collects (Figure 4.18). One wall of the pocket is formed by root cementum and the other by inflamed fibrous and granulation tissue which has replaced destroyed periodontal fibres and alveolar bone. The epithelium of the gingival sulcus, which is normally attached to the tooth at the enamel–cemental junction, extends apically along the

Desquamative Gingivitis

Desquamative gingivitis is a clinical descriptive term for a condition in which the attached gingiva and sometimes adjacent alveolar mucosa is bright red, shiny and frequently painful. It can be distinguished from uncomplicated chronic gingivitis since the marginal gingiva is usually spared and the lesions fail to respond to improvements in oral hygiene. In most cases desquamative gingivitis appears to be a variant of either atrophic lichen planus or mucous membrane pemphigoid. The presence of lichenoid striations on the gingiva or elsewhere in the mouth, or bulla formation, aids clinical differentiation. The microscopical and immunocytochemical features are described in Chapter 5.

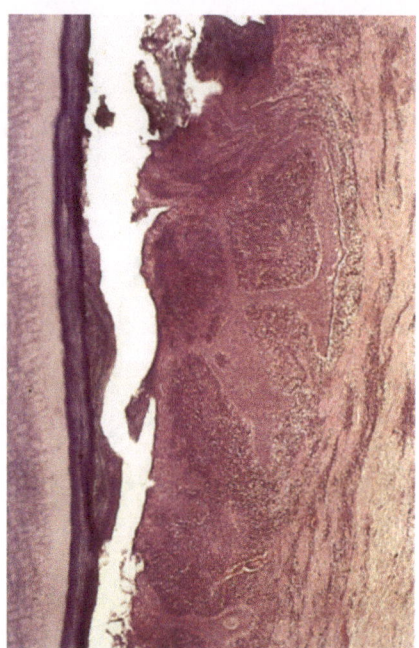

Figure 4.19 Higher magnification of Figure 4.18 showing a pocket. One wall is formed from root cementum and attached calculus and the soft tissue wall consists of hyperplastic epithelium and underlying inflamed corium.   H & E × 40

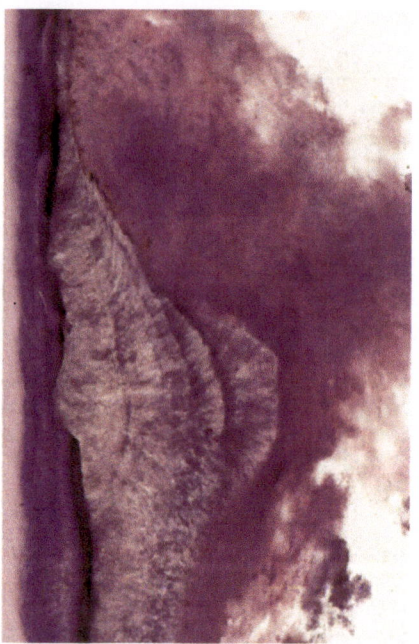

Figure 4.20 Calculus and plaque. Calculus consists of irregular, superimposed deposits of calcified material. This is covered by masses of mainly filamentous organisms (dental plaque).   H & E × 200

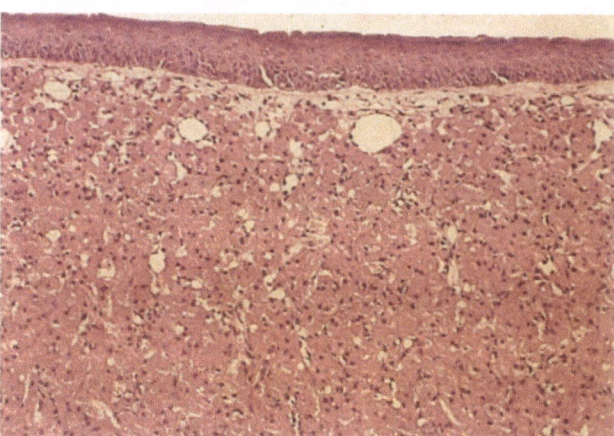

Figure 4.21 Congenital epulis. Microscopy shows a dense mass of granular cells beneath a thin epithelium.   H & E × 40

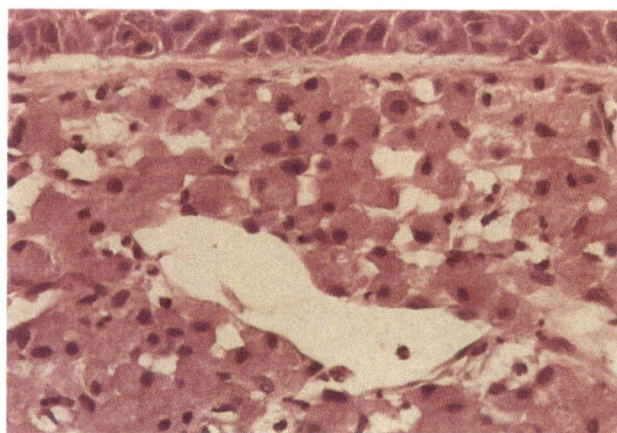

Figure 4.22 Congenital epulis. Higher magnification showing prominent capillaries and large granular cells.   H & E × 400

cementum, covering the inflamed tissues and forming the floor of the pocket. There are dense masses of inflammatory cells in the wall of the pocket, plasma cells and lymphocytes predominating (Figure 4.19). Although bone loss is a feature of chronic periodontal disease, the process is usually very slow; it has been estimated that the rate of loss of alveolar bone in uncomplicated periodontal disease is only one millimetre in five years. Therefore it is hardly surprising that frank osteoclastic resorption of the alveolar bone is rarely seen.

The bacterial plaque in periodontal pockets frequently calcifies to form firmly adherent subgingival calculus (Figure 4.20). This is a source of continuous irritation to the periodontal tissue and accelerates damage.

The Epulides

Epulis is a clinical term describing a localized swelling of the gingiva. By convention it is applied to the lesions described here, although a wide variety of benign and malignant tumours and other lesions can present as nondescript epulides and these possibilities should be considered when examining a specimen with the clinical diagnosis of epulis.

Congenital Epulis

This lesion is seen in newborn infants and is some ten times commoner in females than in males. It presents as a smooth swelling, usually in the maxillary incisor region.

Microscopically, the lesion consists of a mass of densely packed granular cells, similar to those of granular cell myoblastoma and separated from the thin overlying epithelium by a narrow cell-free zone (Figure 4.21). There is

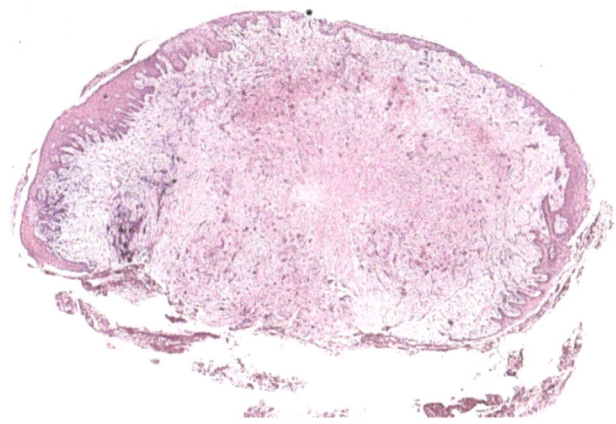

Figure 4.23 Giant cell epulis. This is a diffuse, cellular lesion with focal collections of multinucleated giant cells and patchy haemosiderin deposits. H & E × 7·5

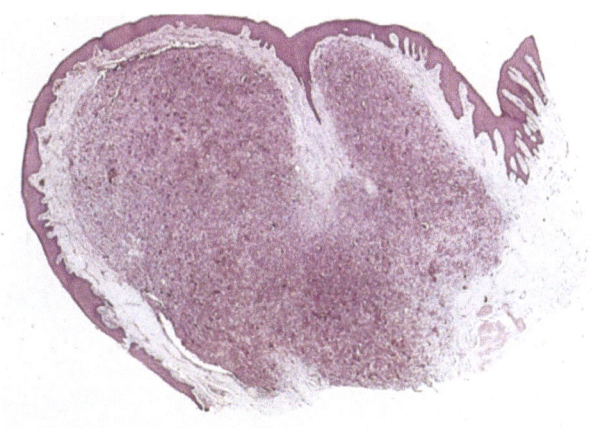

Figure 4.25 Giant cell epulis. This specimen shows a discrete, densely cellular lesion. H & E × 11·5

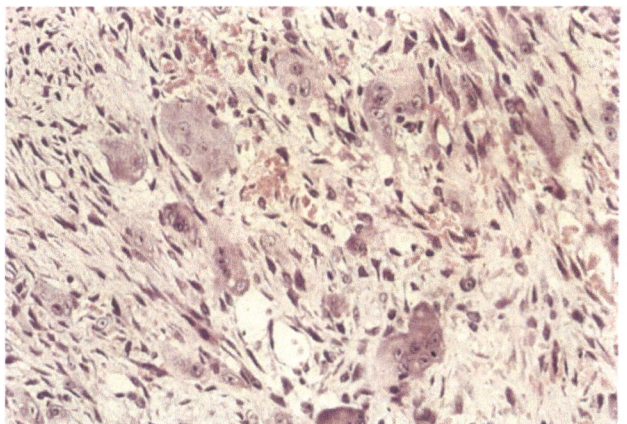

Figure 4.24 Giant cell epulis. Higher magnification showing pale staining, patchily distributed multinucleated giant cells in a stroma containing spindle cells and areas of haemorrhage. H & E × 200

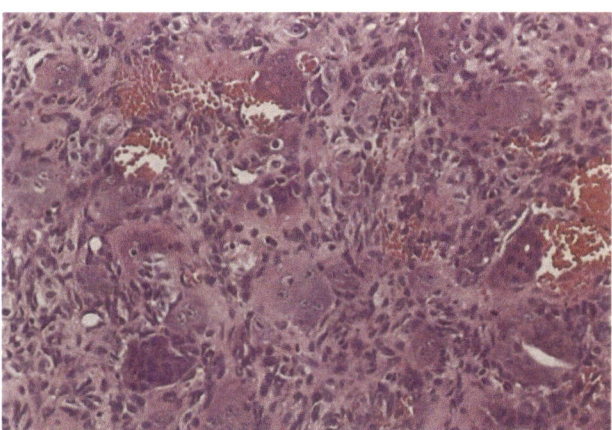

Figure 4.26 Giant cell epulis. Higher magnification shows many multinucleated giant cells and plump spindle-shaped cells. H & E × 200

no hyperplasia of the epithelium such as is seen in granular cell myoblastoma. The round or oval eosinophilic granular cells have a small vesicular nucleus with a well defined central nucleolus (Figure 4.22). The stroma is scanty, but numerous capillaries may be present[8, 9].

Giant Cell Epulis

This relatively common lesion presents as a deep red or maroon swelling of the gingiva, usually in the mandible, and arising most frequently anterior to the first permanent molars. Microscopically, it consists of one or more islets of multinucleated giant cells in a matrix of spindle cells, very similar to the intraosseous or central giant cell granuloma (Figures 4.23–4.27). Small areas of haemorrhage are common. The islets are situated in the corium at a small distance from the epithelium. Although it may recur if not completely removed, the giant cell epulis is essentially a local gingival lesion. Occasionally, however, a central giant cell granuloma may perforate the cortex and present as an epulis and the same may happen with an intra-osseous lesion ('brown tumour') of hyperparathyroidism, so these possibilities should be borne in mind[10].

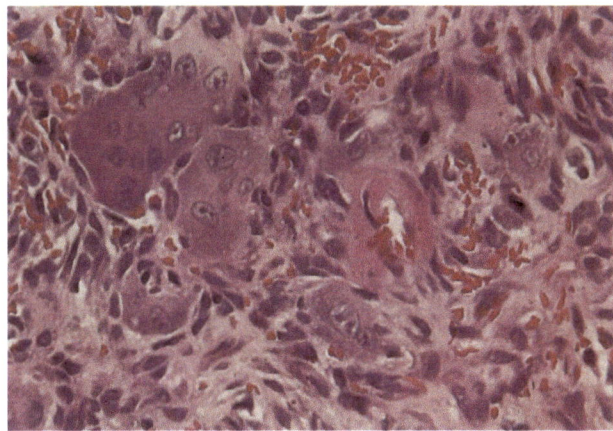

Figure 4.27 Giant cell epulis. Occasional cells with mitoses may be seen. H & E × 400

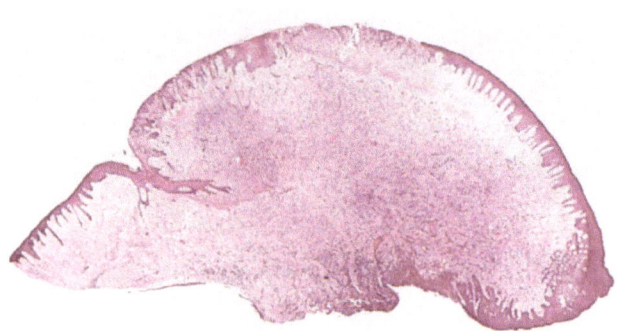

Figure 4.28   Fibrous epulis. The lesion is a severely inflamed, mainly collagenous fibrous overgrowth.   H & E × 10

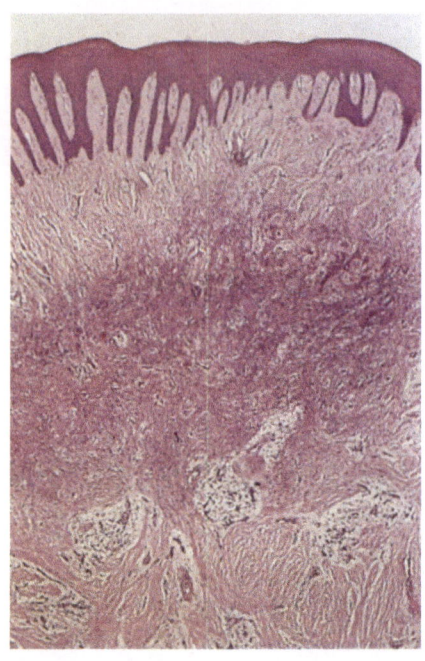

Figure 4.30   Fibrous epulis. This lesion is much more fibroblastic and contains areas of dystrophic calcification and osseous metaplasia.   H & E × 40

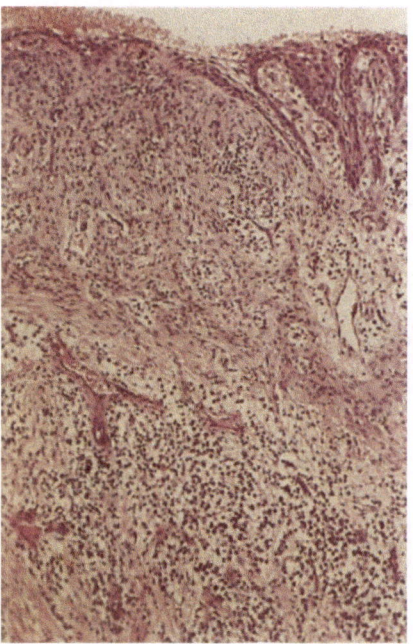

Figure 4.29   Fibrous epulis. Higher magnification showing fibroblastic tissue towards the surface and heavy chronic inflammatory infiltration of the deeper tissue.   H & E × 100

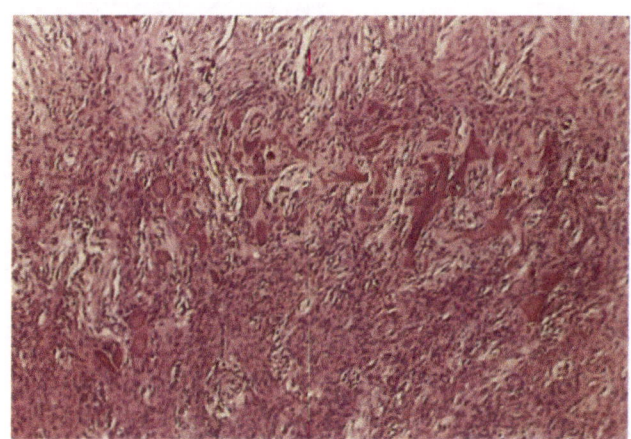

Figure 4.31   Fibrous epulis, showing spheroidal and irregular calcifications. H & E × 100

Fibrous Epulis

This is a common lesion that appears as a firm sessile or pedunculated swelling of the gingiva, usually involving an interdental papilla. Some lesions are relatively pale, others are inflamed and may show superficial ulceration.

Microscopically, the lesion consists of fibrous tissue in which there is variable inflammation and fibroblastic proliferation (Figures 4.28–4.30). Areas of diffuse or focal dystrophic calcification and osseous metaplasia are common and sometimes extensive (Figures 4.30–4.32)[11]. This new bone formation should not be confused with an involucrum or with neoplastic bone. In some cases the fibrous epulis is a much more collagenous lesion, consisting of sparsely cellular coarse fibrous tissue.

The covering epithelium is often inflamed and ulcerated, particularly in the actively growing fibroblastic lesions. It is usually normal or slightly hyperplastic in the more collagenous lesions.

Pregnancy Epulis

This lesion, which is structurally identical to pyogenic granuloma (page 132) is sometimes seen in the second and third trimesters of pregnancy. It appears to be a localized exacerbation of the generalized gingivitis frequently appearing at that time.

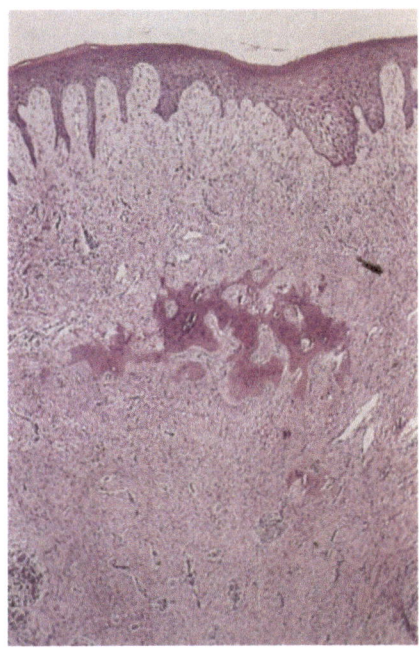

Figure 4.32 Fibrous epulis. The bone in this fibroblastic lesion is more mature than that in Figure 4.30.   H & E × 40

References

1. Raeste, A.-M., Collan, Y. and Kilpinen, E. (1978). Hereditary fibrous hyperplasia of the gingiva with varying penetrance and expressivity. *Scand. J. Dent. Res.*, **86**, 357

2. Giansanti, J. S., McKenzie, W. T. and Owens, F. C. (1973). Gingival fibromatosis, hypertelorism, antimongoloid obliquity, multiple telangiectases and *café au lait* pigmentation: a unique combination of developmental anomalies. *J. Periodontol.*, **44**, 299

3. Hassell, T. M. (1981). *Monographs in Oral Science. Vol. 9*. Epilepsy and the oral manifestations of phenytoin therapy, chapter 7, p. 116. (Basel, München, Paris, London, New York, Sydney: S. Karger)

4. Palmer, R. M. and Eveson, J. W. (1981). Plasma cell gingivitis. *Oral Surg.*, **51**, 187

5. Newman, H. N. (1982). Infection and the periodontal ligament. In: *The Periodontal Ligament in Health and Disease*, chapter 15, p. 335. B. K. B. Berkovitz, B. J. Moxham and H. N. Newman (eds.). (Oxford, New York, Toronto, Sydney, Paris, Frankfurt: Pergamon Press)

6. Page, R. C. and Schroeder, H. E. (1976). Pathogenesis of inflammatory periodontal disease. *Lab. Inv.*, **33**, 235

7. Seymour, G. J., Powell, R. N. and Davis, W. I. R. (1979). The immunopathogenesis of progressive inflammatory periodontal disease. *J. Oral Pathol.*, **8**, 249

8. Fuhr, A. H. and Krogh, P. H. J. (1972). Congenital epulis of the newborn: centennial review of the literature and report of a case. *J. Oral Surg.*, **30**, 30

9. Kay, S., Elzay, R. P. and Willson, M. A. (1971). Ultrastructural observations on a gingival granular cell tumor (congenital epulis). *Cancer*, **27**, 674

10. Giansanti, J. S. and Waldron, C. A. (1969). Peripheral giant cell granuloma: a review of 720 cases. *J. Oral Surg.*, **27**, 787

11. Southham, J. C. and Venkataraman, B. K. (1973). Calcification and ossification in epulides in man (excluding giant cell epulides). *Arch. Oral Biol.*, **18**, 1243

5

The Oral Mucosa

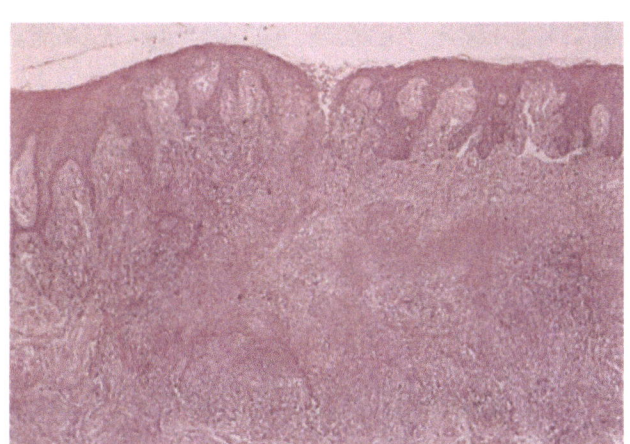

Figure 5.1 Tuberculosis. There is superficial ulceration and the corium contains acute and chronic inflammatory cell infiltrate and epithelioid granulomas. H & E × 40

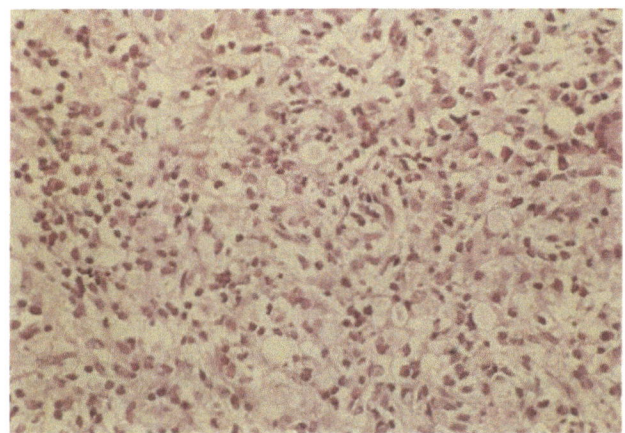

Figure 5.3 Lepromatous leprosy. Sheets of large, pale-staining foamy macrophages (lepra cells) are intermingled with scattered smaller macrophages and lymphocytes. H & E × 250

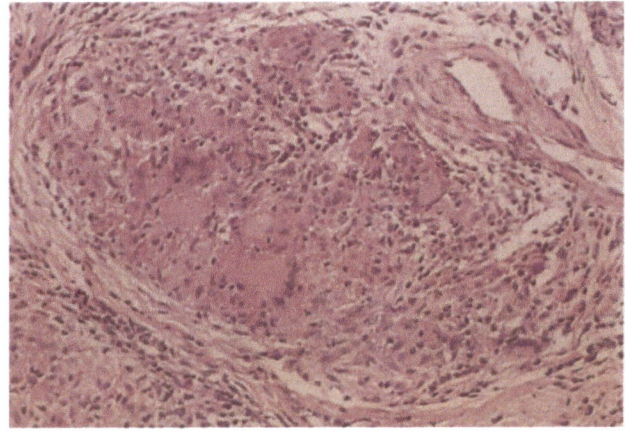

Figure 5.2 Tuberculosis. Higher magnification showing non-caseating epithelioid granulomas with multinucleated giant cells. H & E × 200

INFECTIVE CONDITIONS

Bacterial Infections

Tuberculosis

Tuberculous lesions are uncommon in the mouth and are usually secondary to open pulmonary tuberculosis. A tuberculous ulcer is the usual presentation, the dorsal surface of the tongue being the typical site[1]. The ulcer tends to be single, painful, and characteristically has irregular, undermined edges and a friable, granular floor. Microscopy shows the corium to be infiltrated by epithelioid granulomas with moderate numbers of Langhans giant cells (Figures 5.1 and 5.2). Extensive caseation is uncommon and it is unusual for tubercle bacilli to be identified either by Ziehl–Neelsen stain or by immunofluorescent techniques. Chest radiographs and sputum culture are much more likely to lead to definitive diagnosis.

Leprosy

Between 20 and 60% of patients with leprosy have facial and oral involvement[2,3]. Perioral lesions are particularly common and scarring may lead to microstomia. Intraoral lesions are usually firm nodules which tend to ulcerate and can cause severe scarring, perforation of the palate and loss of the uvula. Gingival lesions are hyperplastic and there is often loosening of associated teeth.

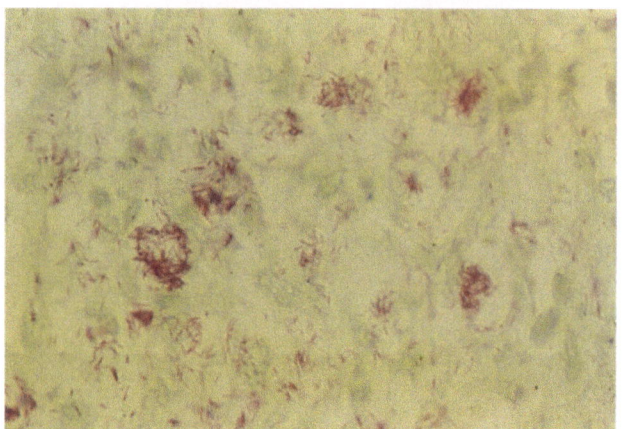

Figure 5.4 Lepromatous leprosy. Many acid-fast bacilli are present in the lepra cells. Triff × 1000

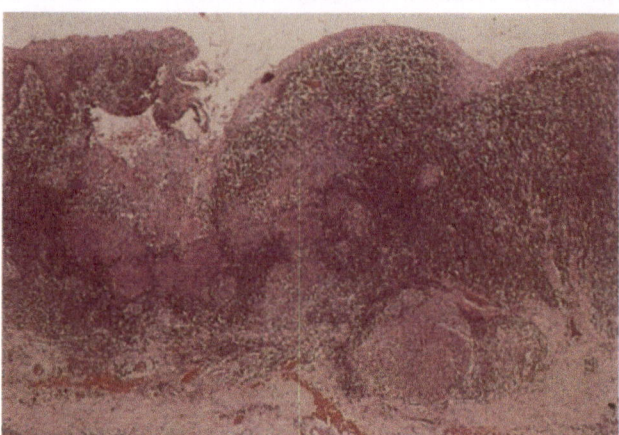

Figure 5.5 Sarcoidosis. There is dense chronic inflammatory cell infiltrate and discrete epithelioid granulomas beneath the ulcerated epithelium. H & E × 40

Microscopically, the tuberculoid form of the disease shows well defined follicular granulomas scattered throughout the corium. The follicles consist of epithelioid cells and multinucleated giant cells surrounded by variable numbers of lymphocytes and dense fibrous tissue. Granulomas or mononuclear cell infiltrates frequently involve the neurovascular bundles, a feature which aids differential diagnosis. Acid-fast bacilli are practically never detected in tuberculoid leprosy. In lepromatous leprosy the lesions consist of dense aggregates of foamy macrophages (lepra cells) and chronic inflammatory cells (Figure 5.3). A modified Ziehl–Neelsen (Triff) stain shows the lepra cells to contain numerous bacilli (Figure 5.4). There is no inflammatory involvement of the nerves.

Sarcoidosis

Although sarcoidosis and Crohn's disease are of undetermined etiology, it is convenient to consider them in this section as the lesions have many histological similarities to chronic bacterial infections.

Oral involvement is not common in sarcoidosis and it is rare for such lesions to be the presenting symptoms of the disease[4]. The facial and perioral skin, oral mucosa or salivary glands may be affected. Although the oral lesions can be extremely variable in appearance, they are typically painless, firm, dark reddish nodules which only rarely ulcerate. Salivary gland lesions may be associated with granulomatous uveitis and facial paralysis (Heerfordt's syndrome; uveoparotid fever).

Microscopically, non-caseating epithelioid granulomas with Langhans type giant cells are seen (Figures 5.5 and 5.6). These lesions are not specific for sarcoidosis and other causes of epithelioid granulomas have to be considered in the differential diagnosis. Lip biopsy may be helpful, since it has been shown that random biopsy of clinically normal minor glands of the lower lip in patients with known sarcoidosis shows non-caseating epithelioid granulomas in nearly 60% of cases[5].

Crohn's Disease

Crohn's disease can affect any part of the gastro-intestinal tract, including the mouth. Oral involvement is particularly common in patients who have extra-intestinal manifestations such as skin or joint lesions[6], but oral lesions have been recorded in the absence of demonstrable gut pathology. Oral lesions include aphthae, swelling of the lips or

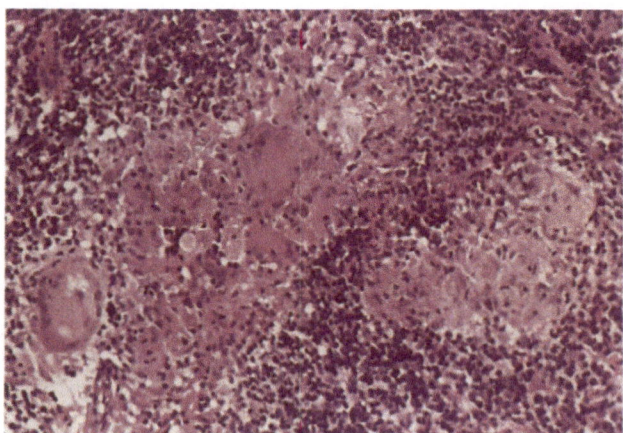

Figure 5.6 Sarcoidosis. Higher magnification shows non-caseating epithelioid granulomas and occasional giant cells. H & E × 200

cheeks, a typical 'cobblestone' appearance of the involved mucosa and persistent linear ulcers[7]. Microscopy shows variable features. In most cases there is oedema of the superficial corium and patchy chronic inflammatory infiltration (Figure 5.7). Chronic inflammatory cells, especially lymphocytes, may be seen aggregated around thin-walled vessels which are probably lymphatics. About 10% of cases show non-caseating, epithelioid granulomas which may be present in the superficial or deep corium and are not infrequently found in the underlying muscle[8] (Figures 5.8 and 5.9).

Lesions that are histologically similar to those of Crohn's disease may be found in the lips in the absence of other signs or symptoms of the disease; this condition is termed cheilitis granulomatosa. When cheilitis granulomatosa appears in conjunction with facial paralysis and a fissured tongue the triad constitutes the Melkersson–Rosenthal syndrome. The relationship, if any, between these conditions and Crohn's disease is not known.

The lesions of Crohn's disease and cheilitis granulomatosa cannot be distinguished from those of sarcoidosis on histological grounds alone. However, the generalized nature of sarcoidosis, in particular the lung and mediastinal lymph node involvement, a positive Kveim test and the presence of multiple immunological abnormalities aid differentiation.

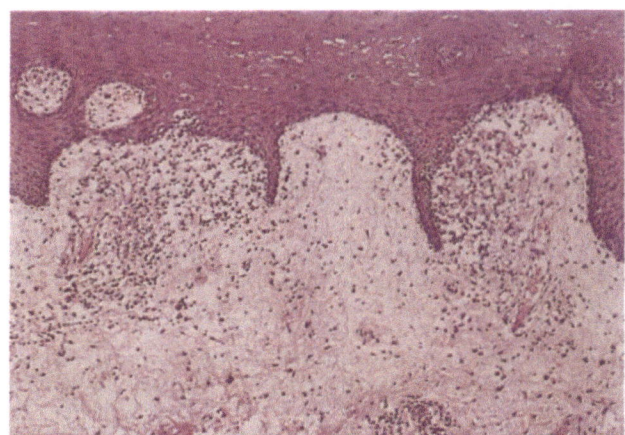

Figure 5.7 Crohn's disease. In this biopsy from the lip there is oedema of the superficial corium and ill defined aggregates of macrophages together with patchy chronic inflammatory infiltration. H & E × 100

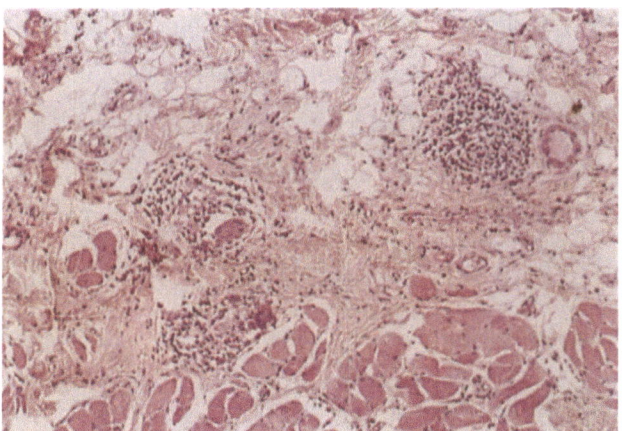

Figure 5.8 Crohn's disease. In the deeper corium there are scattered poorly defined epithelioid granulomas and giant cells. H & E × 100

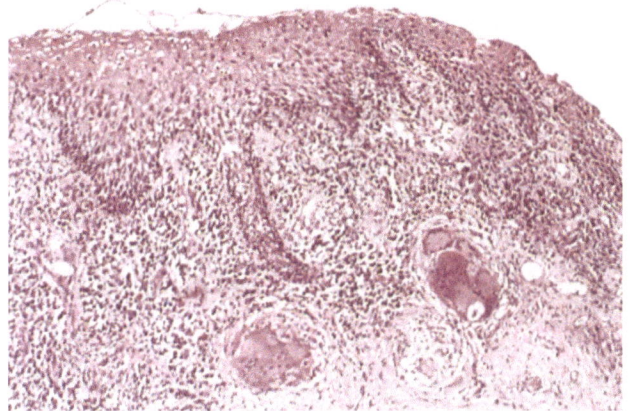

Figure 5.9 Crohn's disease. Gingival biopsy showing dense chronic inflammatory cell infiltration and large multinucleated giant cells. H & E × 100

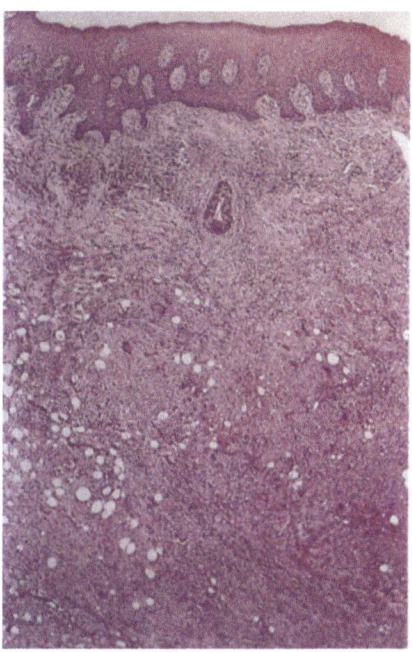

Figure 5.10 Syphilis. In this late stage lesion in the palate there are sheets of epithelioid cells, chronic inflammatory cells and scattered multinucleated giant cells. H & E × 40

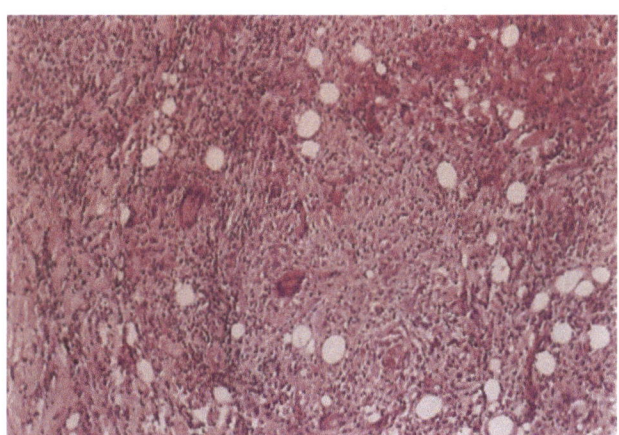

Figure 5.11 Syphilis. Higher magnification showing ill defined epithelioid granulomas and giant cells. H & E × 100

Syphilis

Oral syphilitic lesions, once not at all uncommon, are now rare[9]. Gummas are the commonest lesions seen in the mouth and the only oral syphilitic lesion likely to be biopsied. They are usually found in the midline of the palate or the tongue and form rubbery nodules up to several centimetres in diameter. These nodules tend to break down centrally, leaving ulcers with sharply demarcated edges.

Microscopy shows coagulative necrosis and extensive granulation tissue with occasional multinucleated giant cells. Sometimes there may be extensive formation of follicular granulomas with epithelioid cells, giant cells and lymphocytes (Figures 5.10 and 5.11). Obliterative endarteritis, if present, aids diagnosis, but this can only be confirmed by serological tests.

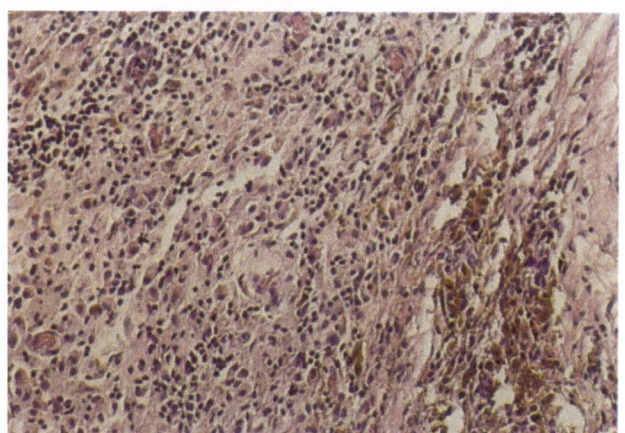

Figure 5.12 Actinomycosis. There are foamy macrophages, mixed inflammatory infiltrate and deposits of haemosiderin in tissue from the edge of the main lesion. H & E × 200

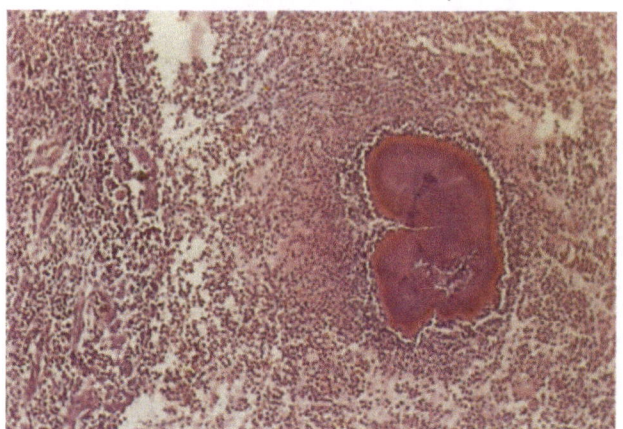

Figure 5.13 Actinomycosis. A colony of actinomyces is surrounded by a mass of neutrophils and macrophages. H & E × 200

Actinomycosis[10,11]

Actinomycosis usually affects previously fit young adults; organisms penetrate the oral mucosa, often following surgical trauma such as extractions, or fracture, and may remain localized or spread to involve adjacent salivary glands, bone or facial skin. An indurated swelling forms and abscesses drain through multiple sinuses.

The typical lesions of actinomycosis are areas of acute suppurative inflammation in which there are discrete colonies of organisms. The organisms are surrounded by numerous leucocytes, foamy macrophages and occasional multinucleated giant cells (Figures 5.12 and 5.13). There is extensive fibrous repair at the periphery of these abscesses, splitting the lesions into locules. The actinomyces form a Gram positive mycelium, frequently with Gram negative lipid 'clubs' in the host tissue at the periphery of the colony.

Occasionally, colonies of actinomyces are seen in lesions such as periapical granulomas and in material that has been curetted from periodontal pockets (page 32). In these situations it is doubtful if the organisms play a significant pathogenic role.

Epithelioid Granulomas in Biopsies of Oral Tissues

The following conditions have to be considered in the differential diagnosis when epithelioid granulomas are detected in biopsy material from the oral tissues:

(1) Tuberculosis
(2) Sarcoidosis
(3) Tuberculoid leprosy
(4) Tertiary syphilis
(5) Fungal infections such as coccidioidomycosis, sporotrichosis and others
(6) Foreign bodies:
  endogenous – keratin
  exogenous – suture material
    zirconium (present in some tooth-pastes)
(7) Crohn's disease and related disorders

The presence of epithelioid granulomas, as in other sites, does not constitute a diagnosis but merely indicates that a further series of clinical and laboratory investigations is required. These may include:

(1) Examination of the specimen in polarized light for the presence of birefringent foreign material
(2) Ziehl–Neelsen and Triff stains for acid and alcohol fast bacilli
(3) Stains for fungi
(4) Serology for syphilis
(5) Kveim test for sarcoidosis

Occasionally an isolated epithelioid granuloma is seen as a chance finding in otherwise normal tissue; such lesions are not rare in gingival tissue removed during routine gingivectomy. There are usually no other features of local or systemic disease in these cases and the significance of the lesions is not clear. It is most likely that they are a reaction to an unidentified foreign body.

Fungal Infections

Apart from candidosis oral mycoses are not common in temperate zones, although over the last few years there has been a steady increase in the frequency and range of these infections, especially in patients receiving cytotoxic drugs or immunosuppressive therapy. The intraoral mycoses most likely to be seen in western countries are candidosis, aspergillosis, histoplasmosis and mucormycosis.

Candidosis[12,13]

Candidal infections of the oral mucosa are common. Most are opportunistic, the infection being superimposed on underlying local or systemic disease. Oral lesions can form part of a wider mucocutaneous disorder.

Candida albicans is present as a commensal in over 40% of apparently normal mouths, but only in the yeast form. The pathogenic phase of the organism is the hyphal form which consists of cell bodies 7–8 µm in diameter, enclosed by a thick refractile wall.

Candidosis appears clinically in the following forms:

Acute candidosis
  Thrush
Chronic candidosis
  Denture-related stomatitis
  Chronic hyperplastic candidosis

Thrush is seen most commonly in infants, pregnant women and debilitated patients, especially those receiving cytotoxic or immunosuppressive treatment. The condition is also common following treatment with broad spectrum antibiotics (so-called antibiotic stomatitis). The lesions consist of creamy yellow, soft plaques which rub off easily to leave an erythematous base which may be painful. These lesions are only rarely biopsied but smears

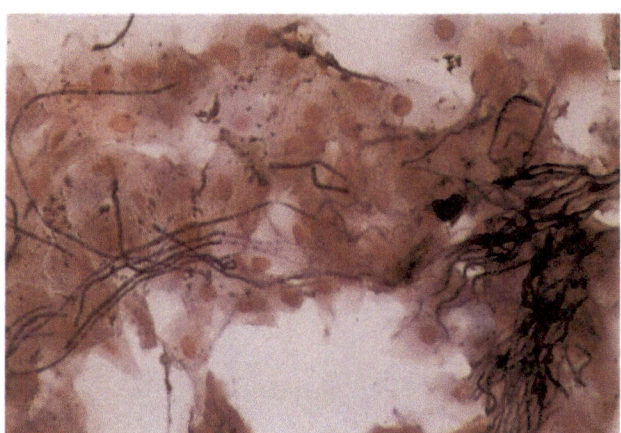

Figure 5.14 Candidosis. This is a smear from a case of thrush, showing squames and a tangled mass of Gram-positive hyphae. Gram × 400

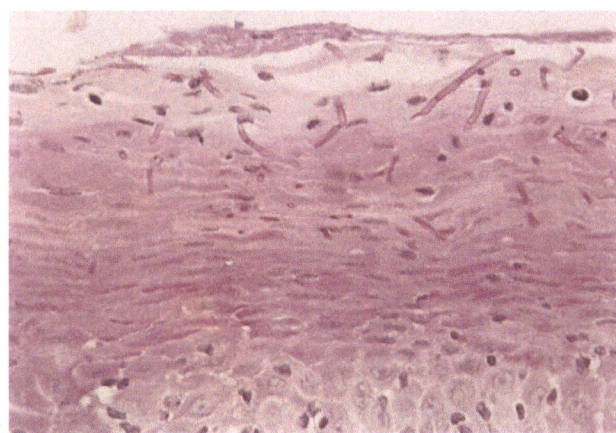

Figure 5.15 Candidosis. There are many hyphae in the parakeratinized epithelial plaque. PAS × 400

from a plaque are frequently taken to confirm the diagnosis. These should be stained with Gram or PAS. Microscopy shows squames, bacteria and the typical branching hyphae of *Candida albicans* (Figure 5.14).

Denture-related stomatitis is not uncommonly seen in individuals who have complete upper dentures, especially when the prosthesis is worn continuously. The condition is usually painless and there is often a related angular cheilitis. Clinically, there is bright erythema limited sharply to the upper denture-bearing area. Organisms can sometimes be seen in scrapings from the involved mucosa, but in many cases the fungus grows in the superficial interstices of the denture acrylic.

Chronic hyperplastic candidosis (Candidal leukoplakia). *Candida albicans* may be associated with firm, white, persistent plaques on the oral mucosa; such lesions are termed candidal leukoplakia or chronic hyperplastic candidosis. These plaques do not rub off and the surrounding mucosa is usually erythematous. Less often the lesion has a speckled appearance. The sites commonly involved in chronic hyperplastic candidosis are the commisures, dorsum of the tongue and palate. Occasionally, chronic hyperplastic candidosis is associated with chronic mucocutaneous candidosis. Hyphae can usually be readily identified in smears from the lesions, but as these plaques have to be differentiated from other white lesions and as epithelial dysplasia is not uncommon in chronic hyperplastic candidosis, this is the form of the disease most likely to be biopsied.

When candida organisms develop pathogenic propensities they appear to become intracellular parasites and cause epithelial hyperplasia in infected tissue. The response is essentially similar in the acute and chronic forms of the disease. The characteristic plaque of candidosis is a hyperparakeratinized layer of epithelium invaded by candidal hyphae (Figure 5.15). The hyphae tend to be orientated at 90° to the surface and extend usually no deeper than the glycogen-rich zone of the epithelium. A particularly distinctive feature is the accumulation of fluid and neutrophils in the superficial parakeratinized layers, often forming microabscesses. The underlying epithelium shows irregular hyperplasia with downgrowths of blunt rete ridges and there may be thinning of the suprapapillary epithelium producing a psoriasiform appearance (Figure 5.16). There is variable but sometimes severe inflammatory infiltration of the corium. Lymphocytes and plasma cells are predominant but acute inflammation, sometimes with striking fibrin exudation, is occasionally seen in the superficial corium (Figure 5.17).

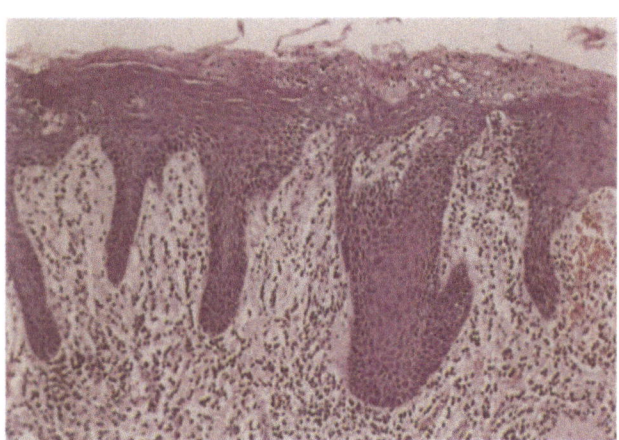

Figure 5.16 Chronic hyperplastic candidosis, showing irregular epithelial hyperplasia and an oedematous epithelial plaque of parakeratinized cells infiltrated by neutrophils and hyphae. H & E × 100

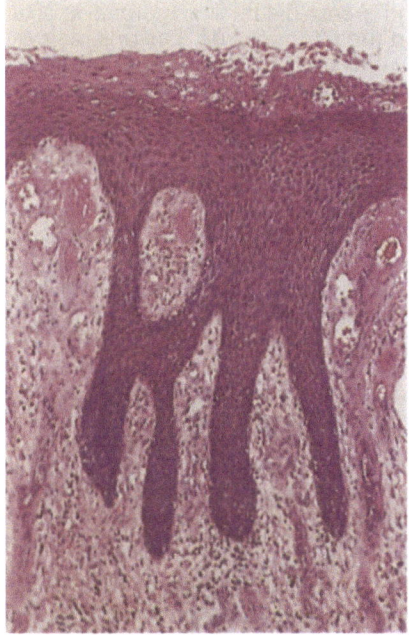

Figure 5.17 Chronic hyperplastic candidosis, showing extensive fibrin exudation from superficial vessels. H & E × 100

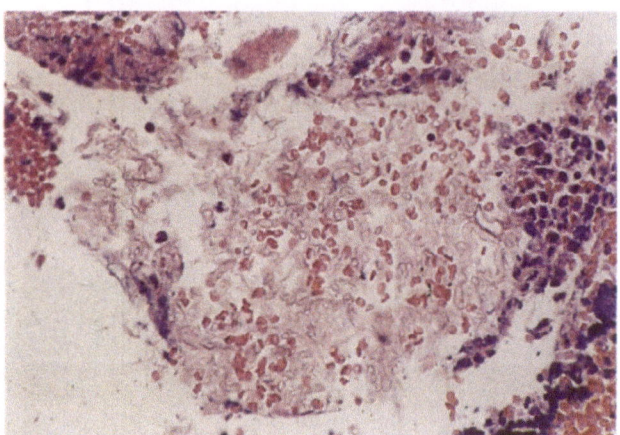

Figure 5.18 Aspergillosis. The lesion contains a mass of hyphae and inflammatory cells.   H & E × 400

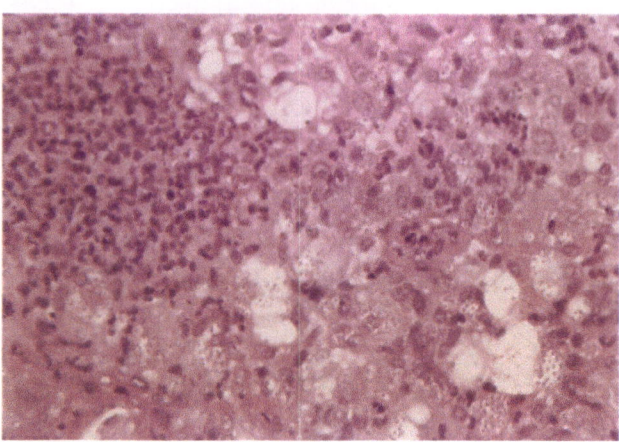

Figure 5.19 Histoplasmosis, showing neutrophil microabscesses and macrophages containing oval spores.   H & E × 400

The presence of high level intra-epithelial micro-abscesses in biopsies of oral mucosa should always make the pathologist suspect that the lesion is candidal in origin. In classical oral candidosis the presence of a thick para-keratotic plaque in which the fungal hyphae can be identified makes diagnosis easy. However, sometimes the plaque has been lost due to friction or during the biopsy procedure and fungal hyphae may not be obvious. Increasing the contrast by racking down the condenser or using PAS stain makes identification of the hyphae much easier.

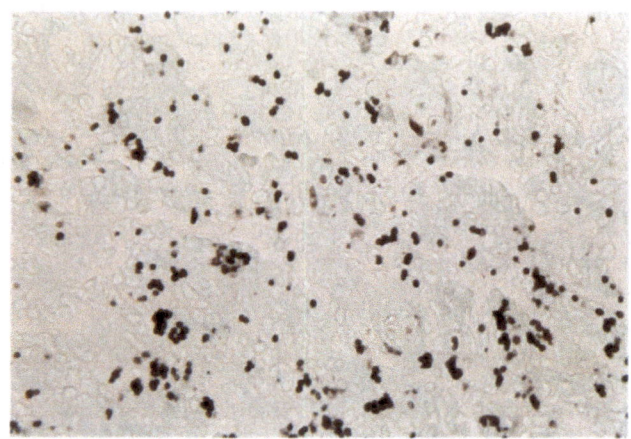

Figure 5.20 Histoplasmosis. Gomori's methenamine silver stain to show spores. × 400

Aspergillosis[14]

Oral lesions in aspergillosis are rare. Infection of the maxillary sinus, usually as part of the disseminated form of the disease, initially causes symptoms of chronic suppurative sinusitis and green, gelatinous material is often present in the nose on the affected side. Lesions may cause erosion of the bony walls of the antrum and spread to involve the orbit and palate, or ultimately the brain. Rare cases have been described involving the tongue and soft palate. Occasionally the fungus is found growing as a ball-like mass in the maxillary sinus without invading tissue.

The microscopical appearances are very variable. In the 'fungus ball' type of lesion there is virtually no inflammatory response, whereas in the disseminated form the typical lesions are tuberculoid granulomas in which there are varying amounts of central necrosis. Histological diagnosis depends on demonstrating the fungus; aspergillus species are septate, dichotomously branching hyphae with occasional chains of chlamydospores (Figure 5.18).

Histoplasmosis

Histoplasmosis is caused by the dimorphous soil saprophyte *Histoplasma capsulatum* which forms oval, budding spores. In primary infections the lungs are the usual site of involvement, which is very often asymptomatic. Severe, disseminated histoplasmosis is uncommon except at the extremes of life and in immunosuppressed patients.

Oral lesions are usually exophytic and involve the buccal mucosa, tongue, gingiva and palate[15]. Superficial ulceration is common; more rarely necrosis is extensive with punched-out ulcers resembling gummas, leading to considerable destruction of the palate, nose and pharynx.

Microscopy shows numerous histiocytes and a mixed inflammatory infiltration. The histiocytes contain oval spores which are 2–4 μm in diameter (Figure 5.19). The clear capsule of these spores stains intensely with PAS, and they can be well demonstrated with silver stains (Figure 5.20). When there are focal areas of necrosis epithelioid granulomas with occasional giant cells may be present, so that the lesions closely resemble those of tuberculosis and tertiary syphilis.

Mucormycosis

Saprophytic zygomycetes can sometimes proliferate in the tissues, usually when the host has some underlying systemic disease such as poorly controlled diabetes, extensive burns, leukaemia or lymphoma, and in immunosuppressed patients. The fungus invades and proliferates in blood vessels which characteristically leads to thrombosis with consequent infarction. The usual sites of invasion are the paranasal sinuses, lungs and gastrointestinal tract. In local lesions of the sinuses there is frequently erosion of the bony walls and spread to the orbit and brain or intraorally to the hard and soft palate[16].

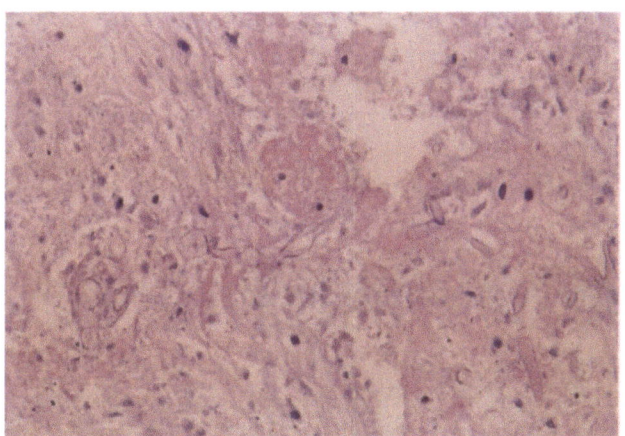

Figure 5.21 Mucormycosis. The organisms form ribbon-like non-septate, irregular hyphae. H & E × 400

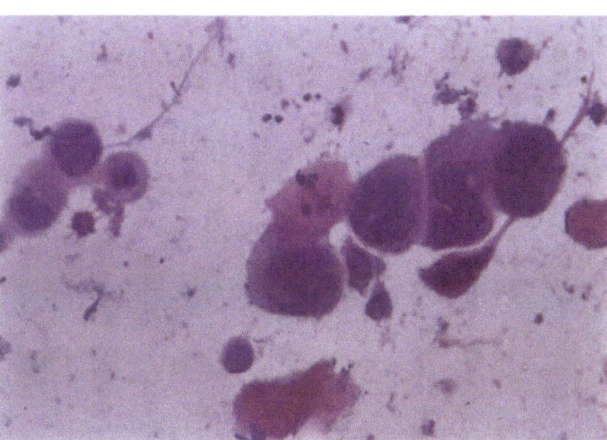

Figure 5.23 Virally damaged epithelial cells. This smear shows loss of inter-cellular adhesion and formation of multinucleated epithelial cells. H & E × 400

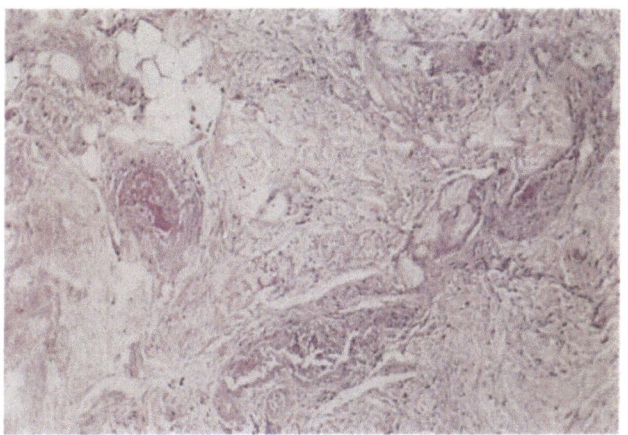

Figure 5.22 Mucormycosis, showing thrombosis and extensive necrosis. H & E × 100

Microscopically, the fungus has broad, nonseptate, irregular hyphae (Figure 5.21). The organisms are found in vessel walls, within thrombi and in the surrounding tissues (Figure 5.22). There is usually extensive necrosis and oedema and intense polymorphonuclear infiltration. Occasionally epithelioid granulomas with giant cells are seen.

Viral Infections

Viral diseases of the mouth are common and include the following:

    Herpes simplex
        Primary herpetic gingivostomatitis
        Recurrent herpes (herpes labialis)
    Herpes zoster
    Chickenpox
    Coxsackie viral infections
        Hand-foot-and-mouth disease
        Herpangina
    Infectious mononucleosis
    Measles
    Verruca vulgaris

It is exceptional for any of these lesions, apart from verruca vulgaris, to be biopsied. However, scrapings from the bases of blisters or ulcers are frequently sent for cytological examination. Such specimens do not show changes that are diagnostic for any particular virus but they can suggest a viral cause for an ulcer or vesicle. Thus, ballooning degeneration is a characteristic feature of virally damaged cells, which also lose their intercellular adhesion and separate from each other. The cytoplasm becomes brightly eosinophilic and homogeneous and some of the cells contain multiple nuclei (Figure 5.23). In zoster, varicella and herpes simplex intranuclear, eosinophilic inclusion bodies may be seen, especially in the balloon cells.

NON-INFECTIVE CONDITIONS

White Patches and Leukoplakia

There has been much confusion over the terminology used to describe the wide variety of intraoral lesions which appear as white patches on the mucosa. These include:

    White sponge naevus
    Smoker's keratosis
    Frictional keratosis
    Chemical burns
    Lichen planus
    Discoid lupus erythematosus
    Thrush and chronic hyperplastic candidosis
    Squamous cell carcinoma
    'Leukoplakia' (idiopathic keratosis).

Initially the term leukoplakia was used to describe any white patch and was often used as a general designation for dysplastic lesions. However, the World Health Organization Collaborating Centre for Oral Precancerous Lesions has defined leukoplakia as 'a white patch or plaque that cannot be characterized clinically or pathologically as any other disease'[17]. Thus leukoplakia is essentially a clinical diagnosis derived by exclusion and the term has no specific histological implications.

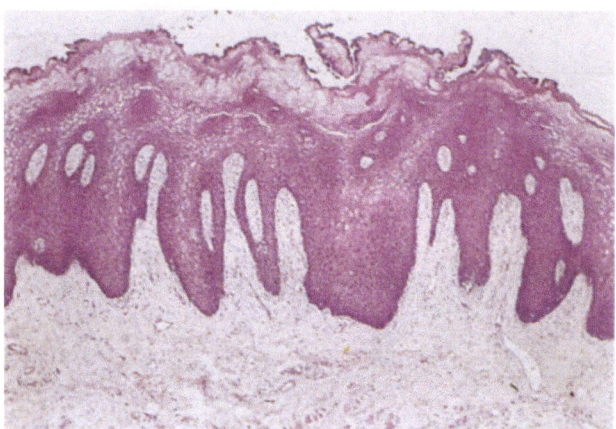

Figure 5.24   White sponge naevus. There is shaggy parakeratosis with bacterial conglomerates in the superficial keratin, and acanthosis and hydropic change in the superficial stratum spinosum.   H & E × 40

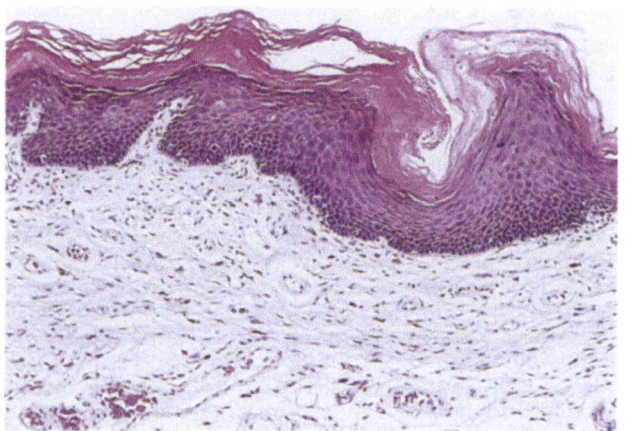

Figure 5.25   Smoker's keratosis. There is irregular hyperkeratosis, epithelial atrophy and mild dysplasia.   H & E × 100

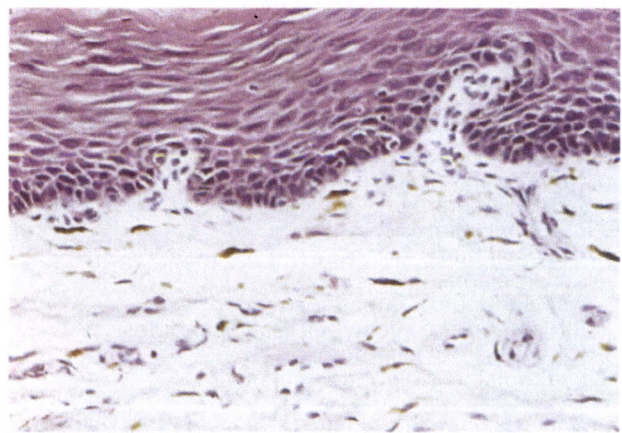

Figure 5.26   Smoker's keratosis. There has been pigmentary incontinence and melanophages are present in the superficial corium.   H & E × 200

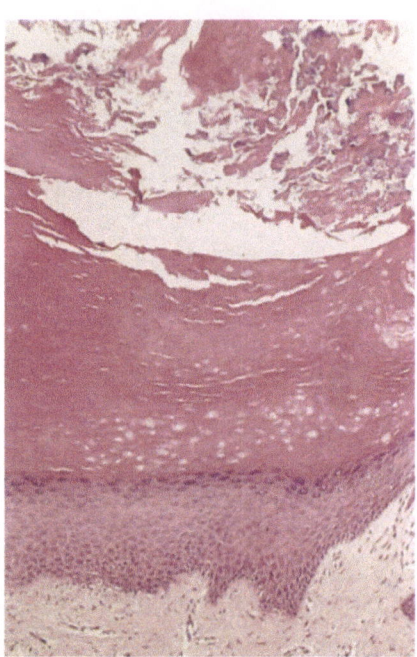

Figure 5.27   Frictional keratosis. The epithelium is atrophic and there is a thick layer of orthokeratin.   H & E × 100

White Sponge Naevus[18]

This inherited condition may be seen as a congenital lesion, or it may not make its appearance until later. Its designation aptly describes the dead white, heaped up, sodden or spongy appearance of the affected area of mucosa, which on microscopy shows parakeratosis and acanthosis with hydropic degeneration of the prickle cells (Figure 5.24). There is no atypia. The lesion may arise in any part of the oral mucosa, and similar lesions may also be present in the rectal or vaginal mucosa.

Smoker's Keratosis

The exact location of smoker's keratosis depends on how the cigarette, pipe or cigar is customarily held in the mouth[19]. In those individuals who allow cigarettes to dangle from their lips and often let the cigarette burn to a very small stub, keratosis of the lips is common[20]. In patients who preferentially hold the cigarette or cigar in one side of the mouth, keratosis is often seen in the buccal mucosa and retromolar region on that side. Keratosis of the palate and nicotinic stomatitis (page 83) are seen typically in habitual pipe smokers.

Microscopy usually shows mild epithelial atrophy and hyperkeratosis (Figure 5.25). On occasion the epithelium is dysplastic. Pigmentary incontinence is common (Figure 5.26).

Frictional Keratosis

This is the commonest type of intraoral white patch and is due to chronic trauma or friction. Cheek and lip sucking and chewing cause linear white patches on the buccal mucosa and lips, sometimes with areas of shredding. Localized lesions may be found opposite sharp edges of teeth, restorations or dentures.

Microscopy shows epithelial hyperplasia or atrophy. There is often a prominent granular cell layer and a thick layer of orthokeratin or, less commonly, parakeratin (Figure 5.27). There is no significant dysplasia and, in the absence of ulceration, inflammation is minimal.

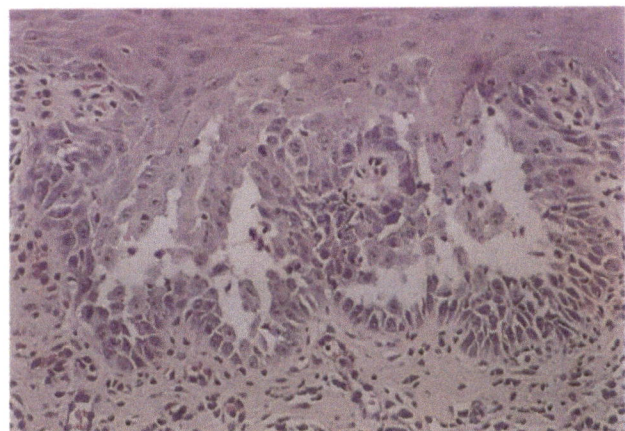

Figure 5.28 Pemphigus vulgaris. There is suprabasal acantholysis and formation of an intraepithelial bulla.   H & E × 200

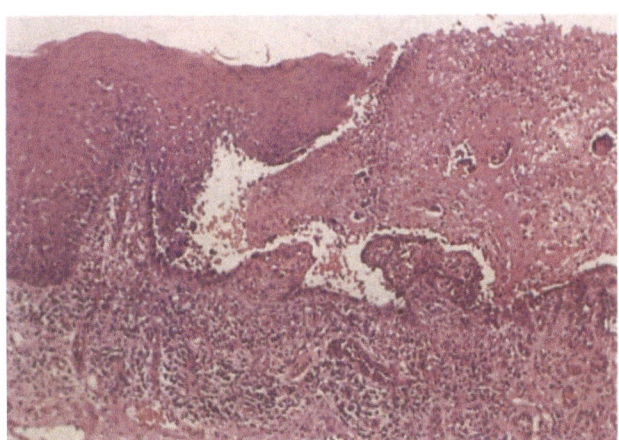

Figure 5.30 Pemphigus vulgaris. The roof of the bulla has been lost but there is a layer of basal keratinocytes covering the inflamed corium.   H & E × 100

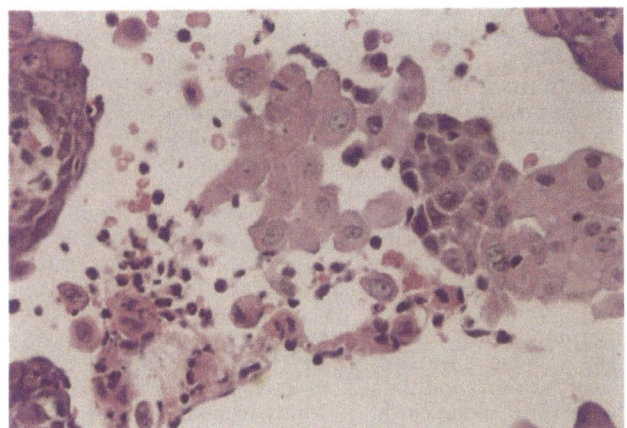

Figure 5.29 Pemphigus vulgaris. Higher magnification, showing acantholytic cells.   H & E × 400

Chemical Burns

Chemical burns of the mouth are common. Those most frequently encountered are due to aspirin tablets that have been held in the buccal sulcus opposite a painful tooth, or crushed into a carious cavity, in a futile attempt to relieve toothache. The mucosa rapidly becomes white and eventually sloughs. Microscopy shows necrotic epithelium,

Mucocutaneous Lesions

Many diseases which are primarily dermatological can also involve the mouth and in some cases the oral lesions precede those of the skin.

Pemphigus

The lesions of pemphigus, which are characterized by the presence of autoantibodies to the intercellular cement substance of stratified squamous epithelium, occur not infrequently in the oral mucosa in pemphigus vulgaris and pemphigus vegetans. Oral lesions, however, are extremely rare in pemphigus foliaceous and pemphigus erythematosus.

Pemphigus vulgaris. This is the most common and the most severe form of the disease and over half the patients first present with oral lesions[21]. Adults of either sex are affected and it is especially common in Jews. The lesions take the form of bullae that arise on previously apparently normal mucosa or skin, especially in areas liable to trauma. The effect of shearing forces on the development of the bullae can be demonstrated by rubbing the skin or mucosa, when they promptly appear (Nikolsky's sign). Once formed, bullae in the mouth rapidly rupture leaving shallow, painful ulcers with irregular tags of mucosa at the margins. The ulcers heal without scarring.

Histologically, pemphigus is characterized by the formation of intraepithelial bullae. First, a cleft forms immediately above the basal layer due to acantholysis of the suprabasal keratinocytes (Figure 5.28). This then expands to form a bulla which is thus contained completely within the epithelium. There is loss of intercellular cohesion and the rounded, acantholytic cells float off into the bulla, which also contains serous fluid and moderate numbers of inflammatory cells, especially eosinophils (Figure 5.29). The acantholysis frequently spreads down the ducts of minor salivary glands. In the corium there is nonspecific inflammatory infiltration, which tends to be more severe in oral mucosa than in skin. Loss of the roof of bullae during the biopsy procedure is very common and microscopy then shows a shallow ulcer with a floor of inflamed corium covered by a thin layer of basal keratinocytes (Figure 5.30). Loss of lateral adhesion leads to separation of these cells and occasional acantholytic suprabasal cells may be seen. The diagnosis can easily be missed in such specimens.

Clinicians frequently use the so-called Tzanck test for the diagnosis of pemphigus. A smear is made from the floor of a bulla and the presence of acantholytic cells, recognizable by their large nuclei, prominent nuclear membrane and narrow halo of pale, homogeneous cytoplasm, is characteristic. As with most cytological techniques, a negative result does not exclude the diagnosis of pemphigus.

Pemphigus vegetans. Involvement of the oral mucous membrane is not uncommon in this less severe variant of pemphigus. Lesions are proliferative or vegetative and the most common oral lesions are granular masses involving the vermilion border of the lips.

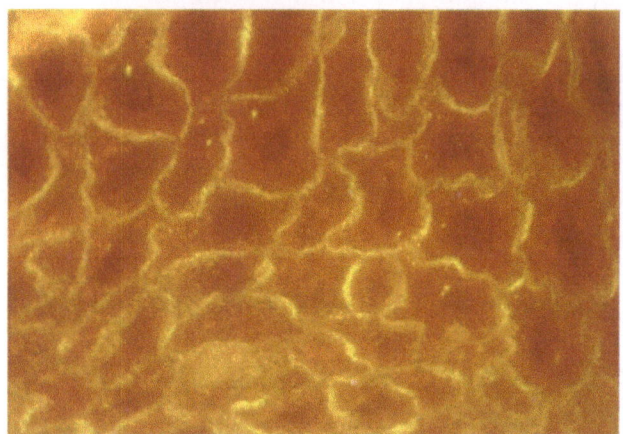

Figure 5.31 Pemphigus vulgaris. Immunofluorescence shows IgG against intercellular cement substance of the oral epithelium. × 550

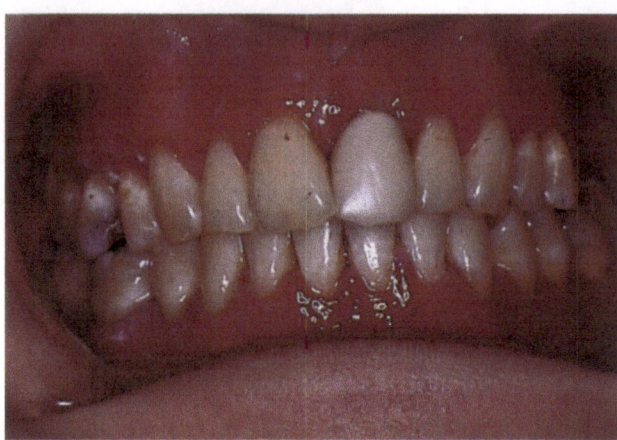

Figure 5.32 Mucous membrane pemphigoid. This illustration shows the disease presenting as desquamative gingivitis. There is severe erythema of the gingivae and related alveolar mucosa, with ruptured bullae.

Microscopically, the early lesions are similar to those of pemphigus vulgaris, but as the lesions age they become heaped up and warty. The edge of an early lesion may show acantholysis but this is often masked by a dense inflammatory infiltrate. There is acanthosis and long, thick rete ridges extend into the oedematous corium. At the tips of the elongated rete ridges there is a dense collection of inflammatory cells, mainly eosinophils.

Differential diagnosis. Benign acantholysis is also seen in Darier's disease, warty dyskeratoma and familial benign chronic pemphigus. Darier's disease and warty dyskeratoma are rare in the mouth and the presence of corps ronds and grains aids diagnosis. In familial benign chronic pemphigus the acantholytic process is less severe but extends higher into the epithelium than in pemphigus vulgaris. Immunohistochemical techniques (Figure 5.31) may be needed to distinguish between the diseases with certainty (Table 1)[22,23]. Acantholysis is occasionally seen in dysplastic lesions of the oral mucosa, but the presence of other features of epithelial atypia should make the diagnosis clear.

Occasionally, multinucleated cells are seen in smears taken from the bullae in pemphigus and have to be distinguished from the multinucleated cells seen in herpes simplex and herpes zoster. In herpetic lesions the giant cells are much more bizarre and have more irregular nuclei than those seen in pemphigus. In addition, there are many other clinical and histological features which aid differentiation of these lesions.

Pemphigoid[24]. There are two forms of pemphigoid, both of which can affect the mouth. Bullous pemphigoid is primarily a disease of skin and oral involvement is relatively uncommon. Mucous membrane pemphigoid (benign mucous membrane pemphigoid; cicatricial pemphigoid; ocular pemphigus) is a commoner bullous disorder and affects mainly mucosae, especially the mouth, eyes and genitalia. The histological features of the two forms of pemphigoid are identical and further discussion is restricted to mucous membrane pemphigoid.

The disease is most often seen in women in the 50–60 years age group and the oral mucosa is the most frequently affected site. The condition tends to be chronic and may be associated with periods of remission and exacerbation. It may eventually become inactive. Involvement of the mucosa of the nose, throat and oesophagus is not uncommon and limited skin involvement is seen in about half the patients. The scarring which is so typical of ocular and genital lesions is only rarely seen in the mouth.

The typical oral presentation is fiery red, painful gingivae – so-called desquamative gingivitis[25] (Figure 5.32). Small bullae with erythematous margins can develop elsewhere in the mouth, especially at sites of irritation, but rapidly burst to leave shallow ulcers with clean-cut edges and erythematous haloes.

Table 1   Immunocytochemical findings in the diagnosis of oral lesions

Disease	Type of staining in tissue	Percentage of cases with positive findings	Significance
Pemphigus	Intercellular antibody deposits	98	Diagnostic
Pemphigoid	Basement membrane antibodies and C3	< 80	Diagnostic
Lichen planus	Cytoid bodies in epithelium or corium. Fibrin deposits at epithelio-mesenchymal junction	> 90	Non-diagnostic
Lupus erythematosus (discoid)	Cytoid bodies in epithelium or corium. IgG or C3 at epithelio-mesenchymal junction in lesions only.	> 80	Non-diagnostic
Lupus erythematosus (systemic)	Deposits of IgG and C3 at epithelio-mesenchymal junction in lesion and normal tissue	> 90	Diagnostic

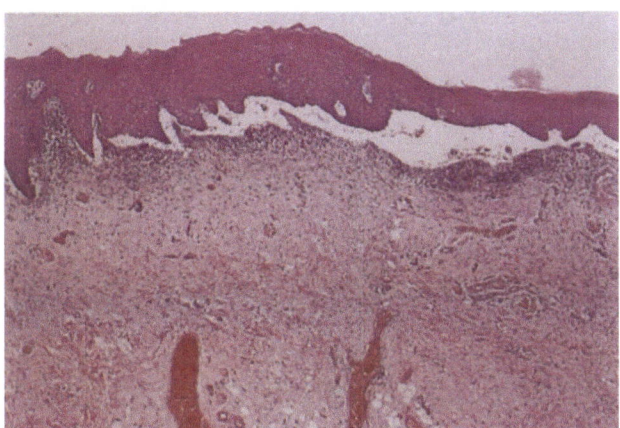

Figure 5.33 Mucous membrane pemphigoid, showing subepithelial bulla formation and mild inflammation of the superficial corium.   H & E × 40

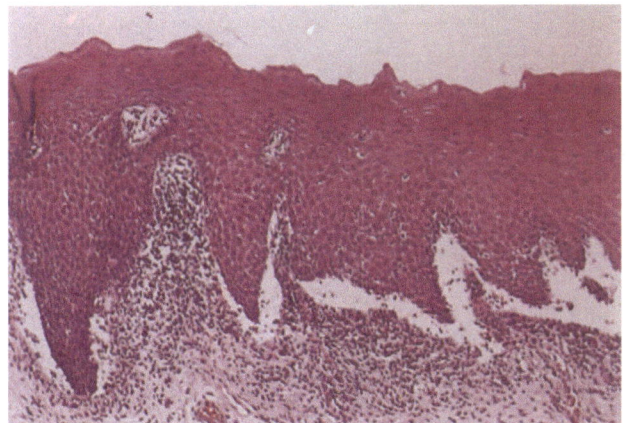

Figure 5.34 Mucous membrane pemphigoid. Higher magnification, showing that the floor of the bulla is formed by inflamed corium. This should be contrasted with Figure 5.30.   H & E × 100

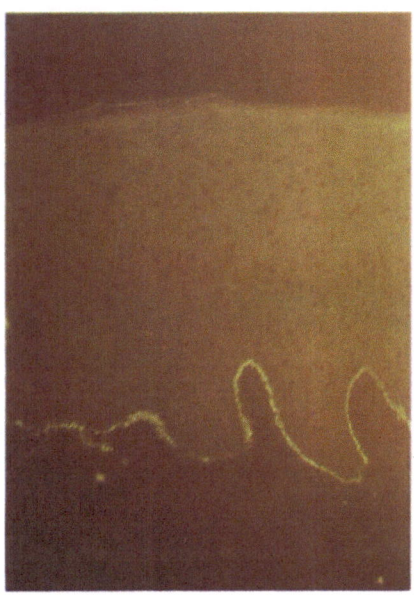

Figure 5.35 Mucous membrane pemphigoid. There is immunofluorescence of the basement membrane zone with anti-C3.   × 100

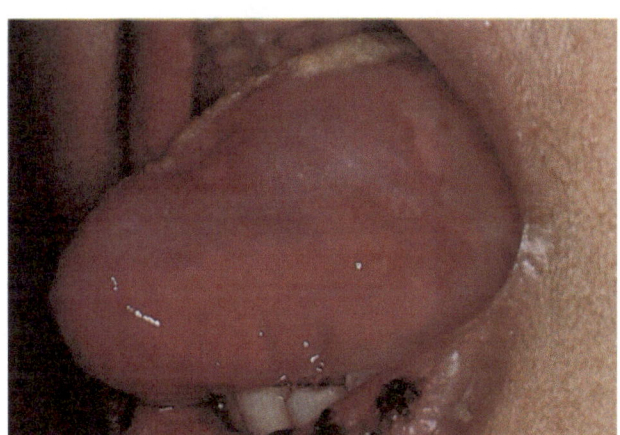

Figure 5.36 Erythema multiforme. There is haemorrhagic crusting of the lips and extensive ill defined erosions in the mouth.

Since the bullae rupture very easily, it is unusual to receive intact lesions for microscopic examination. If an intact bulla is examined it will be seen to be subepithelial, due to separation at the epithelio-mesenchymal junction (Figures 5.33 and 5.34). The bulla contains serosanguineous fluid and occasional inflammatory cells. The corium is densely infiltrated with acute and chronic inflammatory cells. In oral biopsies the specimen often consists of inflamed corium denuded of epithelium. In such circumstances a definitive diagnosis cannot be made but the appearances are at least suggestive of pemphigoid. Occasionally there may be regeneration of epithelium across the floor of an intact bulla, giving the lesion a pseudo-intraepithelial appearance.

Differential diagnosis. The diseases most likely to cause confusion in the histological diagnosis of mucous membrane pemphigoid are lichen planus, pemphigus vulgaris and erythema multiforme.

Lichen planus may present as an ulcerative lesion which closely resembles pemphigoid and it is in addition a common cause of desquamative gingivitis. The presence of severe basal cell liquefaction can cause the formation of microvesicles in lichen planus and, since there is a plane of weakness between the epithelium and connective tissue, this can lead to separation during the biopsy procedure. The characteristic subepithelial band-like infiltrate of lymphocytes in lichen planus and the basal cell degeneration aid differentiation, but this can be difficult when there has been extensive ulceration. Immunofluorescent studies[22] may be of value (Table 1).

Pemphigoid may be confused with pemphigus when large areas of the overlying epithelium have been lost. However, in pemphigus scattered basal keratinocytes may be still adherent to the corium and acantholytic cells are usually found. Again, it may be necessary to resort to immunofluorescent tests (Figure 5.35) to make a definitive distinction (Table 1).

The lesions may closely resemble bullous erythema multiforme, but in the latter condition the presence of constitutional symptoms and the characteristic skin lesions serve to prevent confusion (Figure 5.36).

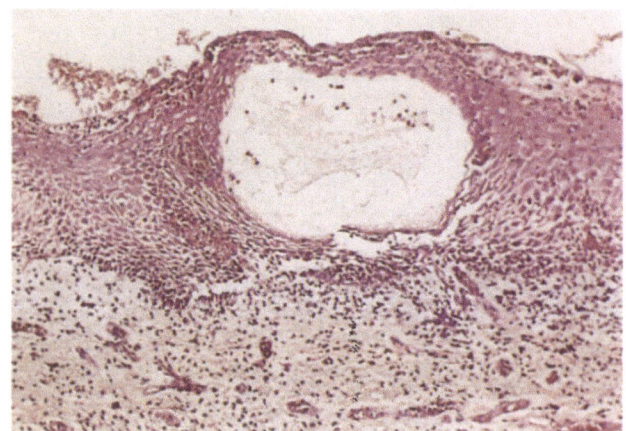

Figure 5.37 Erythema multiforme. The epithelium shows an intraepithelial bulla and patchy inflammation and oedema of the superficial corium.   H & E × 100

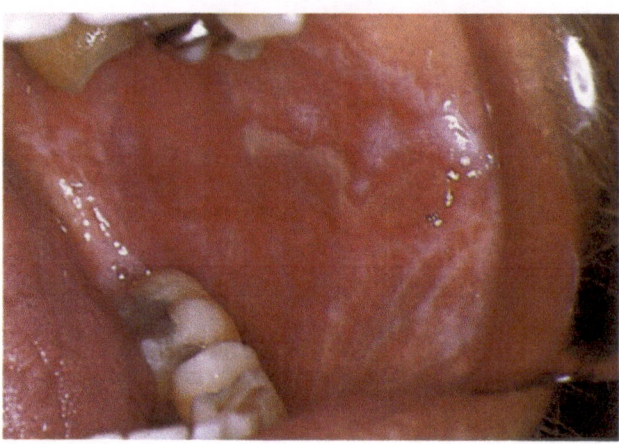

Figure 5.39 Lichen planus. This illustration shows typical reticular lichen planus of the buccal mucosa with an extensive area of linear ulceration.

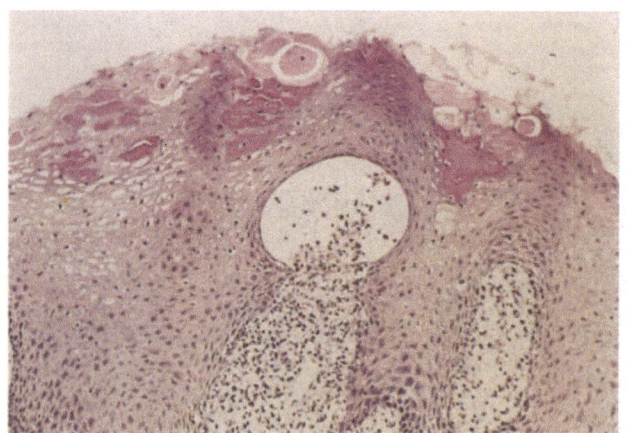

Figure 5.38 Erythema multiforme. There is a subepithelial bulla and fibrin accumulation in the superficial epithelium.   H & E × 100

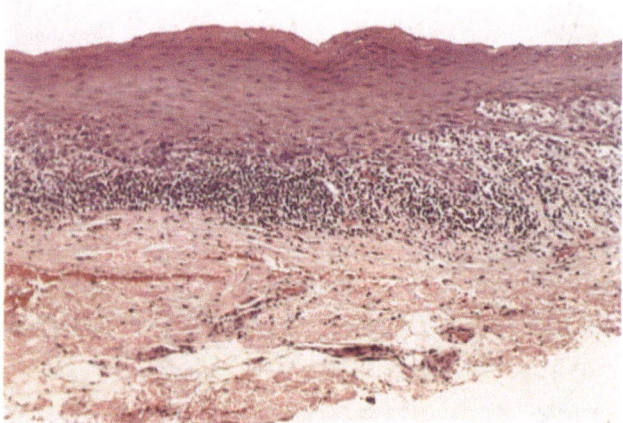

Figure 5.40 Lichen planus. There is hyperkeratosis, irregular acanthosis, and a dense, band-like infiltrate of lymphocytes in the superficial corium.   H & E × 100

Erythema Multiforme

The clinical and histological manifestations of this muco-cutaneous disorder are extremely variable, with the lesions presenting as macules, papules or bullae of varying sizes. The disorder is often confined to the mouth. In more severe forms there may be ocular, genital, respiratory and joint involvement and the patient may suffer from a toxic, febrile illness (Stevens–Johnson syndrome).

In the mouth, there are ill defined symmetrical, reddish areas which form blisters or shallow ulcers. Lesions are commonest in the anterior parts of the mouth and on the lips, where thick, haemorrhagic crusts form (Figure 5.36). The disease usually lasts 4–6 weeks, but recurrences are common[26].

The histological features of erythema multiforme are much less characteristic in the oral mucosa than in skin[27]. The main value of biopsy is to exclude other lesions such as pemphigus, pemphigoid and lichen planus which can closely resemble erythema multiforme clinically. In the epithelium there may be inter- and intracellular oedema

and the formation of microvesicles, and there may also be extensive accumulation of mononuclear and polymorpho-nuclear leukocytes. There is oedema of the superficial and deep corium and variable, but often severe, inflammatory infiltration of the superficial corium (Figure 5.37). Occasionally there is frank separation at the epithelio-mesenchymal junction with subepithelial bulla formation (Figure 5.38). Vascular dilatation and congestion are common and sometimes pronounced. There are no character-istic immunocytochemical features.

Lichen Planus

Since lichen planus is one of the commonest muco-cutaneous diseases, this is a very common provisional diagnosis accompanying specimens taken from muco-cutaneous disorders and sent for histological examination. In its classical form lichen planus is relatively easy to recognize, both clinically and histologically. However such lesions are rarely biopsied. The atypical cases which are biopsied often show atypical histological features and

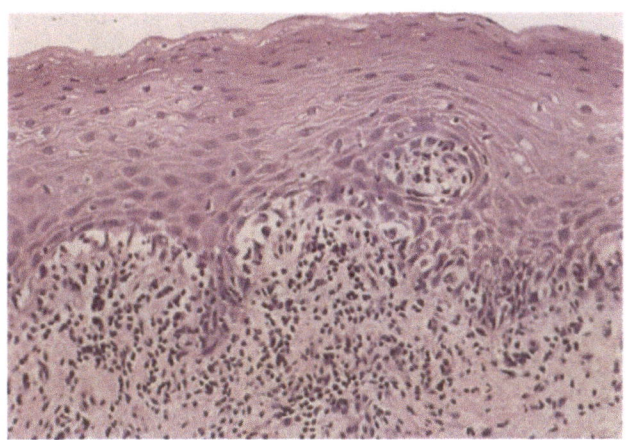

Figure 5.41   Lichen planus. Higher magnification, showing patchy basal cell liquefaction.   H & E × 200

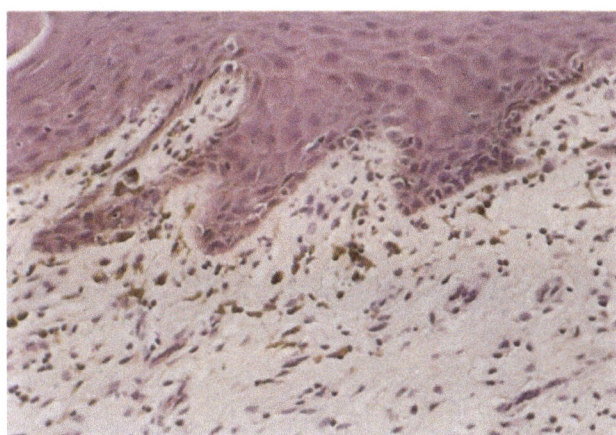

Figure 5.43   Lichen planus. There are pigment-laden macrophages in the superficial corium of this involutional lesion.   H & E × 200

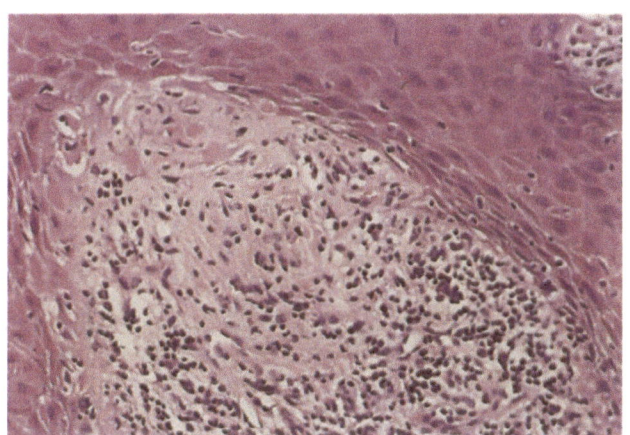

Figure 5.42   Lichen planus, showing Civatte bodies in the superficial corium. H & E × 200

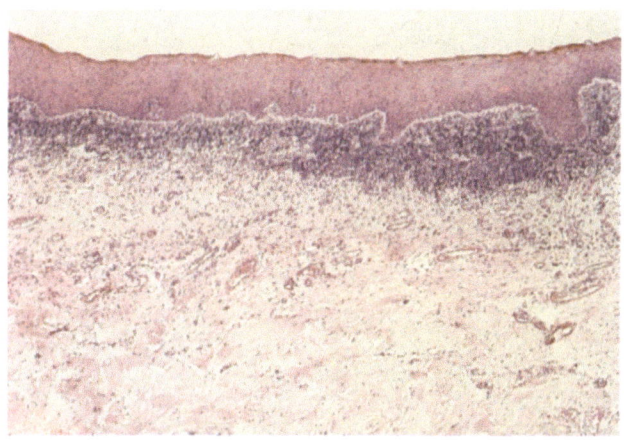

Figure 5.44   Lichen planus. In this lesion there is a relatively flat epithelio-mesenchymal junction and a prominent basement membrane. The characteristic band-like infiltrate of lymphocytes is also seen.   H & E × 40

definitive diagnosis is difficult or impossible. Under such circumstances the pathologist has to issue the familiar 'Consistent with but not diagnostic of . . .' type of report.

Oral lesions tend to be symmetrically distributed, the buccal mucosa and tongue being the commonest sites[28]. When the gingivae are involved the appearances are usually those of desquamative gingivitis. The commonest clinical presentation is a fine lace-like pattern of slightly raised white striations – so-called reticular lichen planus (Figure 5.39). In papular lichen planus the lesions are small, discrete papules which sometimes merge to form solid white plaques. In atrophic lichen planus the mucosa is thin, red and shiny and it may break down to form shallow ulcers which are often called erosions. A bullous form is described clinically, but in many instances lesions thought to be bullae are simply slough over an area of mucosal ulceration. Occasionally squamous cell carcinomas appear to arise in areas of long-standing lichen planus, especially the atrophic form.

The histological features of classical lichen planus of oral mucosa are similar to those seen in skin lesions. There is hyperorthokeratosis with a prominent granular cell layer, or parakeratosis. The epithelium is acanthotic and shows a 'saw-tooth' rete ridge pattern. There is liquefaction of cells in the basal layer and a band-like infiltrate, consisting mainly of lymphocytes, is present in the superficial corium (Figures 5.40 and 5.41). Civatte, or colloid, bodies may be present in the epithelium or the corium (Figure 5.42). The basal cell liquefaction leads to pigmentary incontinence and pigment-laden macrophages are sometimes prominent, especially in involutional lesions (Figure 5.43). Pigmentary incontinence, however, is not specific and may be seen in lupus erythmatosus and smoker's keratosis especially. The typical saw-tooth pattern of rete ridges is often absent in mucosal specimens, where there is frequently a relatively flat epithelio-mesenchymal junction (Figure 5.44). This is especially the case in atrophic lesions. When there has been ulceration secondary inflammatory changes are superimposed on the lesion. The inflammatory infiltrate then consists of lymphocytes, plasma cells, neutrophils and macrophages and its band-like disposition may be lost close to areas of ulceration.

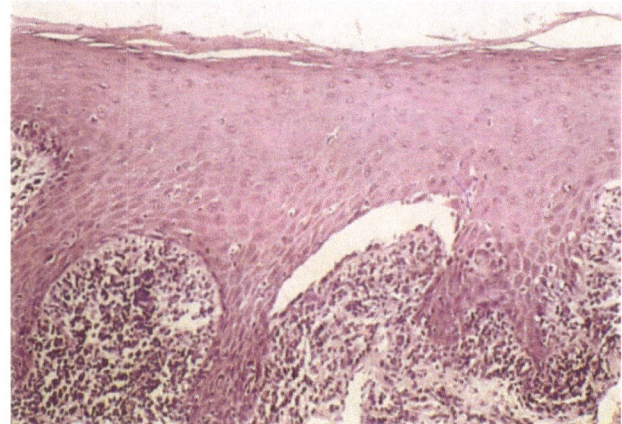

Figure 5.45 Lichen planus. Microscopic subepithelial vesiculation is not uncommon. H & E × 200

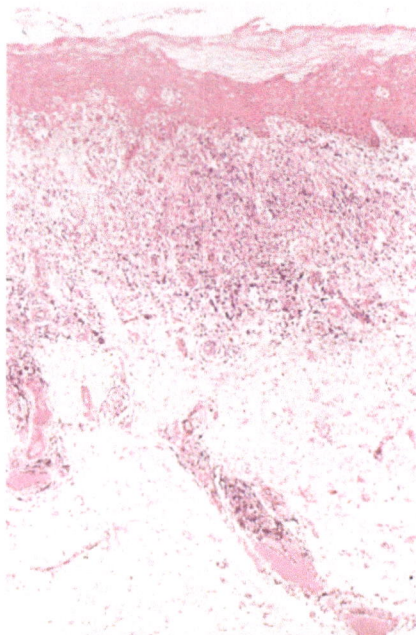

Figure 5.47 Discoid lupus erythematosus. There is irregular epithelial hyperplasia and patchy chronic inflammatory infiltration of the superficial corium. In the deeper corium the inflammatory infiltrate has a mainly perivascular distribution. H & E × 40

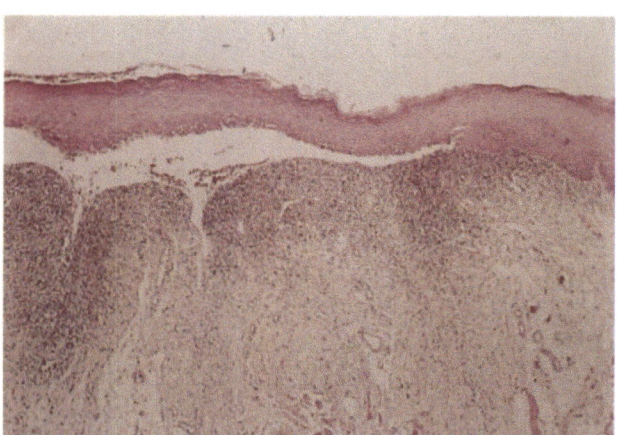

Figure 5.46 Lichen planus. In this example there has been extensive separation of the epithelium from the corium, simulating pemphigoid. However, the band-like inflammatory infiltrate of lichen persists. H & E × 40

Lupus Erythematosus

Oral lesions of chronic discoid lupus erythematosus are much less frequent than those of skin[29]. On the other hand, oral involvement is common in the systemic form of the disorder. In many instances, however, the oral lesions in systemic lupus erythematosus appear to be non-specific and are probably secondary to such factors as neutropenia, uraemia or general debility. Patients may have an associated Sjögren's syndrome which in itself predisposes to oral ulceration and candida infection.

Chronic discoid lupus erythematosus. This variety is seen most often in the 20–40 years age group, especially in women. It is characterized by periods of remission and exacerbation, but often the disease eventually seems to burn out. Progression to systemic lupus erythematosus is rare. Oral lesions are present in about a quarter of patients with skin involvement but can arise in the absence of detectable skin lesions. The buccal mucosa, lips and palate are the commonest sites. The lesions tend to be irregular, well defined atrophic areas with surrounding, radially arranged, prominent capillaries. White plaques and areas of scarring may be seen within the central part of the lesion or radiating from the periphery as a striated halo.

Microscopy shows parakeratosis or hyperkeratosis and alternating areas of epithelial atrophy and hyperplasia[30] (Figures 5.47 and 5.48). Extensive, narrow downgrowths of the rete ridges are common (Figure 5.49) and there may be striking pseudoepitheliomatous hyperplasia. Follicular plugging, related to the openings of minor salivary gland ducts, has been described but in practice is rarely seen. There is basal cell liquefaction which occasionally leads to microscopic subepithelial vesiculation (Figure 5.50). The basement membrane is strongly PAS-positive and may show irregular thickening. Pigment-containing macrophages are not uncommon in the papillary corium. There is variable, predominantly lymphocytic, chronic inflammatory cell infiltration of the corium, the infiltrate being most dense superficially. In the deeper corium the infiltrate tends to have a perivascular distribution (Figure 5.47).

Microscopic subepithelial bulla formation is not uncommon, presumably due to extensive basal cell liquefaction (Figure 5.45). Sometimes surgical trauma leads to separation of large areas of corium and epithelium and the appearances may then simulate pemphigoid (Figure 5.46).

The immunocytochemical changes are characteristic but not diagnostic (Table 1).

Differential diagnosis. Because of the frequency with which lichen planus presents with atypical histological features, it may be difficult to separate it microscopically from white patches of unknown cause. The symmetrical distribution of the lichenoid lesions aids clinical distinction. Sometimes moderate degrees of dysplasia are present in areas of lichen planus and occasionally these are severe enough to raise the question of malignancy. This can be a difficult problem in interpretation, since a number of reported cases suggest an increased risk of squamous cell carcinoma developing in lichen planus. One of the most important and difficult differential diagnoses is lupus erythematosus; this is considered below. If there is extensive epithelial separation and the lesion closely resembles mucous membrane pemphigoid, immunofluorescent studies of biopsy tissue or blood often allow a definitive diagnosis to be made.

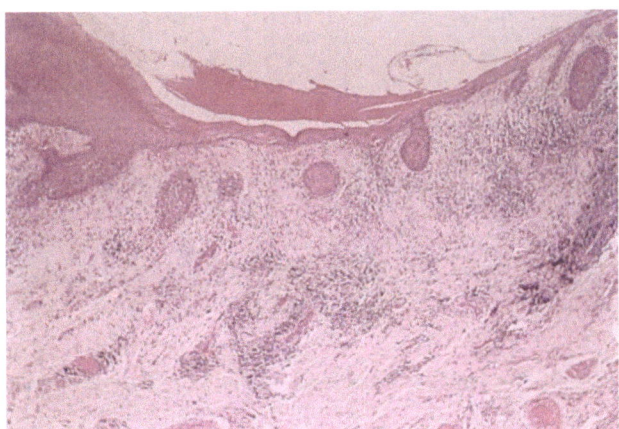

Figure 5.48 Discoid lupus erythematosus. In this example there is severe epithelial atrophy and hyperkeratosis. H & E × 40

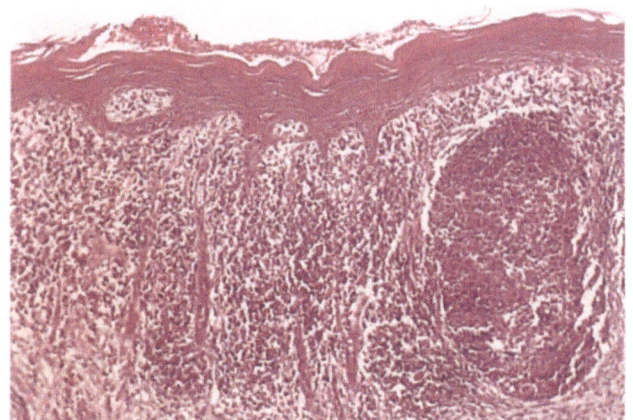

Figure 5.49 Discoid lupus erythematosus. There are narrow downgrowths of the rete ridges and dense chronic inflammatory cell infiltration. H & E × 100

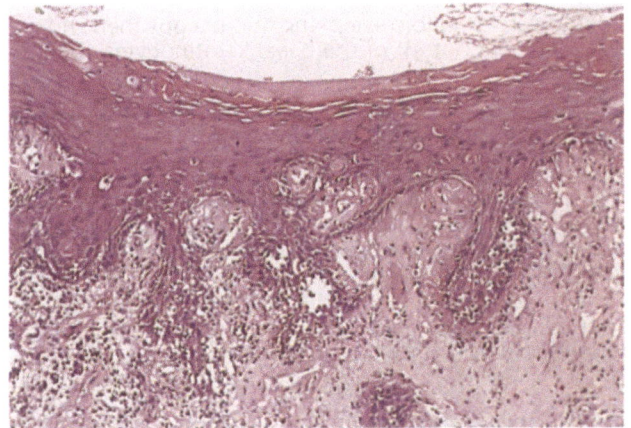

Figure 5.50 Discoid lupus erythematosus. showing extensive basal cell liquefaction and basement membrane thickening. H & E × 100

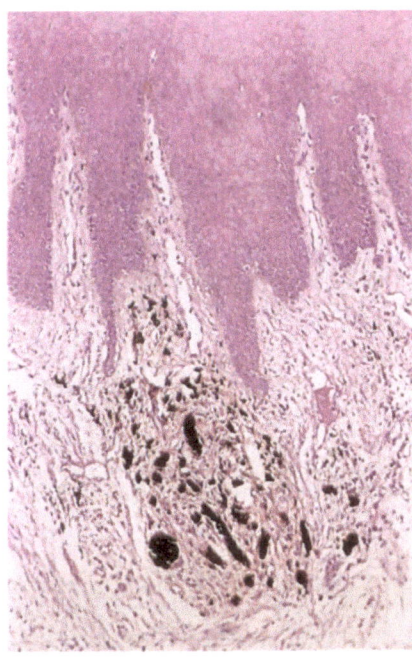

Figure 5.51 Amalgam tattoo. There are dense black granular deposits of amalgam with minimal reactive changes in the surrounding tissues. H & E × 100

Differential diagnosis. The differential diagnosis of oral discoid lupus erythematosus is difficult. The disease most likely to cause confusion is lichen planus and at times it is not possible to differentiate between the conditions on the basis of conventional histology. The pseudoepitheliomatous hyperplasia alternating with areas of epithelial atrophy and the patchiness of the inflammatory infiltrate, especially the extension into the deeper corium in a perivascular distribution, are the most significant differences. Immunocytochemical examination may be useful (Table 1). Occasionally discoid lupus erythematosus presents clinically as a nondescript white patch, and since in atrophic areas there may be moderate and sometimes severe epithelial dysplasia, this, together with the presence of pseudoepitheliomatous hyperplasia, can lead to an erroneous diagnosis of a premalignant or malignant lesion. But at the same time, there does appear to be an increased tendency for the development of squamous cell carcinoma in discoid lesions, especially those of the lower lip.

Systemic lupus erythematosus. The mucosal lesions are non-specific and can be vesicles, areas of epithelial atrophy or frank ulcers. They are rarely biopsied as other signs and symptoms of the disease usually point to the diagnosis, confirmed by immunological tests. The histological changes also lack specific features. They include epithelial spongiosis, basal cell liquefaction and lymphocytic infiltration of the corium, especially perivascularly. Secondary inflammatory changes due to ulceration are common. Systemic lupus erythematosus can be distinguished from discoid lesions by immunocytochemical methods (Table 1).

Pigmented Lesions

Amalgam Tattoo

This relatively common lesion usually results from fragments of silver amalgam filling material fracturing from a restoration during tooth removal and becoming embedded in the extraction wound[31] (Figure 5.51). After healing, the lesion is seen as a discrete area of bluish-black

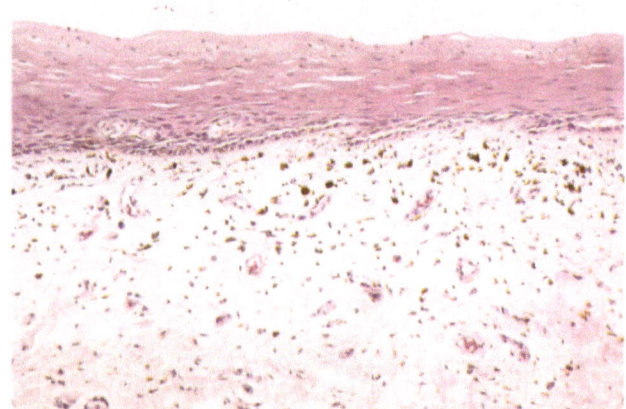

Figure 5.52 Oral melanotic macule. There are many melanophages in the superficial corium. The overlying epithelium is normal.   H & E × 200

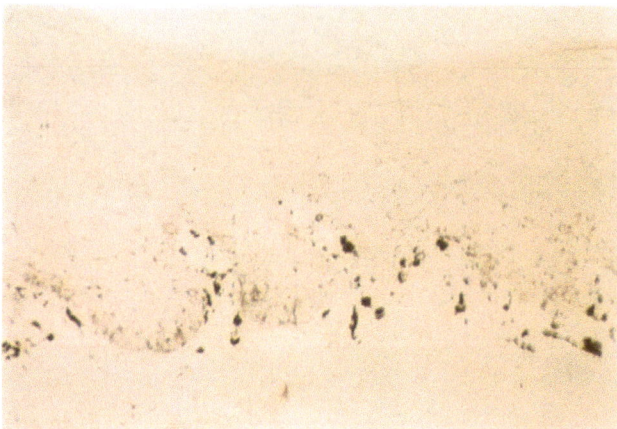

Figure 5.54 Oral melanotic macule, showing the distribution of melanin. Fontana × 200

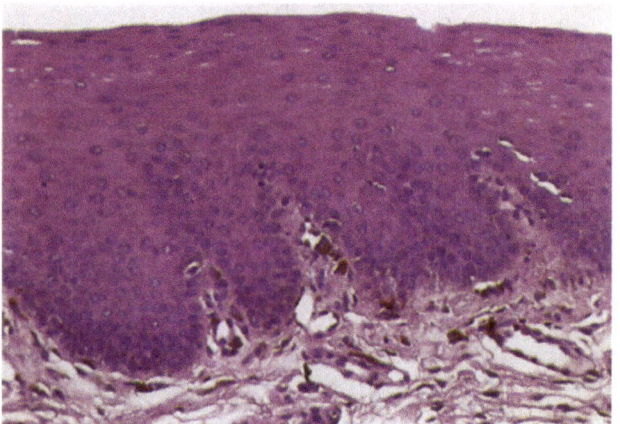

Figure 5.53 Oral melanotic macule. There is increased melanin in the basal and, to a lesser extent, suprabasal keratinocytes and in melanophages in the superficial corium.   H & E × 200

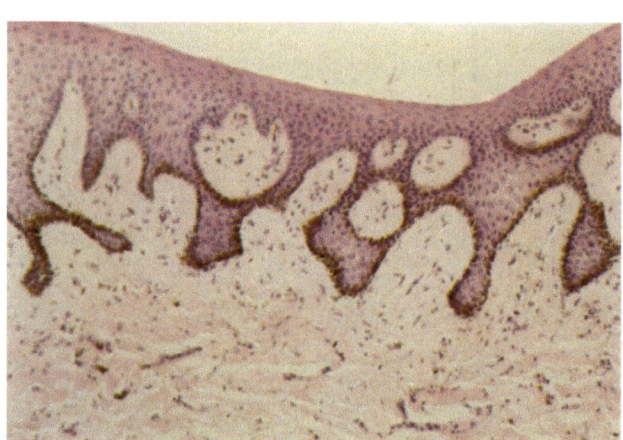

Figure 5.55 Racial pigmentation. There is a high content of melanin in the basal keratinocytes.   H & E × 100

discolouration, usually on the alveolus or the gingiva. Microscopically, there are dark, refractile fragments of material and a variable inflammatory response, sometimes with multinucleated foreign body giant cells. Small granules of material are distributed along collagen fibres, sometimes at a considerable distance from the main focus.

Oral Melanotic Macule

Small pigmented macules in the oral mucosa usually appear as solitary or multiple lesions and are most commonly seen in young and middle-aged adults[32]. Although they can present anywhere in the mouth, the vermilion border of the lips, particularly the lower lip, and gingivae are the commonest sites. The macules are usually well defined and vary from greyish-brown to black. These lesions are usually only biopsied when melanoma is suspected.

Microscopically there may be increased melanotic pigmentation of the basal cell layer, the superficial corium (in melanophages) (Figure 5.52) or a combination of both (Figures 5.53 and 5.54).

Racial Pigmentation

Dark, and especially black, skinned people often have areas of intraoral melanotic pigmentation. The gingivae are the most commonly involved sites. Occasionally these pigmented areas are biopsied and microscopy then shows a high melanin content of the basal keratinocytes (Figure 5.55).

Addison's Disease

Melanotic pigmentation of skin and mucous membrane is an early feature of Addison's disease. The cheeks and lateral borders of the tongue are the intraoral sites most commonly affected. Microscopy shows features identical to those of racial pigmentation.

Other pigmented lesions that may be biopsied include the benign naevi and melanoma, and the melanotic neuroectodermal tumour of infants.

Miscellaneous Lesions

Geographical Tongue

This condition, which affects 1–2% of the population, consists of areas of depapillation on the dorsal surface of the tongue[33]. The lesions have well defined, slightly raised, yellowish, serpiginous margins and tend to spread centrifugally whilst healing centrally. They are usually painless but may occasionally give rise to a burning sensation. Similar lesions may appear elsewhere in the mouth – so-called geographical stomatitis.

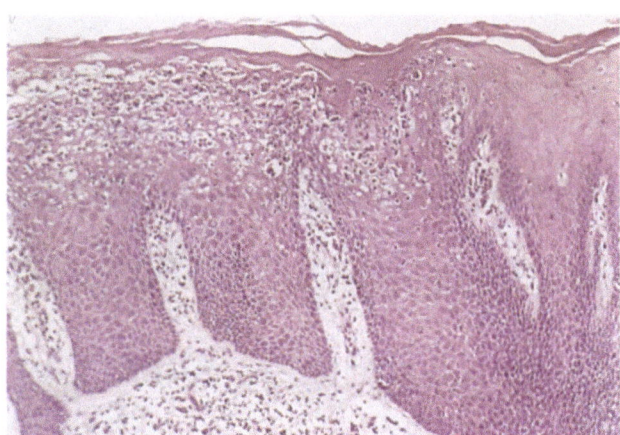

Figure 5.56 Geographical tongue. The normal papillation has been lost and there is extensive infiltration of the epithelium by neutrophils. H & E × 100

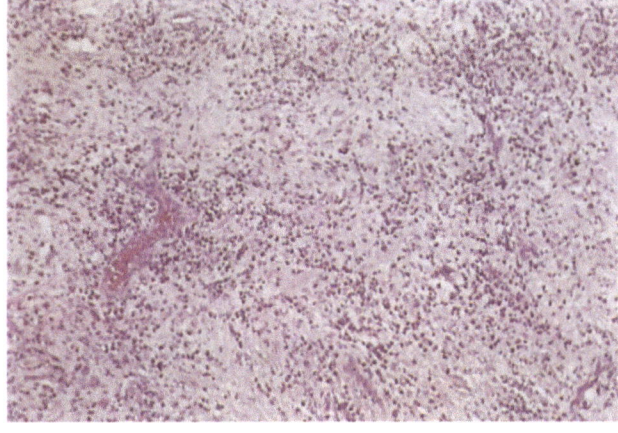

Figure 5.58 Traumatic eosinophilic granuloma. A field from the area just below a mucosal ulcer, showing a dense infiltrate of eosinophils and histiocytes. H & E × 40

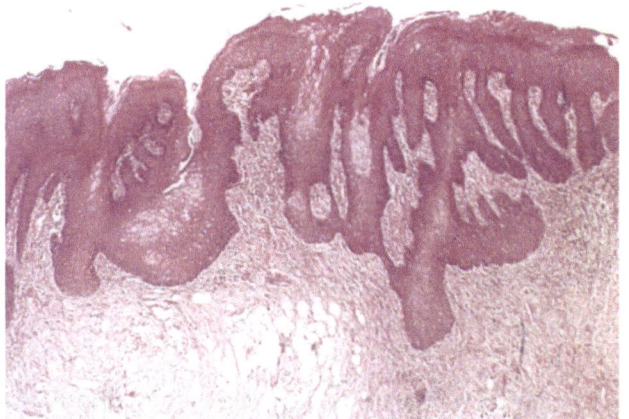

Figure 5.57 Median rhomboid glossitis. There is loss of papillation and a thick layer of parakeratosis. The underlying epithelium shows acanthosis with branching and anastomosis of the rete ridges. H & E × 40

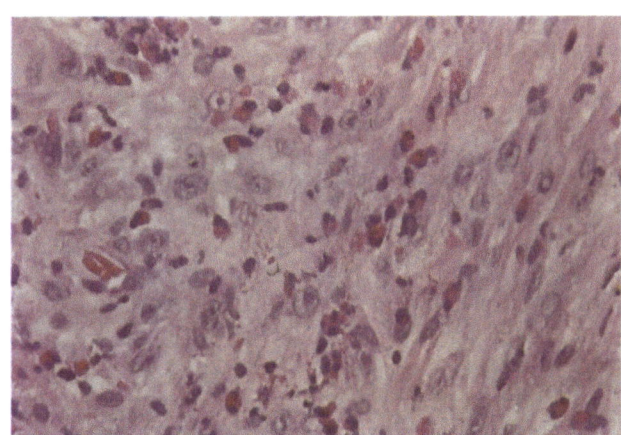

Figure 5.59 Traumatic eosinophilic granuloma. Higher magnification from Figure 5.58. H & E × 400

Microscopy shows loss of papillae, mild acanthosis and spongiform pustules in the superficial layers of the epithelium (Figure 5.56). There is usually mild inflammatory infiltration of the superficial corium.

The histological changes in geographical tongue resemble those of psoriasis and Reiter's syndrome. Differentiation of these lesions depends on the clinical features. Geographical tongue also resembles candidosis, especially when the parakeratotic plaque has been lost and hyphae are difficult to find (page 52). The inflammatory infiltration of the corium is usually much less severe in geographical stomatitis than in candidosis.

Median Rhomboid Glossitis

Median rhomboid glossitis usually appears as a dark red, smooth, roughly rhomboidal area located in the midline of the tongue anterior to the sulcus terminalis. Occasionally the surface is nodular and fissured. It is usually asymptomatic but sometimes causes soreness or a burning sensation. The lesion was thought to be a developmental abnormality, but it appears to be very uncommon in children and many now believe that candidal infection is implicated in the aetiology[34,35].

Microscopy shows loss of the normal papillae and parakeratosis, which may be extensive. There is acanthosis with branching and anastomosis of the rete ridges (Figure 5.57). Neutrophils are frequently present in the superficial layers of the epithelium and candidal hyphae can be identified in over 85% of cases. There is variable lymphocytic and plasma cell infiltration of the corium and there is usually increased vascularity. Occasionally the epithelium may show mild to moderate dysplasia, but it is very rare for malignancy to develop in the dorsum of the tongue.

Traumatic Eosinophilic Granuloma

This is a benign, self-limiting condition in which there is localized ulceration and induration of the oral mucosa. Although the histological picture is dominated by eosinophils and histiocytes there is no association with eosinophilic granuloma of bone.

The lesion is seen most commonly in the tongue and there is frequently a history of preceding trauma[36]. Microscopy shows ulceration and many eosinophils and histiocytes in the underlying corium. The histiocytes may be somewhat pleomorphic and mitoses may be present. In addition there may be fibroblastic proliferation and areas of muscle damage (Figures 5.58 and 5.59). Although the histological features are sometimes suggestive of malignancy the lesion usually heals spontaneously without scarring[37].

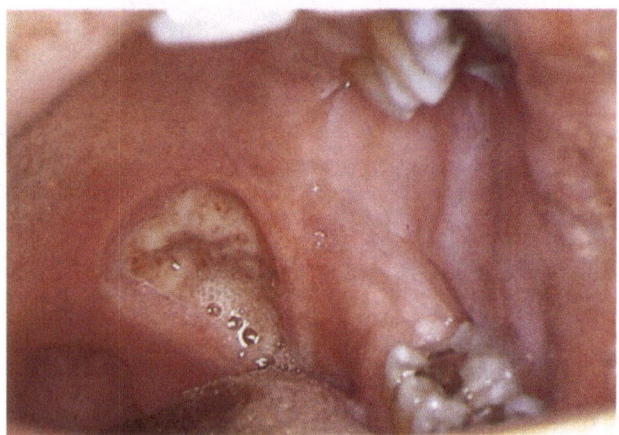

Figure 5.60 Major aphtha. This large painful ulcer of the palate healed after several months, leaving a scar.

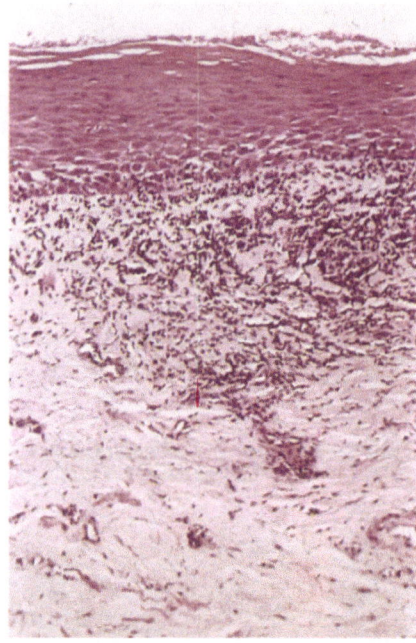

Figure 5.62 Submucous fibrosis. In this early lesion there is mild epithelial atrophy, chronic inflammatory infiltration and fibroelastic change in the deeper corium. H & E × 100

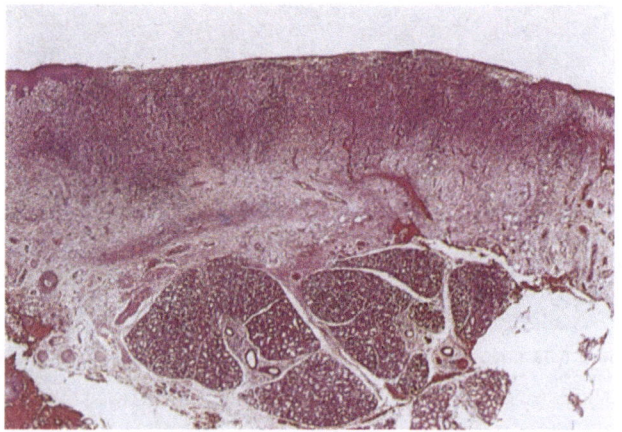

Figure 5.61 Major aphtha. Biopsy specimen shows ulceration and heavy, non-specific chronic inflammation. H & E × 8

Recurrent Aphthous Stomatitis[38]

This is a very common disorder in which there are one or more persistently recurrent, painful ulcers in the oral mucosa. It usually begins in childhood or adolescence, but attacks tend to become less frequent after the third decade. If the condition first appears in adult life a systemic predisposing cause should be suspected.

In the common form of the disease (minor type) several small, painful ulcers develop on the nonkeratinized mucosa and heal without scarring within 7–10 days. Major aphthae (periadenitis mucosa necrotica recurrens) are much less common and are characterized by the formation of usually single ulcers which are large (up to two or more centimetres in diameter), painful and which may persist for several months before finally healing with scarring (Figure 5.60). Local, painful lymphadenopathy is common. In the herpetiform type of the disease there are many (30 or more) pinhead-sized ulcers which often coalesce.

Aphthae are usually idiopathic but may be associated with systemic diseases which include: gastrointestinal disorders such as ulcerative colitis and coeliac disease; haematological abnormalities such as iron, vitamin B_{12} or folate deficiencies, either occult or overt and Behçet's

syndrome. Occasionally ulceration is related to the menstrual cycle, with ulcers appearing in the luteal phase.

Minor aphthae are virtually never biopsied, since their nature is clearly indicated by the clinical history, the macroscopic appearance of the ulcers and their rapid healing. Major aphthae, on the other hand, can be extremely recalcitrant to treatment; the scarring at the margin of the ulcer leads to induration and, in the absence of a clear-cut history or evidence of scarring elsewhere in the mouth, the lesion is easily confused with squamous cell carcinoma. Biopsy is therefore often carried out for these major aphthae. Microscopically, there is non-specific ulceration, usually with heavy acute inflammatory infiltration of the superficial corium (Figure 5.61). Chronic inflammatory cells, especially lymphocytes, predominate in the deeper corium.

Smears are sometimes taken from minor aphthae in order to exclude a viral cause for the ulceration. They show acute and chronic inflammatory cells, bacteria and debris, but no evidence of virally damaged cells.

Submucous Fibrosis

Oral submucous fibrosis is a slowly progressive disease seen almost exclusively in Indians and Pakistanis[39]. It causes dense fibrosis mainly in the buccal mucosa, soft palate, tongue and lips. Initially there are subepithelial blisters which rupture to leave shallow but painful ulcers. Microscopy shows chronic inflammation and fibroelastic change, consisting of hyalinization of collagen and the appearance of coarse irregular elastic fibres, in the superficial corium (Figure 5.62). This is followed by atrophy of the epithelium and frequently dysplasia (Figure 5.63). Bands of hyaline scar tissue extend into the underlying muscles. This can lead to trismus and difficulty in mastication, speech and swallowing. There is strong evidence that submucous fibrosis is a premalignant condition and about a third of the patients eventually develop squamous cell carcinoma.

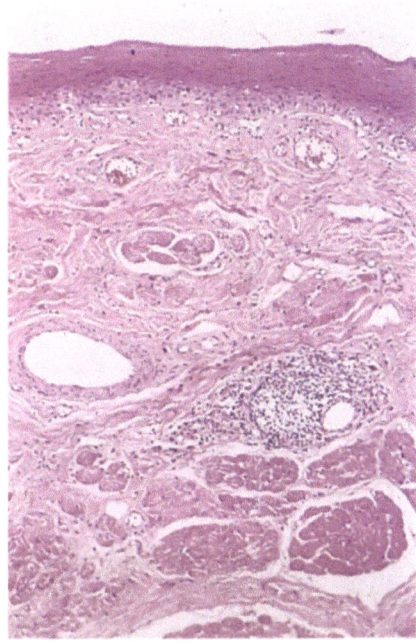

Figure 5.63 Submucous fibrosis. A late stage lesion, showing severe epithelial atrophy and mild-to-moderate dysplasia. Fibroelastic change extends into the underlying, degenerating muscle bundles. H & E × 100

References

1. Prabhu, S. R., Daftary, D. K. and Dholakia, H. M. (1978). Tuberculous ulcer of the tongue: report of a case. *J. Oral Surg.*, **36**, 384

2. Reichart, P. (1976). Facial and oral manifestations in leprosy. *Oral Surg.*, **41**, 385

3. Southam, J. C. and Venkataraman, B. K. (1973). Oral manifestations of leprosy. *Brit. J. Oral Surg.*, **10**, 272

4. van Maarsseveen, A. C. M. Th., van der Waal, I., Stam, J., Veldhuizen, R. W. and van der Kwast, W. A. M. (1982). Oral involvement in sarcoidosis. *Int. J. Oral Surg.*, **11**, 21

5. Nessan, V. J. and Jacoway, J. R. (1979). Biopsy of the minor salivary glands in the diagnosis of sarcoidosis. *N. Engl. J. Med.*, **30**, 922

6. Greenstein, A. L., Janowitz, H. D. and Sachar, D. B. (1976). The extra-intestinal complications of Crohn's disease and ulcerative colitis. *Medicine*, **55**, 401

7. Bernstein, M. L. and MacDonald, J. S. (1978). Oral lesions in Crohn's disease: report of two cases and update of the literature. *Oral Surg.*, **46**, 234

8. Basu, M. K., Asquith, P., Thompson, R. A. and Cooke, W. T. (1975). Oral manifestations of Crohn's disease. *Gut.*, **16**, 249

9. Meyer, I. and Shklar, G. (1967). The oral manifestations of acquired syphilis. *Oral Surg.*, **23**, 45

10. Brown, J. R. (1973). Human actinomycosis: a study of 181 subjects. *Human Pathol.*, **4**, 319

11. Stenhouse, D., MacDonald, D. G. and MacFarlane, T. W. (1975). Cervico-facial and intraoral actinomycosis: a five-year retrospective study. *Brit. J. Oral Surg.*, **13**, 172

12. Walker, D. M. (1975). Candidal infection of the oral mucosa. In: *Oral Mucosa in Health and Disease*. A. E. Dolby (ed.). (Oxford: Blackwell Scientific Publications)

13. Cawson, R. A. (1976). Infections of the oral mucous membrane. In: *Scientific Foundations of Dentistry*. B. Cohen and I. R. H. Kramer (eds.). (London: William Heinemann Medical Books Ltd)

14. Young, R. C., Bennett, J. E., Vogel, C., Carbone, P. P. and DeVita, V. T. (1970). Aspergillosis. *Medicine*, **49**, 147

15. Young, L. L., Dolan, C. T., Sheridan, P. J. and Reeve, C. M. (1972). Oral manifestations of histoplasmosis. *Oral Surg.*, **33**, 191

16. Berger, C. J., Disque, F. C. and Topazian, R. G. (1978). Rhinocerebral mucormycosis: diagnosis and treatment. *Oral Surg.*, **40**, 27

17. World Health Organization Collaborating Centre for Oral Precancerous Lesions (1978). Definition of leukoplakia and related lesions: an aid to studies on oral precancer. *Oral Surg.*, **46**, 518

18. Bánóczy, J., Sugár, L. and Frithiof, L. (1973). White sponge nevus: leukoedema exfoliativum mucosae oris: a report on forty-five cases. *Swed. Dent. J.*, **66**, 481

19. Pindborg., J. J. (1980). *Oral Cancer and Precancer*. (Bristol: John Wright and Sons Ltd)

20. Berry, H. H. and Landwerlen, J. R. Cigarette smoker's lip lesion in psychiatric patients. *J. Amer. Dent. Ass.*, **86**, 657

21. Zegarelli, D. J. and Zegarelli, E. V. (1977). Intraoral pemphigus vulgaris. *Oral Surg.*, **44**, 384

22. Daniels, T. E. and Quandra-White, C. (1981). Direct immunofluorescence in oral mucosal disease: a diagnostic analysis of 130 cases. *Oral Surg.*, **51**, 38

23. Dabelsteen, E. (1978). Distribution of complement and immunoglobulin in oral pemphigus lesions. *Acta Derm. Venereol. (Stokh.)*, **58**, 540

24. Scully, C. and Lehner, T. (1980). Disorders of immunity. In: *Oral Manifestations of Systemic Disease*. J. H. Jones and D. K. Mason (eds.). (London, Philadelphia, Toronto: W. B. Saunders & Co. Ltd)

25. Fine, R. M. and Weathers, D. R. (1980). Desquamative gingivitis: a form of cicatricial pemphigoid? *Brit. J. Dermatol.*, **102**, 393

26. Lozada, F. and Silverman, S. (1978). Erythema multiforme: clinical characteristics and natural history of fifty patients. *Oral Surg.*, **46**, 628

27. Buchner, A., Lozada, F. and Silverman, S. (1980). Histopathologic spectrum of oral erythema multiforme. *Oral Surg.*, **49**, 221

28. Pindborg, J. J. (1980). Diseases of the skin. In: *Oral Manifestations of Systemic Disease*. J. H. Jones and D. K. Mason (eds.). (London, Philadelphia, Toronto: W. B. Saunders & Co. Ltd)

29. Schiödt, M., Halberg, P. and Hentzer, B. (1978). A clinical study of thirty-two patients with oral discoid lupus erythematosus. *Int. J. Oral Surg.*, **7**, 85

30. Andreasen, J. O. and Poulsen, H. E. (1964). Oral manifestations in discoid and systemic lupus erythematosus. II. Histologic investigation. *Acta Odontol. Scand.*, **22**, 389

31. Buchner, A. and Hansen, L. S. (1980). Amalgam pigmentation (amalgam tattoo) of the oral mucosa. *Oral Surg.*, **49**, 139

32. Buchner, A. and Hansen, L. S. (1979). Melanotic macule of the oral mucosa: a clinicopathologic study of 105 cases. *Oral Surg.*, **48**, 244

33. Hume, W. J. (1975). Geographic stomatitis: a critical review. *J. Dent.*, **3**, 25

34. Farman, A. G., Van Wyk, C. W., Staz, J., Hugo, M. and Dreyer, W. P. (1977). Central papillary atrophy of the tongue. *Oral Surg.*, **43**, 48

35. Wright, B. A. (1978). Median rhomboid glossitis: not a misnomer. *Oral Surg.*, **46**, 806

36. Shapiro, L. and Juhlin, E. A. (1970). Eosinophilic ulcer of the tongue. *Dermatologica*, **140**, 242

37. Burgess, G. H., Mehregan, A. H. and Drinnan, A. J. (1977). Eosinophilic ulcer of the tongue: report of two cases. *Arch. Dermatol.*, **113**, 644

38. Greenspan, J. S. (1983). Infections and non-neoplastic diseases of the oral mucosa. *J. Oral Path.*, **12**, 139

39. Pindborg, J. J., Bhonsle, R. B., Murti, P. R., Gupta, P. C., Daftary, D. K. and Mehta, F. S. (1980). Incidence and early forms of oral submucous fibrosis. *Oral Surg.*, **50**, 40

6

Bone

Inflammatory Diseases

Despite the fact that extraction of teeth leaves large areas of bone exposed to the oral fluids and bacteria, serious inflammation of the bone is infrequent in otherwise healthy individuals. The commonest complication of a healing extraction wound is the so-called dry socket or focal osteitis.

Focal Osteitis

In this condition the blood clot that usually fills the socket after tooth extraction does not undergo the normal sequence of organization and subsequent replacement by new bone. Instead, it breaks down to leave the bone of the socket exposed to oral bacteria. There is then a mixed bacterial infection of the empty, or 'dry', socket. This leads to necrosis of the bone of the socket wall, with the formation of small sequestra (Figure 6.1). Healing is slow, with granulation tissue gradually filling the wound from the sides and base, and resorption or shedding of the sequestra. This is followed, as in normal healing, by replacement of the granulation tissue by bone.

Dry socket may very occasionally appear following an uncomplicated extraction, but it is usually associated with difficult or traumatic extractions where there has been more than the usual degree of tissue damage.

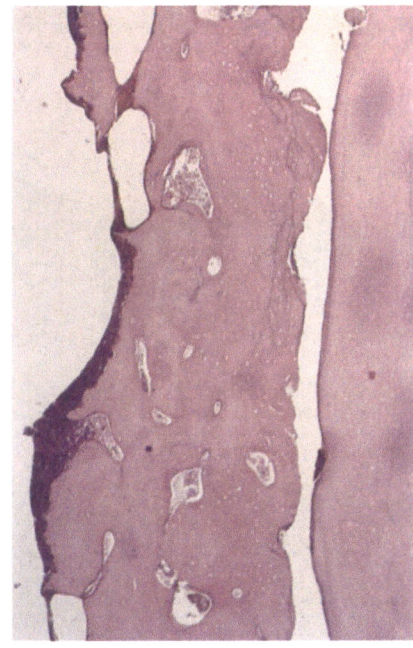

Figure 6.1 Focal osteitis. The necrotic bone of the socket wall (lamina dura) is to the left and a fragment of retained root at right. H & E × 40

Osteomyelitis[1]

Osteomyelitis of the jaws can be classified as:

Suppurative osteomyelitis – acute
                               chronic

Sclerosing osteomyelitis – focal
                               diffuse

Chronic osteomyelitis with proliferative periostitis.

Suppurative Osteomyelitis

This type of osteomyelitis is usually a complication of dental infection, or of a fracture or gunshot wound. It is much less frequently due to haematogenous spread from some distant focus of infection. Radiographs show radiolucent areas in which slightly radiopaque sequestra may be seen (Figure 6.2). The histological features are similar to those seen in other bones. The medullary spaces become

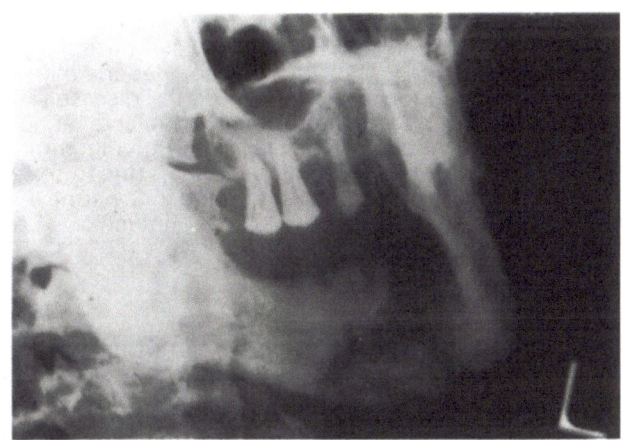

Figure 6.2 Suppurative osteomyelitis following tooth extraction. The radiograph shows a large, irregular radiolucent area and several radiopaque foci.

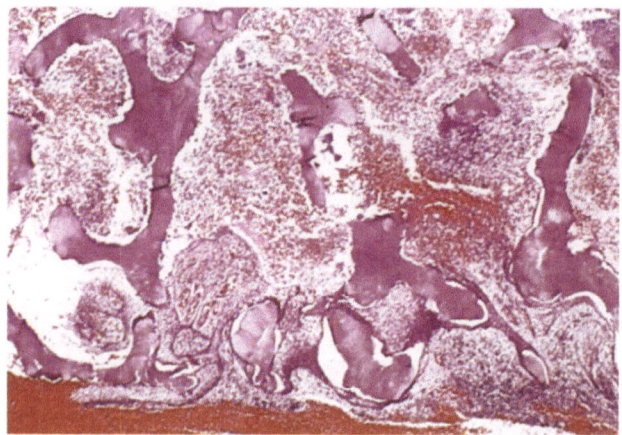

Figure 6.3 Suppurative osteomyelitis. The bone is necrotic and the marrow spaces are filled with neutrophils and colonies of filamentous organisms. H & E × 40

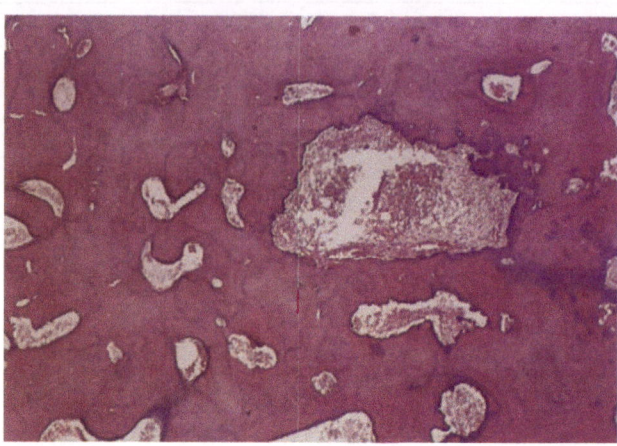

Figure 6.5 Chronic focal sclerosing osteomyelitis. There is a dense mass of poorly vital bone with focal areas of acute inflammatory infiltration. H & E × 40

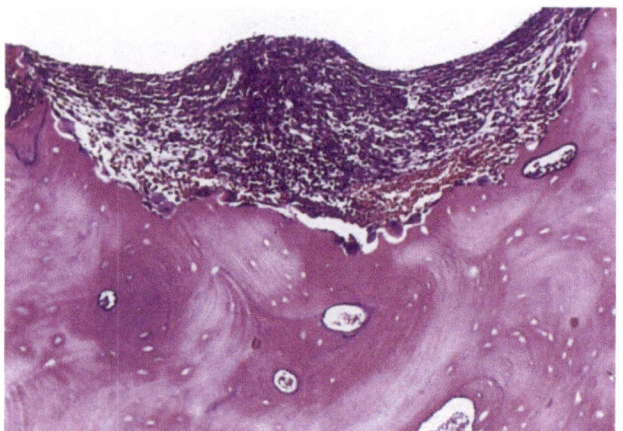

Figure 6.4 Suppurative osteomyelitis. In the necrotic bone the osteocyte lacunae are empty. There is patchy osteoclastic resorption. H & E × 100

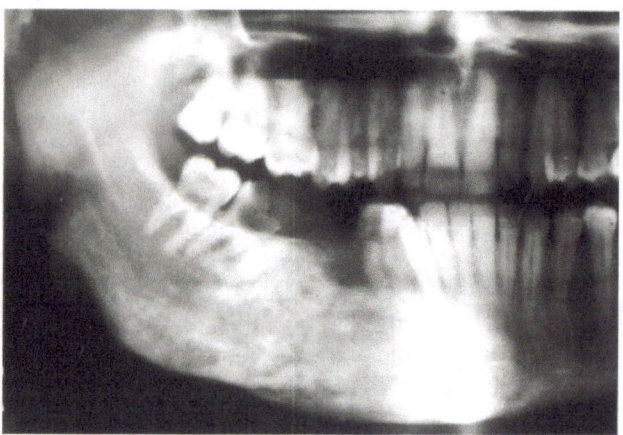

Figure 6.6 Chronic diffuse sclerosing osteomyelitis. The radiograph shows irregular diffuse areas of radiopacity in the mandible.

filled with acute inflammatory cells and occasionally lymphocytes and plasma cells (Figure 6.3). The adjacent bone is necrotic with loss of viable osteocytes and there is osteoclastic resorption (Figure 6.4). As the disease progresses there is sequestration of dead bone and variable new bone formation, but a well-formed involucrum is unusual in the jaws. If the infection remains uncontrolled it becomes chronic, with cloacae forming in the bone and sinuses appearing in the overlying skin or mucosa.

Sclerosing Osteomyelitis

Chronic focal sclerosing osteomyelitis is an uncommon response of the bone to low grade infection. It is almost invariably seen in individuals below the age of 20 years, usually in relation to a carious mandibular first molar tooth. Radiographs show a densely radiopaque mass at the apex of the tooth or alone in the jaw if the offending tooth has been removed. Microscopy shows dense masses of poorly vital or non-vital bone with scanty, fibrous medullary spaces. There is usually patchy, mild chronic inflammatory cell infiltration or focal collections of polymorphs in areas of acute exacerbation (Figure 6.5).

Chronic diffuse sclerosing osteomyelitis appears as a response to low grade infection of the periodontal tissues in patients with longstanding periodontal disease. Accordingly the patients are usually elderly, and may be dentate or edentulous. The disease can be asymptomatic or there may be ill defined pain and bad taste related to draining sinuses. The condition is seen most frequently in the mandible, where radiographs show diffuse, irregular areas of radiopacity, closely resembling the cotton wool pattern of Paget's disease (Figure 6.6). Microscopy shows inflamed fibrous marrow spaces and irregular, coarse bony trabeculae which often have prominent resting and reversal lines resembling the mosaic pattern of Paget's disease (Figure 6.7). It is usual to find areas of continuing new coarse woven bone formation. In areas of acute exacerbation neutrophils are abundant.

There are a number of diseases resembling sclerosing osteomyelitis both radiographically and histologically, including Paget's disease, benign cementoblastoma and gigantiform cementoma. In Paget's disease the cement lines are more generalized and less regular than in sclerosing osteomyelitis and inflammatory changes are usually less severe. In some cases, however, the distinction cannot be made on the histological appearances alone. Chronic

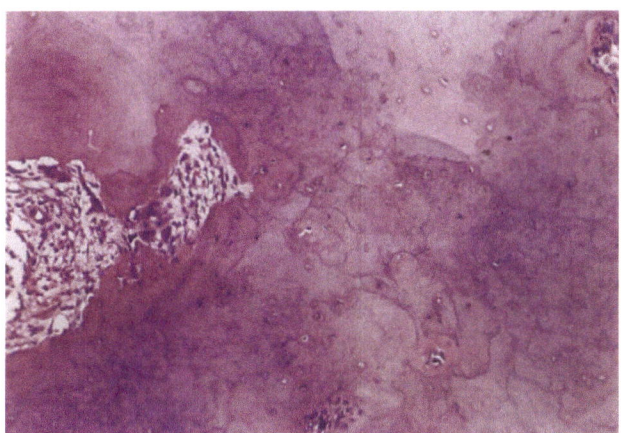

Figure 6.7 Chronic diffuse sclerosing osteomyelitis. There is a dense mass of poorly vital bone with a pagetoid pattern of haematoxyphilic resting and reversal lines.   H & E × 100

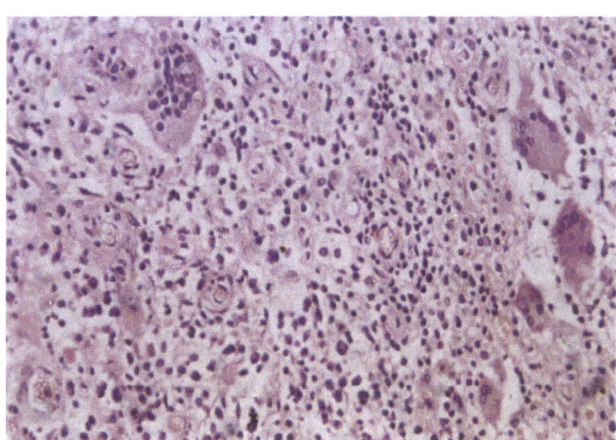

Figure 6.9 Giant cell periostitis with hyaline change. The heavily inflamed periosteum contains scattered multinucleated giant cells.   H & E × 200

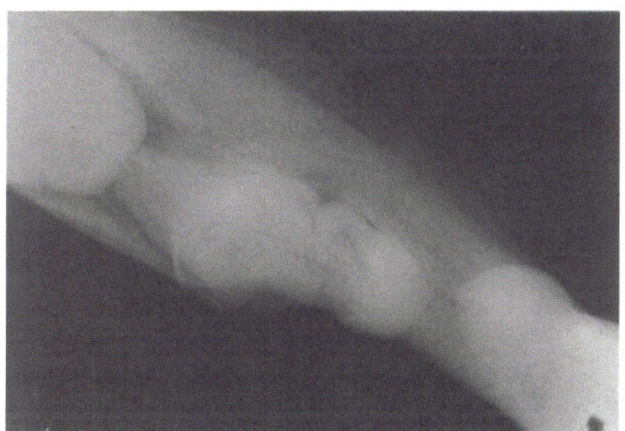

Figure 6.8 Chronic osteomyelitis with proliferating periostitis. The radiograph shows faint radiopaque lines on the outer surface of the jaw.

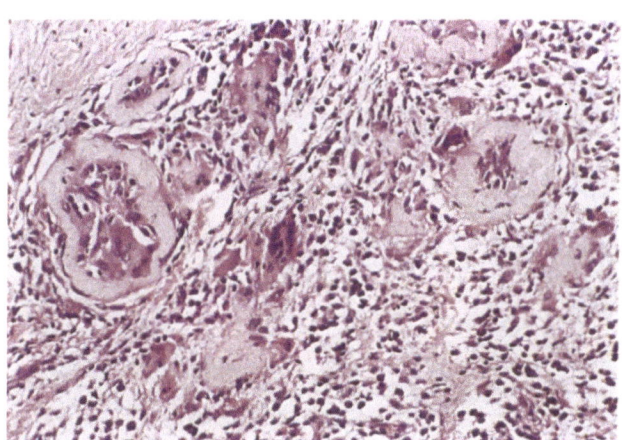

Figure 6.10 Giant cell periostitis with hyaline change. Solid hyaline areas and ring-like hyaline structures are seen. Multinucleated giant cells are associated with the hyaline structures.   H & E × 200

focal sclerosing osteomyelitis is easily confused with benign cementoblastoma radiographically but does not show a peripheral uncalcified zone histologically (which is typical of cementoblastoma), and the reversal lines are less pronounced. The distinction between chronic sclerosing osteomyelitis and gigantiform cementoma is considered on page 123.

Chronic Osteomyelitis with Proliferative Periostitis

This is a non-suppurative, productive periostitis of the jaws that appears in response to low grade, chronic irritation and results in bony and soft tissue swelling. It is typically seen in young people as a non-tender but often painful swelling, usually in the mandible. Constitutional symptoms are mild.

Radiographs often show a carious tooth, usually the lower first molar, as the causative agent. The bone shows cortical thickening with marrow space obliteration. The condition is sometimes seen in relation to infection around an unerupted tooth (folliculitis). A thin radiopaque line, or sometimes a series of parallel radiopaque lines, may be seen on the outer surface of the jaw (Figure 6.8). This appearance has to be distinguished from other diseases in which subperiosteal new bone formation is a significant feature. These include osteosarcoma, Ewing's tumour, leukaemia, syphilis, metastatic neuroblastoma and fracture callus.

Microscopy shows subperiosteal new bone formation and marrow fibrosis with variable chronic inflammatory cell infiltration.

Giant Cell Periostitis with Hyaline Change

This is an uncommon but distinctive lesion of unknown etiology. Patients usually wear dentures. The lesion arises most frequently in the alveolar ridge and related buccal mucosa of the mandible as a painful swelling which may be associated with a localized defect in the underlying bone.

Microscopy shows acute and chronic inflammatory cell infiltration and multinucleated giant cells. Some of the giant cells are patchily distributed throughout the inflamed tissue (Figure 6.9) and others are related to pale-staining hyaline material. This hyaline material can be in the form of rings or more solid areas (Figure 6.10). Giant cells may be found within rings as well as peripherally. Granular dystrophic calcification is common and occasionally there

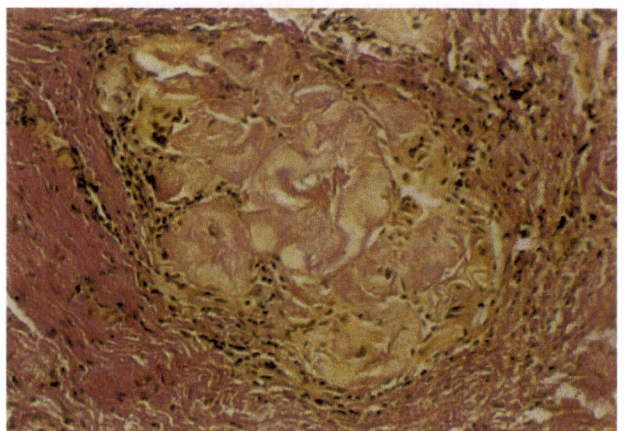

Figure 6.11   Giant cell periostitis with hyaline change. The hyaline rings stain for collagen.   Van Gieson × 200

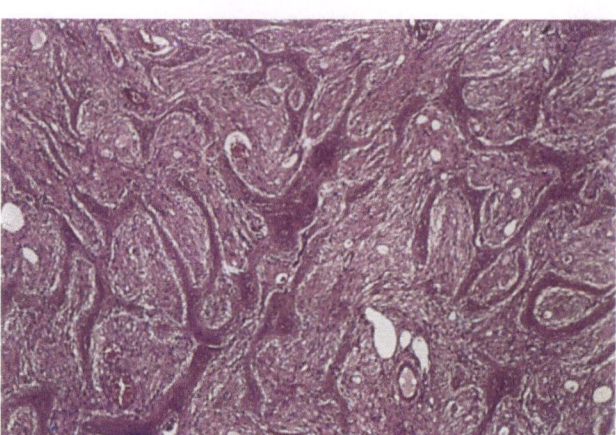

Figure 6.14   Fibrous dysplasia. In this early lesion there are slender trabeculae of metaplastic bone in a cellular fibrous stroma.   H & E × 40

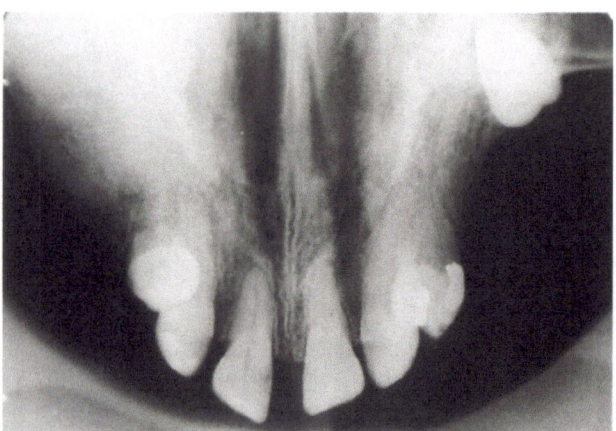

Figure 6.12   Fibrous dysplasia. The radiograph shows expansion and diffuse radiopacity of the maxilla.

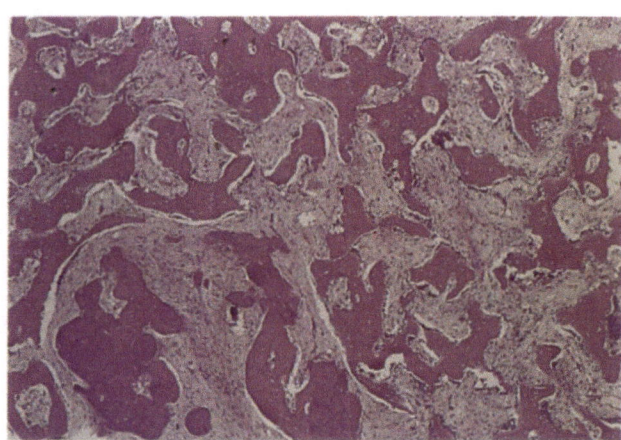

Figure 6.15   Fibrous dysplasia. In this later lesion the bone is lamellar in character and the fibrous stroma is less cellular.   H & E × 40

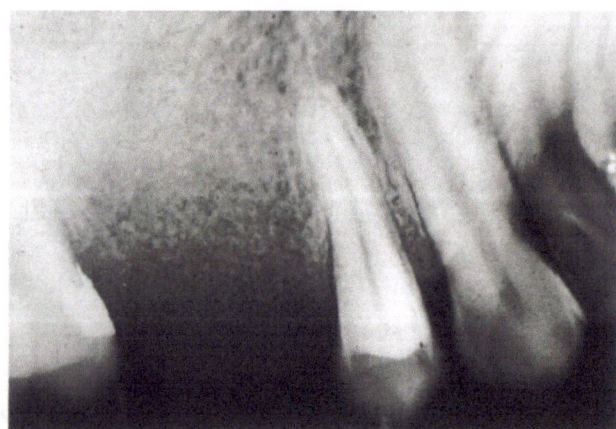

Figure 6.13   Fibrous dysplasia. This intra-oral radiograph shows the typical diffuse ground glass appearance of the bone.

may be more extensive calcification around and within the hyaline rings. Sometimes similar areas are seen in periapical granulomas.

This lesion has been termed *giant cell hyaline angiopathy* in the belief that the hyaline rings are due to degenerative changes in blood vessel walls. However, this seems unlikely, as many of the ring-like structures enclose connective tissue in which blood vessels can be identified. In addition, many of the rings are incomplete[2].

The lesion has also been considered to be a foreign body reaction to leguminous material and termed *pulse granuloma*[3]. It has been postulated that the hyaline rings are the remnants of the cellulose walls of starch cells. However, the hyaline material is generally much thicker than the walls of starch cells and, in addition, stains for collagen (Figure 6.11). Electron microscopy has shown the hyaline material to be fibrillar and probably degraded collagen.

The lesion appears to be an inflammatory reaction in the periosteum and until the etiology is determined the descriptive term used here seems an appropriate designation.

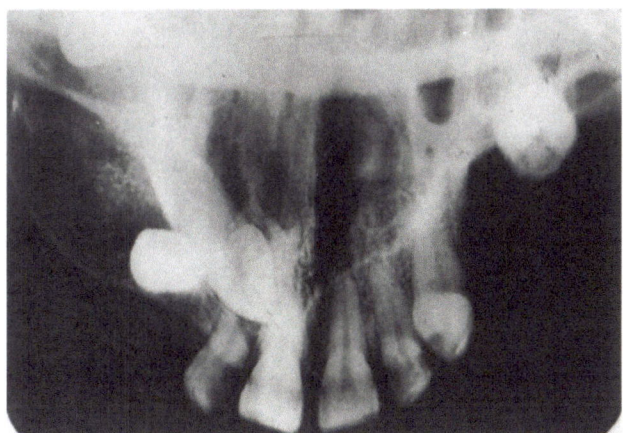

Figure 6.16 Ossifying fibroma. The radiograph shows expansion of the maxilla and a well defined area of radiolucency containing small radiopaque foci.

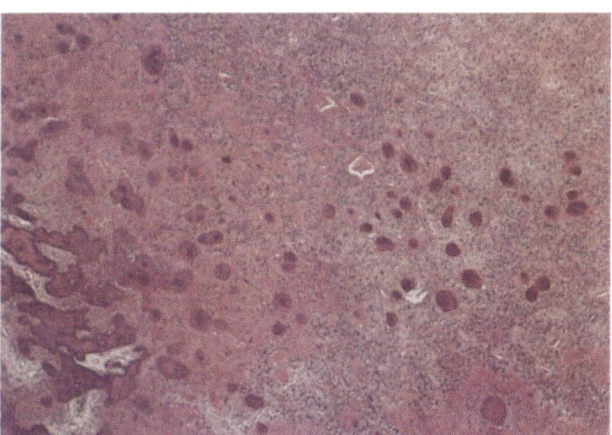

Figure 6.18 Ossifying fibroma. There are foci of calcification of varying size. The stroma is mainly collagenous on the left and highly cellular on the right. H & E × 40

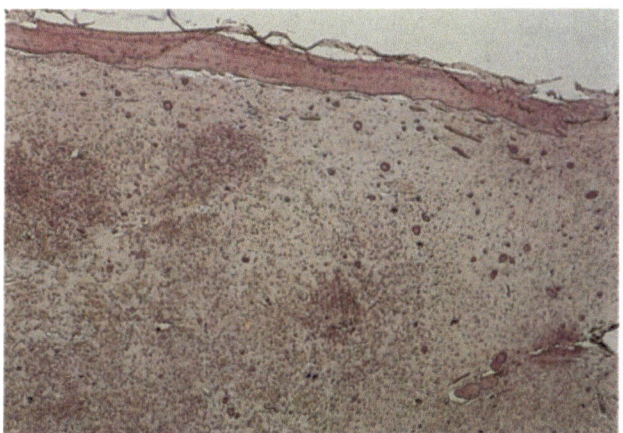

Figure 6.17 Ossifying fibroma. This is the periphery of the lesion, showing a rim of normal bone and a well circumscribed mass of fibrocellular tissue containing scattered foci of spheroidal calcification. H & E × 32

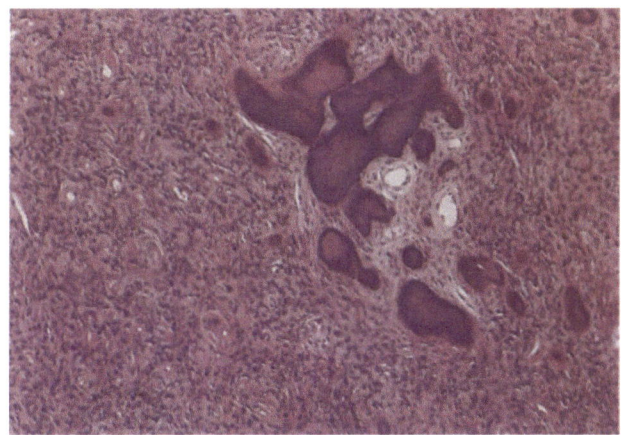

Figure 6.19 Ossifying fibroma. Higher magnification showing the cellular fibroblastic stroma and irregular calcifications. H & E × 100

Dysplasias

Fibrous Dysplasia

The jaws may be affected in monostotic fibrous dysplasia or they may be involved in the polyostotic form of the disease. The maxilla is affected more frequently than the mandible, the lesions usually producing painless, bony-hard swellings that can lead to facial asymmetry. There is active growth in children and young adults, but the lesions usually stabilize after skeletal maturation. Pathological fracture is very rare. Polyostotic lesions are occasionally part of Albright's syndrome.

The radiographic appearances are not constant. There may be bony expansion and a cyst-like radiolucency containing irregular radiopaque areas or, more commonly, diffuse radiopacity with a poorly defined edge (the so-called ground glass appearance) (Figures 6.12 and 6.13).

Microscopy shows replacement of normal bone by fibrous tissue of varying degrees of cellularity in which primitive bone is laid down. The new bone is deposited in the form of irregular, usually thin, trabeculae, often with a V or W configuration (Figure 6.14). There may be rows of osteoblasts on the borders of the bone and moderate numbers of osteoclast-like giant cells may be present, usually in the stroma. At first the bony trabeculae are

formed of osteoid, but they undergo calcification as they mature (Figure 6.15). Sometimes the calcified deposits take the form of concentrically lamellated, spheroidal foci of varying size which may fuse to form large masses of calcified material[4, 5].

Ossifying Fibroma

The clinical features of ossifying fibroma are similar to those of fibrous dysplasia, but there is a tendency to progressive growth and the lesion appears circumscribed on radiography[6]. The lesion grows slowly and may cause facial deformity, the mandible being the site of predilection. It usually appears radiographically as a well defined radiolucency with a thin osteosclerotic margin, containing variable amounts of calcified material (Figure 6.16).

The lesion is sometimes shelled out or it may be removed with a margin of sound bone (Figure 6.17). Larger lesions are apt to be removed piecemeal. Microscopy shows histological features which are frequently indistinguishable from fibrous dysplasia, the differentiation being made on the delimitation of the lesion or evidence of progressive growth in an adult. In some lesions there may be extensive calcification in the form of small spherical deposits or large, often acellular, masses (Figures 6.18 and 6.19).

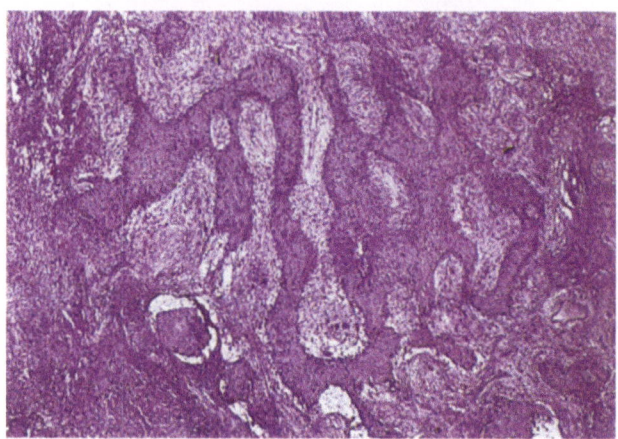

Figure 6.20 Juvenile ossifying fibroma. There are trabeculae of metaplastic bone lined by plump osteoblasts and a stroma composed of interlacing whorls of spindle-shaped cells. H & E × 40

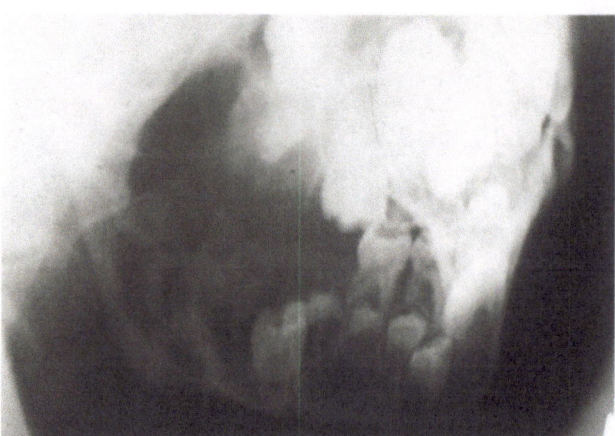

Figure 6.22 Cherubism. The radiograph shows a multilocular cystic lesion of the ramus, angle and body of the mandible. There was a similar lesion in the jaw on the opposite side.

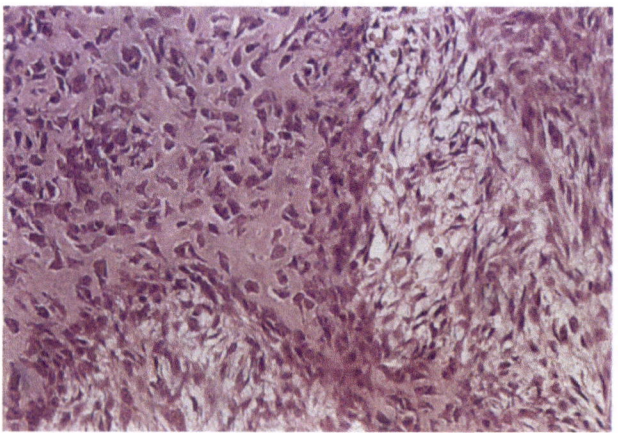

Figure 6.21 Juvenile ossifying fibroma. Higher magnification. H & E × 200

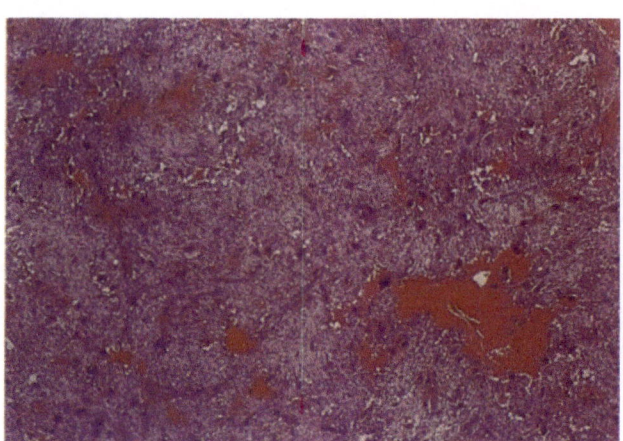

Figure 6.23 Cherubism. There are many multinucleate giant cells patchily distributed throughout the vascular, fibroblastic stroma. H & E × 40

The lesion has to be differentiated from cementifying fibroma and this can only be done with any certainty when a clear relationship between the lesion and the root of a tooth can be demonstrated, as the histological features are generally considered to be identical. Occasionally ossifying fibromas in younger individuals show rapid growth and microscopy shows a very active cellular stroma, with plump spindle-shaped cells in which mitotic figures may not be hard to find (Figures 6.20 and 6.21). These lesions have been called juvenile or aggressive ossifying fibromas and need to be distinguished from fibroblastic osteosarcomas. In juvenile ossifying fibroma the new bone formation is much more regular than in osteosarcoma and there is much less cellular pleomorphism. Abnormal mitoses are not seen[7].

Cherubism (Familial Fibrous Dysplasia)

Affected children with this familial disease are apparently normal at birth, but between the ages of 2 and 4 there appear bilateral swellings of the mandible and maxilla which may cause considerable facial deformity and the typical cherubic facies[8]. The lesions usually stabilize or grow only slowly between about 7 years and puberty, after which time they tend to regress. Patients may have bilateral submandibular lymphadenopathy and occasionally other cervical nodes are enlarged. Radiographs show expansion of the involved bones by a multilocular radiolucency and in the maxilla the sinuses may be obliterated (Figure 6.22).

Microscopy shows that normal bone has been replaced by whorled fibrous tissue in which multinucleated giant cells can be seen (Figure 6.23). These giant cells are particularly conspicuous around the thin walled vessels which are commonly present and sometimes they appear to lie within vascular spaces. Some vessels have a perivascular cuff of pale eosinophilic material which has been shown to be collagen[9] (Figures 6.24 and 6.25). Areas of haemorrhage and haemosiderin deposition are usually seen, but metaplastic bone formation is rare. The enlarged cervical lymph nodes show reactive hyperplasia.

Cherubism cannot be diagnosed solely on the basis of the histological appearances, since parts of the lesions can be identical to central giant cell granuloma and the brown tumour of hyperparathyroidism. However, the characteristic clinical appearances and the familial incidence are usually sufficient to aid distinction. In cherubism the blood chemistry is normal.

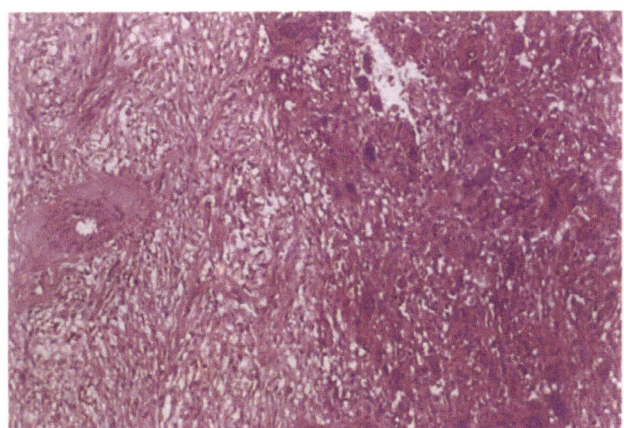

Figure 6.24 Cherubism. This field is much less cellular and contains a blood vessel which shows the characteristic perivascular cuff of collagen.   H & E × 100

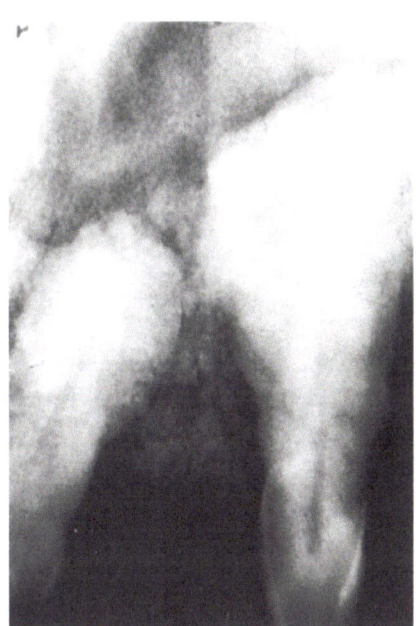

Figure 6.26 Paget's disease. Radiograph showing gross hypercementosis of the tooth roots.

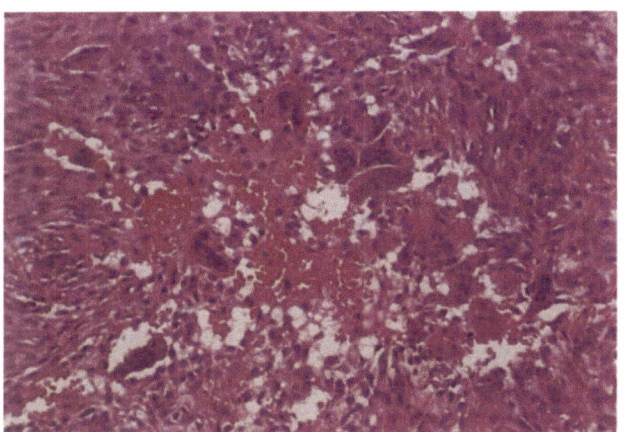

Figure 6.25 Cherubism. Higher magnification showing multinucleated giant cells close to stromal microcysts and areas of haemorrhage.   H & E × 200

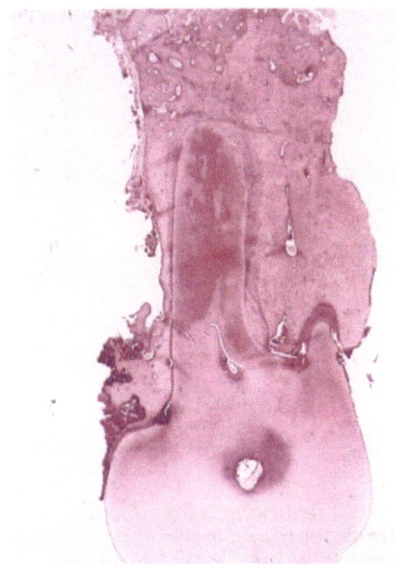

Figure 6.27 Paget's disease. This decalcified section of a molar tooth shows gross hypercementosis.   H & E × 3·5

Paget's Disease of Bone

The jaws are not commonly involved in Paget's disease, but as a number of other lesions in this site can resemble Paget's disease both radiographically and histologically it is often considered in differential diagnosis[10].

Jaw involvement is usually part of the polyostotic form of the disease and the maxilla is involved more frequently than the mandible. It is usual for the radiographic changes of Paget's disease to be generalized throughout an affected jaw and the commonest appearance is the presence of radiopaque areas due to replacement of normal trabecular bone by dense, granular bone. A less common presentation is focal areas of radiolucency. Radiographs of the teeth may show loss of lamina dura, generalized or localized hypercementosis (Figure 6.26), or resorption and replacement of roots by pagetoid bone.

The microscopic features of Paget's disease are the same in the jaws as in other bones, that is, irregular osteoclastic resorption and replacement of bone by cellular fibroblastic tissue in which there is a striking increase in vascularity (Figures 6.27 and 6.28). New bone is laid down by osteoblastic activity and the uncoordinated osteoblastic and osteoclastic activity leads to the characteristic

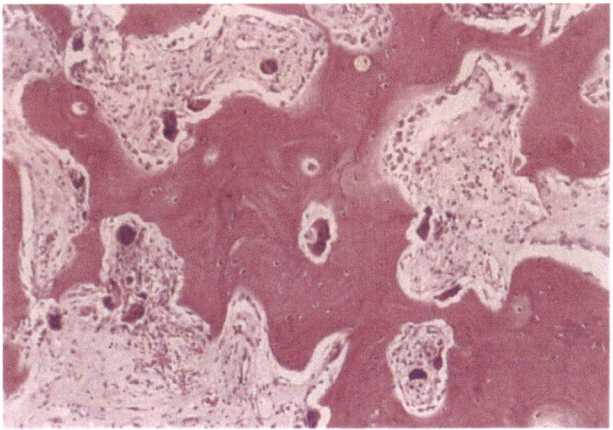

Figure 6.28 Paget's disease, showing irregular bone resorption and apposition. H & E × 100

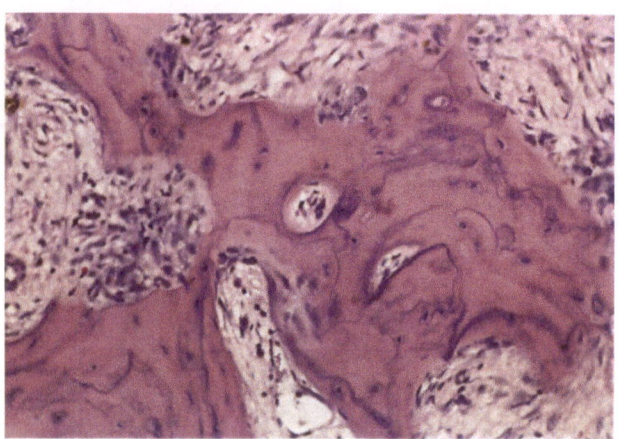

Figure 6.29 Paget's disease. Higher magnification showing the characteristic 'mosaic' pattern of reversal lines.   H & E × 200

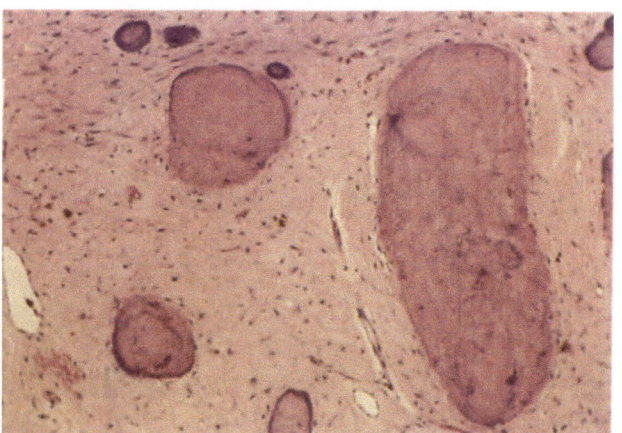

Figure 6.30 Paget's disease. Quiescent area consisting of acellular masses of bone of varying size and sparsely cellular fibrous tissue.   H & E × 100

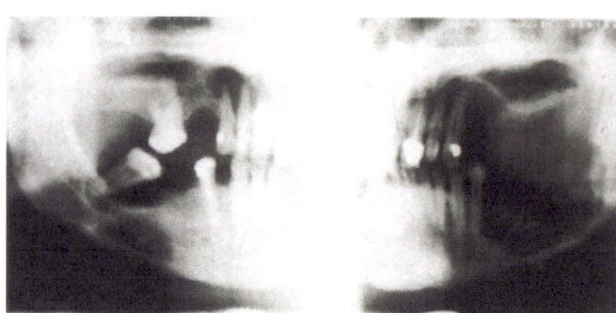

Figure 6.31 Eosinophilic granuloma. The radiograph shows a large area of bone destruction in the left mandible and less severe destruction around the right lower molar and the right upper lateral incisor and canine teeth.

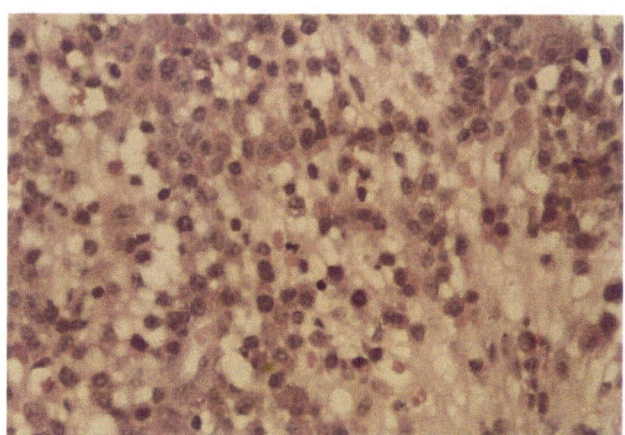

Figure 6.32 Eosinophilic granuloma. There are sheets of large histiocytes in which several mitoses can be seen.   H & E × 250

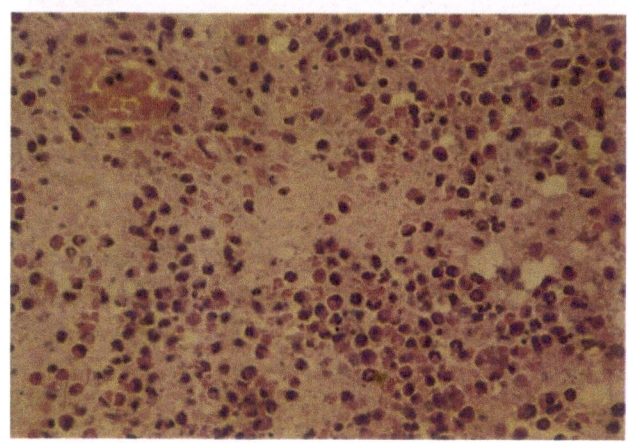

Figure 6.33 Eosinophilic granuloma, showing a dense aggregation of eosinophils.   H & E × 250

mosaic pattern of resting and reversal lines (Figure 6.29). A similar pattern of prominent cement lines can be seen in chronic sclerosing osteomyelitis and benign cementoblastoma. Gigantiform cementoma can resemble Paget's disease radiographically but the blood chemistry is normal. In quiescent lesions the new bone may form acellular spheroidal masses (Figure 6.30).

Miscellaneous Lesions of Bone

Eosinophilic Granuloma of Bone

This non-neoplastic, lytic bone lesion, which is thought to arise from cells of the mononuclear phagocyte system and eosinophils, may be solitary or multifocal. About a quarter of patients with the multifocal form have the classical triad of multiple osteolytic lesions, especially in the skull, diabetes insipidus and exophthalmos (Hand–Schüller–Christian disease)[11,12].

The lesions are commonly seen in the calvarium and facial bones and cause swelling and pain. Although pathological fracture is not uncommon in long bones it is rare in the jaws. The cortex may be perforated with consequent extension of the lesion into the soft tissues. Swelling and gingival ulceration are especially characteristic and loose, painful teeth or failure of healing of an extraction socket may be the primary presentation.

The radiographic features of jaw lesions are those of frank destruction with no new bone formation within the lesion or at its periphery (Figure 6.31). The margins are well defined and involved teeth appear to 'float' in soft tissue.

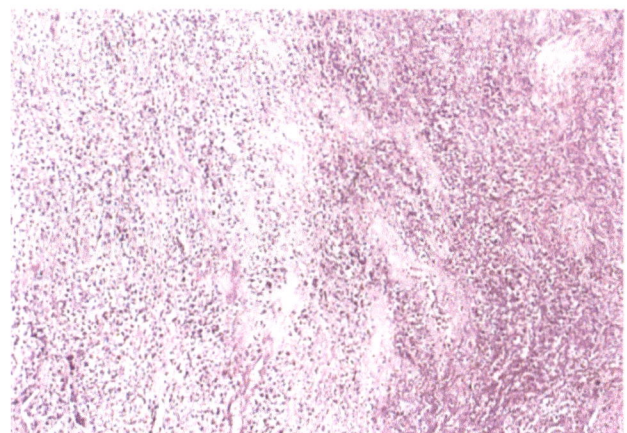

Figure 6.34 Stewart type of midline granuloma. There are sheets of pale-staining cells and extensive areas of necrosis.   H & E × 40

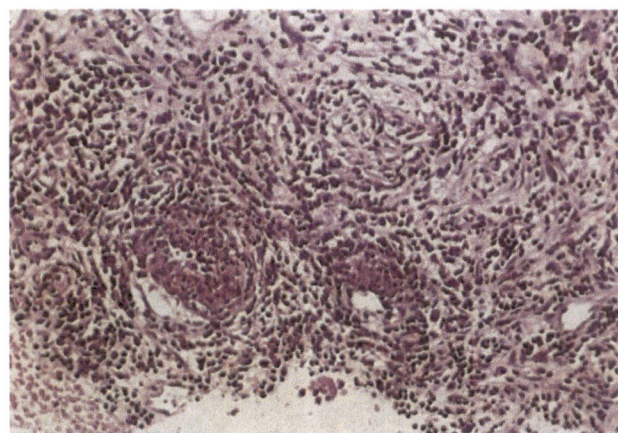

Figure 6.36   Wegener's granulomatosis. Severe vasculitis in tissue removed from an inflamed maxillary antrum.   H & E × 100

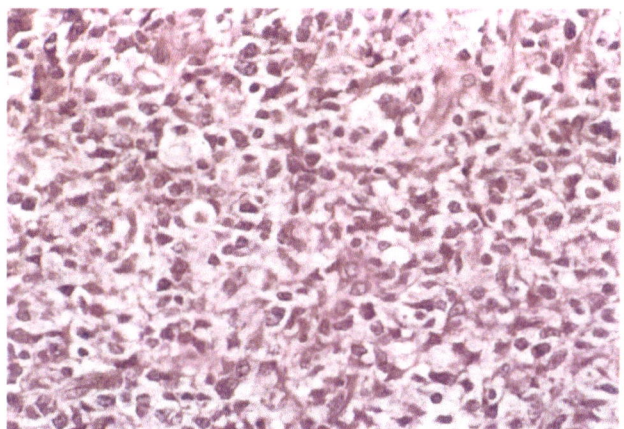

Figure 6.35   Stewart type of midline granuloma. Higher magnification showing large atypical cells with pale cytoplasm.   H & E × 200

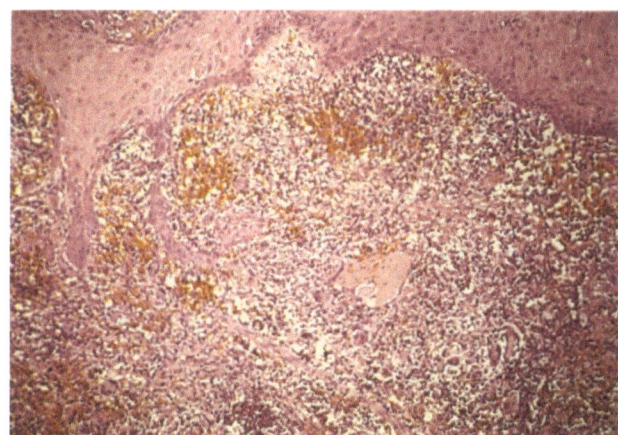

Figure 6.37   Wegener's granulomatosis. In this gingival biopsy there is epithelial proliferation, dense inflammatory infiltration and areas of haemorrhage.   H & E × 40

Microscopy shows that lesions consist mainly of moderately large histiocytes with oval, vesicular nuclei in which mitoses are sometimes seen (Figure 6.32). Multinucleated giant cells may be present and there is an infiltrate of eosinophils, neutrophils and chronic inflammatory cells (Figure 6.33). The eosinophils may be scanty or numerous and in some cases form eosinophil microabscesses. Foci of haemorrhage and necrosis may be present.

Non-healing Midline Granuloma

Although the exact nature and definition of this rare clinical syndrome are controversial, two forms are generally recognized: the Stewart type and Wegener's granulomatosis.

The Stewart type is characterized clinically by slow but progressive destruction of the midline facial structures. In many cases the initial microscopic diagnosis is nonspecific granulation tissue. However, it is becoming increasingly recognized that many, if not most, of these lesions are atypical forms of lymphoma[13]. The main diagnostic features are the presence of widespread necrosis and atypical cells which are large, pleomorphic and may be undergoing mitosis (Figures 6.34 and 6.35). These atypical cells, which are possibly histiocytic, may be masked by the heavy inflammatory infiltrate.

In Wegener's granulomatosis there is much less destruction of the facial tissues, but pulmonary and renal lesions develop, and it is these which largely determine the prognosis.

The typical histological feature of Wegener's granulomatosis is said to be giant cell granulomas in which there is variable necrosis. However, giant cells may be scarce in oral lesions and non-specific chronic inflammation and vasculitis in small arteries and veins may be a more frequent finding (Figure 6.36).

A rare but possibly pathognomonic type of gingivitis can be an early indication of Wegener's granulomatosis[14,15]. There is localized or generalized gingival enlargement in either jaw and the gingival surface is granular, purplish red and mottled. Microscopy of the gingiva shows heavy, mixed inflammatory infiltration of the corium and frequently extensive hyperplasia of the overlying epithelium (Figure 6.37). There may be dense focal aggregates of neutrophils and eosinophils forming microabscesses, and areas of recent and old haemorrhage are common. Multinucleated giant cells, which are a particularly characteristic feature, may be scanty and it may be necessary to examine many sections to detect their presence (Figure 6.38). The vasculitis so typical of Wegener's granulomatosis in other sites is not usually seen in gingival lesions.

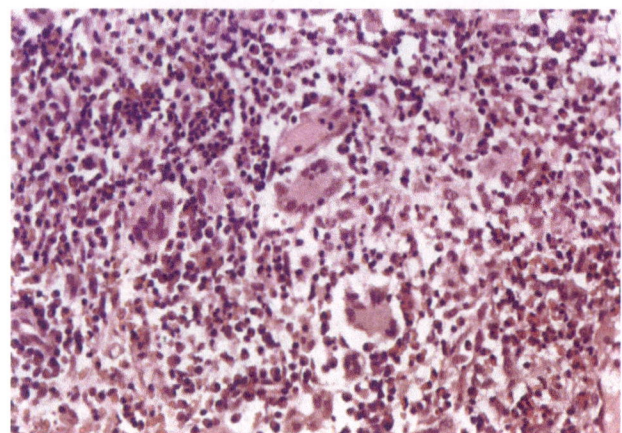

Figure 6.38 Wegener's granulomatosis. Higher magnification showing groups of multinucleated giant cells and acute and chronic inflammatory cells.   H & E × 200

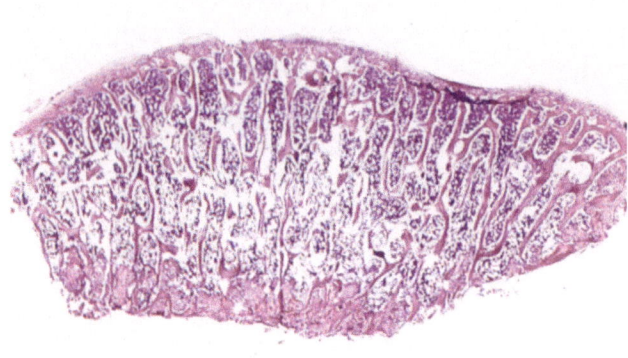

Figure 6.40 Osteoarthrosis. Condylectomy specimen showing irregular erosion of the superficial cartilage.   H & E × 9

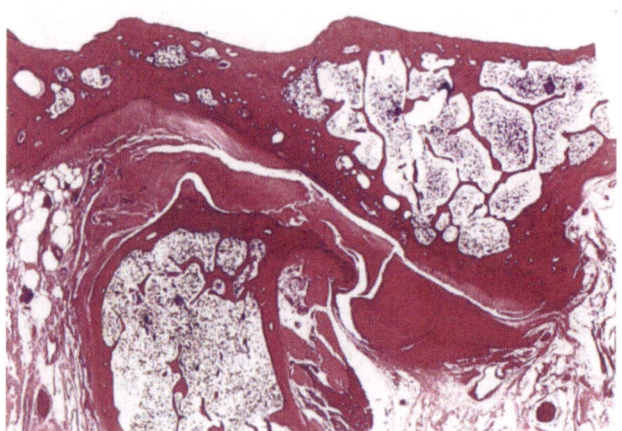

Figure 6.39 Osteoarthrosis. *In situ* specimen showing advanced osteoarthrosis. There is osteophytic lipping and flattening of the articular surface.   H & E × 4 ..

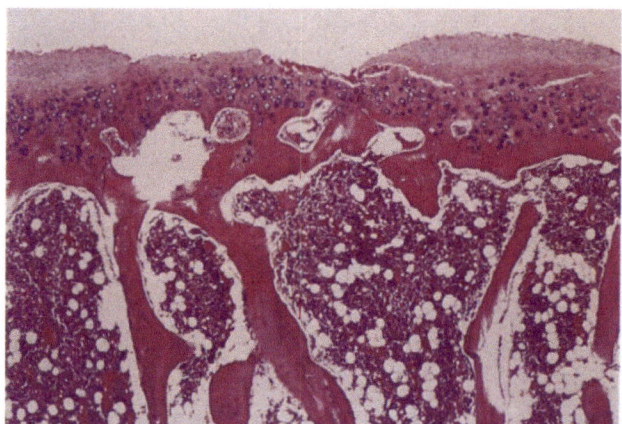

Figure 6.41 Osteoarthrosis. Higher magnification showing erosion of cartilage and horizontal fissures.   H & E × 40

The Temporomandibular Joint

Organic disease in the temporomandibular joint is not common, symptoms referred to the joint usually being associated with the temporomandibular pain-dysfunction syndrome. The syndrome is characterized by pain, clicking or a grating sensation in the joint and trismus. Sometimes the condition is treated by shaving off the articular surface of the condyle or even removing the entire condyle. The surgical specimens from this type of procedure may show no histological abnormalities or mild degenerative changes only.

Osteoarthrosis

Although degenerative changes in the temporomandibular joint have been detected in as many as 40% of patients over the age of 45, most cases are asymptomatic. Patients may complain of clicking in the joint, mild limitation of movement and pain.

There is flattening of the condyle and enlargement with osteophytic lipping (Figure 6.39). The articular surface is irregular and there may be perforation of the disc. The earliest histological change is an alteration in the arrangement of the cells of the fibrous covering of the articular surface, with cells becoming clumped together. There are erosions in the surface of the articular cartilage which extend as vertical cracks into the subchondral bone. Horizontal fissures may develop between the cartilage and the underlying bone (Figures 6.40 and 6.41). Cartilage cells show degenerative changes and in focal areas there may be complete destruction of cartilage. There are reparative reactions in the bone leading to eburnation and osteophytic lipping. Changes in the meniscus include cracks and fissures, dystrophic calcification and hyalinization. In advanced cases there may be complete destruction of the disc.

Rheumatoid Arthritis

Between 50 and 60% of patients with rheumatoid arthritis have involvement of the temporomandibular joint, although it is rarely severe enough to cause pain or limitation in mouth opening. In juvenile rheumatoid arthritis, however, damage to the condylar growth centre can lead to micrognathia and severe malocclusion.

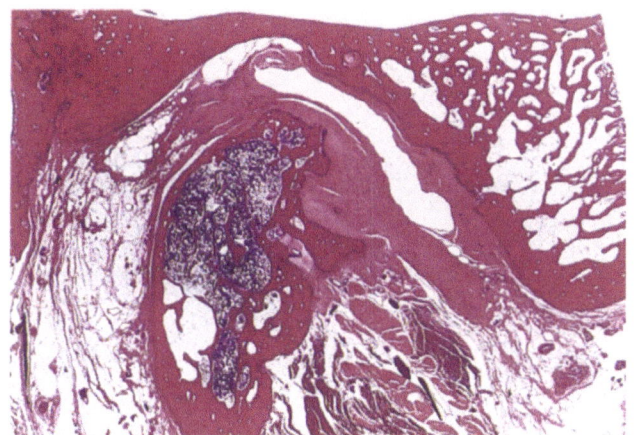

Figure 6.42 Rheumatoid arthritis. *In situ* specimen of a late lesion, showing adhesions between the articular surface and the disc, and partial ankylosis. H & E × 4

The histological features are similar to those seen in other joints. There is heavy chronic inflammatory infiltration and thickening of the synovium, and formation of vascular pannus which may erode the articular surface and underlying bone. Adhesions may form between the articular surface and the disc (Figure 6.42). In advanced lesions the disc may be eroded and destroyed and there may be fibrous ankylosis.

Infective Arthritis

Infective arthritis of the temporomandibular joint is rare but can be caused by a wide variety of organisms, including streptococci, staphylococci, gonococci and tubercle bacilli. Infection may be haematogenous, from a distant focus, or it may be due to direct spread from an adjacent infective focus. Healing frequently results in fibrous ankylosis and in severe cases there may be bony ankylosis. The histological features are the same as in other joints.

References

1. Shafer, W. G., Hine, M. K. and Levy, B. M. (1983). *A Textbook of Oral Pathology*, 4th Edn. (Philadelphia, London, Toronto, Mexico City, Rio de Janeiro, Sydney, Tokyo: W. B. Saunders Company)

2. McMillan, M. D., Kardos, T. B., Edwards, J. L., Thorburn, D. N., Adams, D. B. and Palmer, D. K. (1981). Giant cell hyalin angiopathy or pulse granuloma. *Oral Surg.*, **52**, 178

3. Mincer, H. H., McCoy, J. M. and Turner, J. E. (1979). Pulse granuloma of the alveolar ridge. *Oral Surg.*, **48**, 126

4. Eversole, L. R., Sabes, W. R. and Rovin, S. (1972). Fibrous dysplasia: a nosologic problem in the diagnosis of fibro-osseous lesions of the jaws. *J. Oral Pathol.*, **1**, 189

5. Lucas, R. B. (1984). *Pathology of Tumours of the Oral Tissues*. 4th Edn. (Edinburgh, London, Melbourne, New York: Churchill Livingstone)

6. Langdon, J. D., Rapidis, A. D. and Patel, M. F. (1976). Ossifying fibroma – one disease or six? An analysis of 39 fibro-osseous lesions of the jaws. *Brit. J. Oral Surg.*, **14**, 1

7. Walter, J. M., Terry, B. C., Small, E. W., Matteson, S. R. and Howell, R. M. (1979). Aggressive ossifying fibroma of the maxilla: a review of the literature and report of case. *J. Oral Surg.*, **37**, 276

8. Wayman, J. B. (1978). Cherubism: a report of three cases. *Brit. J. Oral Surg.*, **16**, 47

9. Hamner, J. E. (1969). The demonstration of perivascular collagen deposition in cherubism. *Oral Surg.*, **27**, 129

10. Smith, B. J. and Eveson, J. W. (1981). Paget's disease of bone with particular reference to dentistry. *J. Oral Pathol.*, **10**, 233

11. Hartman, K. S. (1980). Histiocytosis X: a review of 154 cases with oral involvement. *Oral Surg.*, **49**, 38

12. Lieberman, P. H., Jones, C. R., Dargeon, H. W. K. and Begg, D. F. (1969). A reappraisal of eosinophilic granuloma of bone, Hand–Schüller–Christian syndrome and Letterer–Siwe syndrome. *Medicine*, **48**, 375

13. Leading Article (1977). Non-healing (mid-line) granuloma. *Lancet*, **1**, 1296

14. Israelson, H., Binnie, W. H. and Hurt, W. C. (1981). The hyperplastic gingivitis of Wegener's granulomatosis. *J. Periodontol.*, **52**, 81

15. Eveson, J. W. and Slaney, A. E. (1982). Non-healing midline granuloma. *Brit. J. Oral Surg.*, **20**, 102

The Salivary Glands
1. Non-neoplastic Conditions

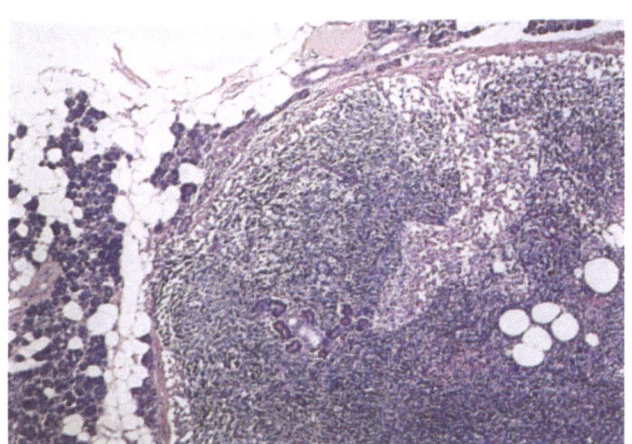

7

Figure 7.1 Intraparotid lymph node. Salivary ducts are seen in the lymphoid tissue. H & E × 45

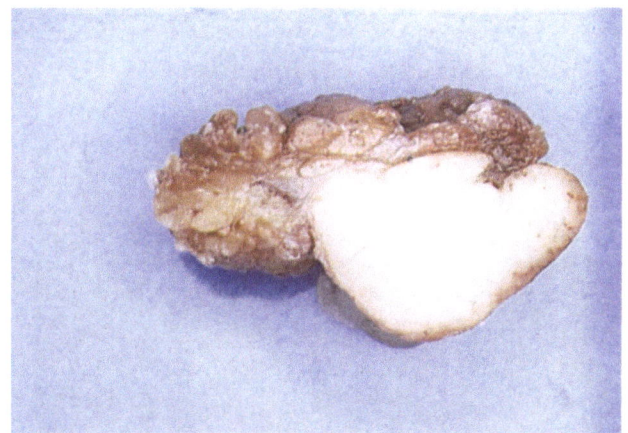

Figure 7.2 Intraparotid lymph node. This hyperplastic node measured 2 × 1·25 cm

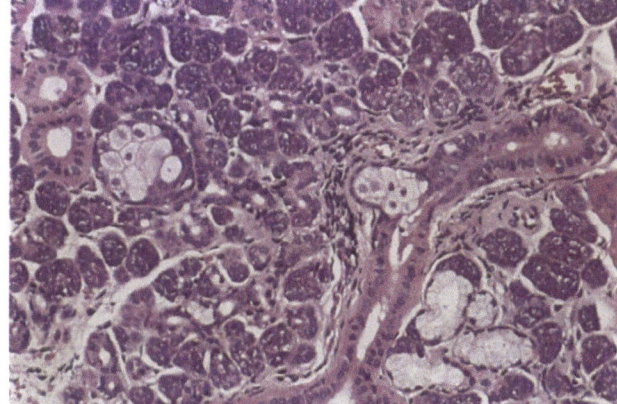

Figure 7.3 Sebaceous glands in the parotid. H & E × 250

DISTRIBUTION AND STRUCTURE

In addition to the three paired major salivary glands, numerous minor glands are distributed throughout the oral tissues. They are plentiful in the posterior part of the hard palate, the soft palate, the lip and the cheek, but are absent from the anterior part of the hard palate and the gingivae[1]. The glands, both major and minor, consist of serous and mucous cells in various combinations, forming acini and arranged in lobules with a duct system.

As well as the usual structure of salivary tissue there are some variable features of interest and importance to the pathologist. Lymph nodes are frequently seen in the substance of the parotid, where they have been included during the development of the gland. Intraglandular nodes are less common in the submandibular and sublingual glands. These nodes may themselves contain salivary tissue (Figure 7.1). Very occasionally an intraglandular node may, as a result of reactive hyperplasia, become large enough to simulate a tumour macroscopically (Figure 7.2).

Sebaceous glands, which develop from the ducts, are frequently present in the parotid, although they are often scanty and may be detected only if looked for in multiple sections (Figure 7.3). They may also be found in the submandibular gland, but are less common there.

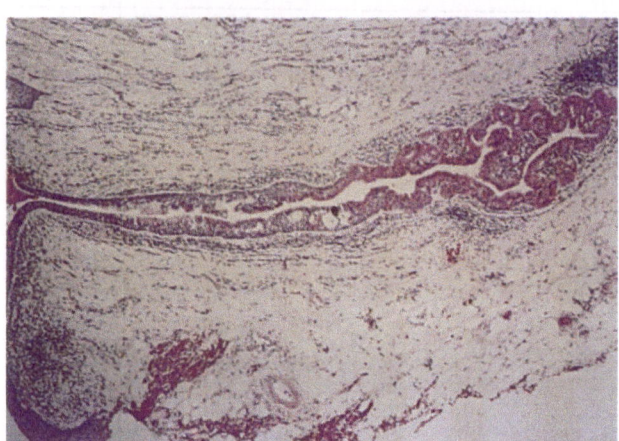

Figure 7.4 Oncocytes in salivary duct. Most of the cells lining this duct of a palatal salivary gland have undergone oncocytic metaplasia. The surface of the palate is on the left, with the duct opening on to it. H & E × 40

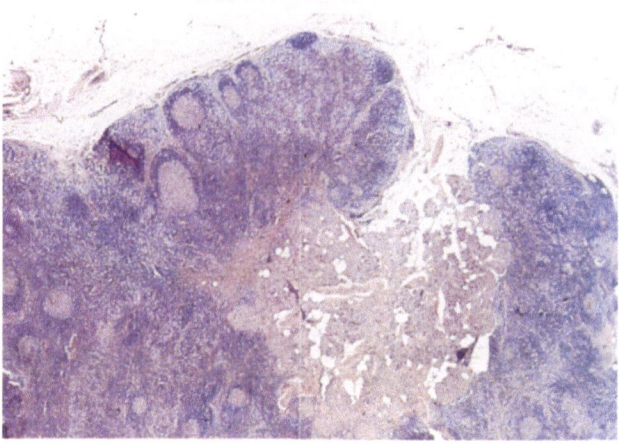

Figure 7.6 Cervical lymph node with included salivary tissue. H & E × 10

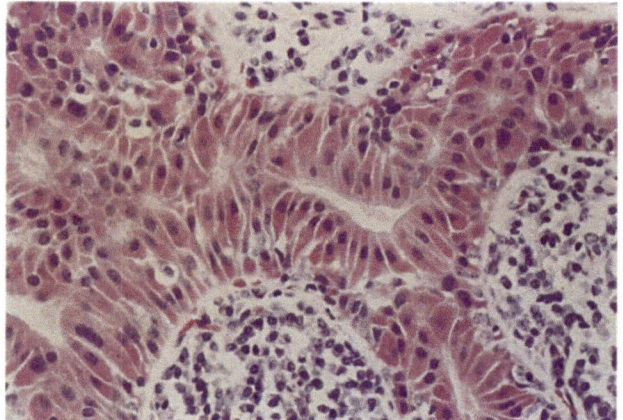

Figure 7.5 A duct adjacent to that shown in Figure 7.4. The lining cells are enlarged, with markedly eosinophilic granular cytoplasm. H & E × 250

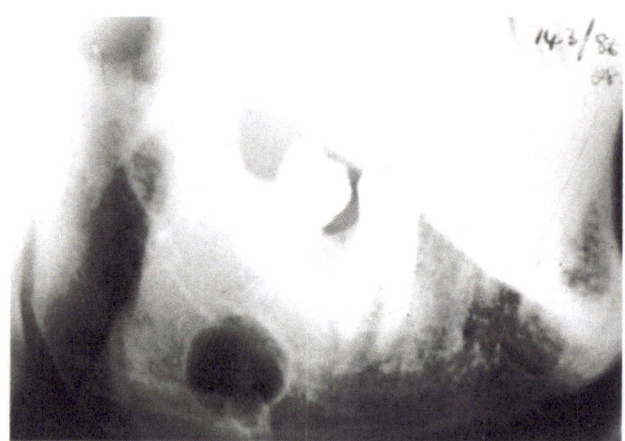

Figure 7.7 Developmental defect in the mandible. A cyst-like radiolucency is seen near the angle of the mandible.

Oncocytic metaplasia is often seen in the salivary glands, especially in the minor glands of the palate. This type of metaplasia occurs in a number of epithelial tissues and is an age-related change, being only occasionally detectable in persons under 50 but present in increasing degree thereafter. Most people over the age of 70 will have oncocytes in various tissues. In the salivary glands the cells of the ducts are most often affected, the acinar cells rather less frequently. The affected cells become enlarged and the cytoplasm is filled with fine eosinophilic granules. The nucleus often remains unchanged, but it may stain more intensely, or become pyknotic (Figures 7.4 and 7.5).

Ectopic salivary tissue has been encountered in a variety of situations, from the hypophysis to the sternoclavicular joint[2]. It is a rare finding in any site, but those from which it has been most frequently reported are the cervical lymph nodes and the mandible (Figure 7.6). In the latter situation salivary tissue may not always, or even often, really be ectopic tissue. It may be an extension of the submandibular gland occupying a depression or cavity in the mandible. Cavities of this type may be developmental anomalies, and they may appear radiographically as cysts in the bone (Figure 7.7).

NON-INFLAMMATORY CONDITIONS

Hyperplasia of Palatal Glands

The palatal glands may very occasionally undergo hyperplasia to such an extent that a palpable palatal swelling results. This is likely to be diagnosed clinically as a pleomorphic adenoma. Microscopic examination, however, shows apparently normal palatal glands present in excessive amount[3].

Oncocytosis

When oncocytes are seen in the salivary glands they are usually present as small scattered groups of cells but, uncommonly, the metaplastic process may spread to involve large areas or even practically the entire gland (Figure 7.8). Apart from the change in the cells the general structure of the gland in oncocytosis remains unaltered. Oncocytic change can also occur in neoplasms and small areas are not rare in pleomorphic adenomas and sometimes in other tumours, but again, as in oncocytosis of the otherwise normal gland, very occasionally large areas of a tumour may be affected.

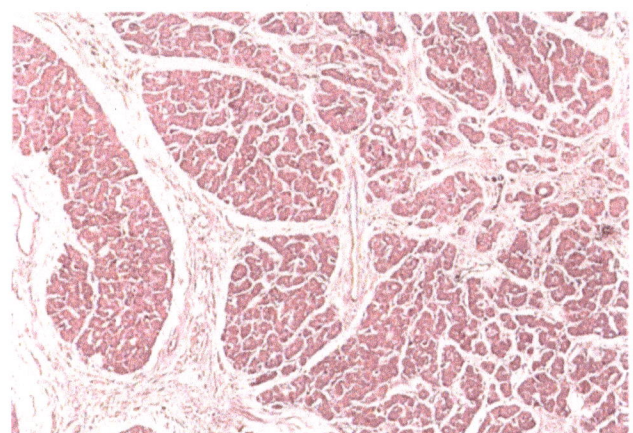

Figure 7.8 Oncocytosis. Practically all the cells of this parotid gland showed oncocytic change, but the general structure of the gland remains unchanged. H & E × 100

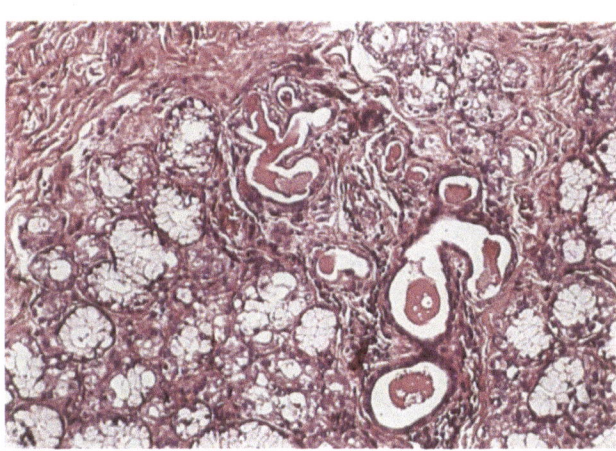

Figure 7.10 Cystic fibrosis. This biopsy of labial salivary glands shows dilatation of the ducts with eosinophilic plugs in the lumens. Some acini are atrophic, in others the cells are swollen. H & E × 300

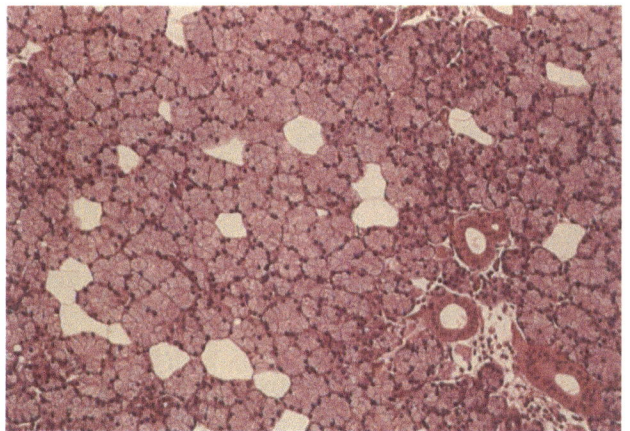

Figure 7.9 Sialosis. The cells of the parotid acini are enlarged and are becoming degranulated. There is also fatty infiltration, but no evidence of inflammation. H & E × 250

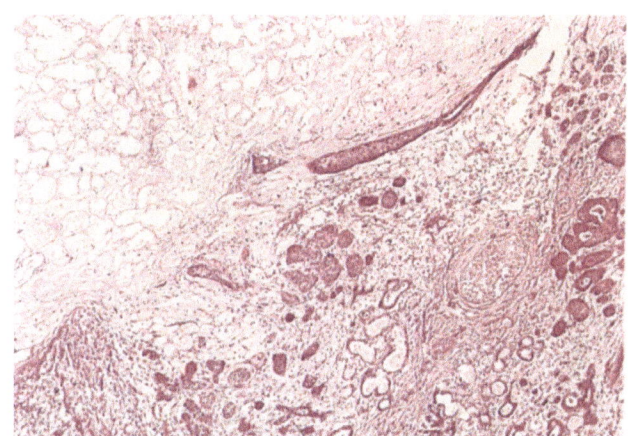

Figure 7.11 Necrotizing sialometaplasia. A palatal lesion, showing the necrotic acini (upper left) and squamous metaplasia in the ducts. There is also chronic inflammatory infiltration. H & E × 100

Sialosis

This recurrent painless bilateral enlargement of the parotid glands, and less commonly the submandibular glands, is seen as an occasional concominant feature in a number of conditions, including chronic alcoholism, hepatic cirrhosis, diabetes mellitus, thyroid insufficiency and other endocrine abnormalities, nutritional deficiencies and following the administration of some drugs, notably phenylbutazone and iodides[4]. There is diminished salivary secretion, but the potassium content of the saliva is increased. The acinar cells are enlarged, their granules disappear, and there is oedema of the interstitial tissues with atrophy of the striated ducts. Fatty infiltration takes place at the same time and progressively replaces the secretory tissue. These two elements, cell change and fatty replacement, vary in their relative proportions from case to case.

A noteworthy feature in the histological diagnosis of sialosis is the absence of any inflammatory features (Figure 7.9).

Cystic Fibrosis

The submandibular, sublingual and the minor salivary glands may be affected in cystic fibrosis but the parotid is rarely, if ever, involved. In the minor glands, dilatation of the ducts is the most prominent feature, with eosinophilic plugs in the duct lumens together with acinar atrophy (Figure 7.10). However, these changes are inconstant and the minor glands may appear normal. Lip biopsy, which has been used in the diagnosis of cystic fibrosis, is thus not always helpful[5].

Necrotizing Sialometaplasia

This condition is seen most commonly in the palate but it may also occur in other parts of the oral mucosa and in other mucosae[6].

In the palate the lesion appears as a single or as bilateral ulcers, or sometimes as a non-ulcerated swelling. It is a painful lesion with a short history, since it is self-limiting and heals spontaneously within a few weeks. However, during the active stage the appearances may suggest a neoplasm and it is likely to be biopsied with this as the provisional diagnosis.

Microscopically, the characteristic features are squamous metaplasia of the excretory ducts of the salivary glands together with hyperplasia of the surface epithelium, and necrosis of the glandular acini. The squamous metaplasia may simulate invasion by well differentiated squamous cell carcinoma or mucoepidermoid tumour, but there is no cellular atypia or mitotic activity. The acinar necrosis may again suggest mucoepidermoid tumour (Figure 7.11). Inflammatory infiltration is practically always present, but it would not seem to be the primary cause of the condition, which still remains unknown.

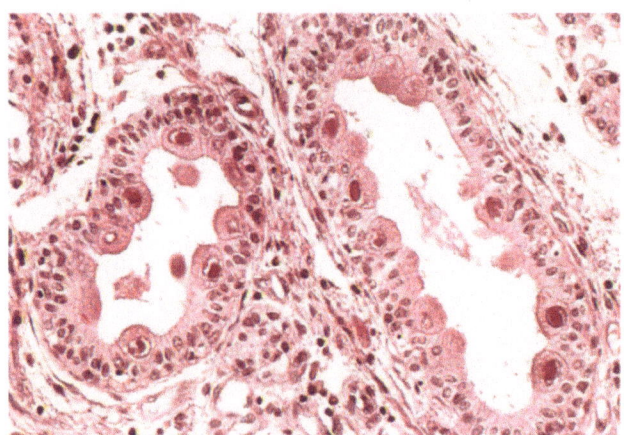

Figure 7.12 Cytomegalovirus in the parotid. The prominent double contoured inclusion bodies are seen in the enlarged duct lining cells. H & E × 250

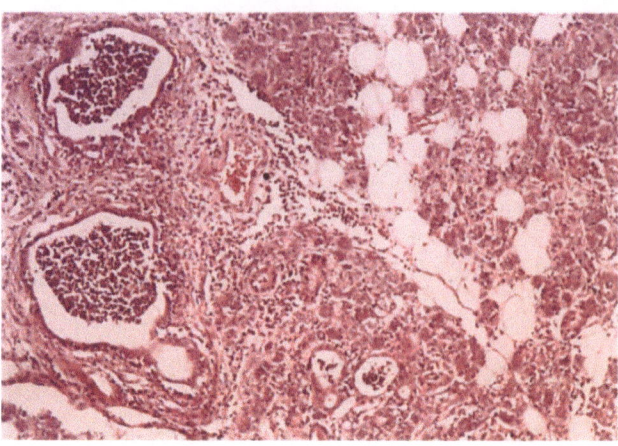

Figure 7.14 Acute parotitis. The parotid ducts are dilated and filled with neutrophils. The acute inflammatory infiltration is beginning to extend into the periductal tissues, but at this comparatively early stage there is as yet little tissue destruction. H & E × 100

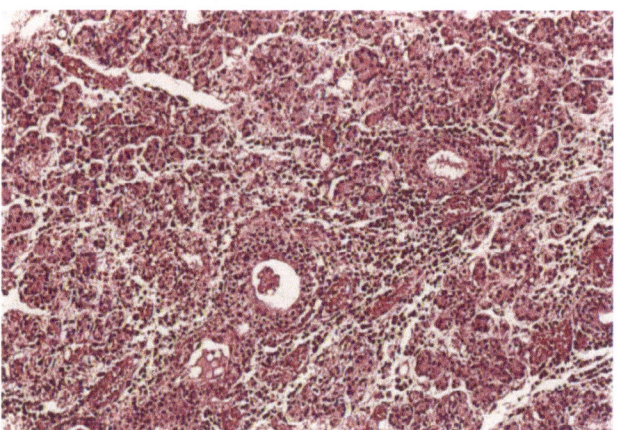

Figure 7.13 Mumps. The acinar and ductal cells are swollen and many are vacuolated. There is lymphocytic and plasma cell infiltration, mainly around the ducts but beginning to spread into the oedematous interacinar connective tissue. H & E × 100

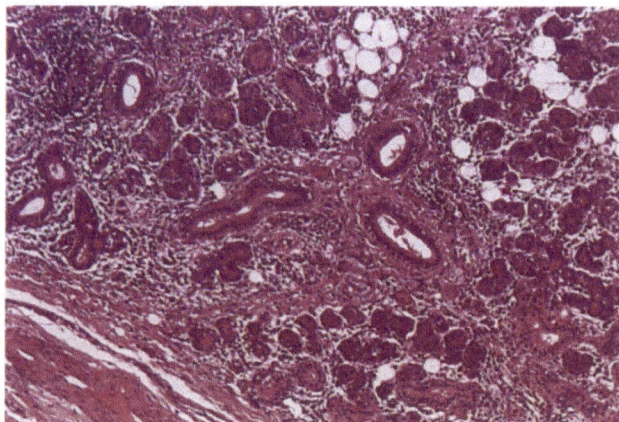

Figure 7.15 Chronic sialadenitis. The submandibular gland shows chronic inflammatory infiltration, patchy fibrosis and atrophy of the secretory tissue. H & E × 100

INFLAMMATORY CONDITIONS

Most of the acute inflammatory lesions of the salivary glands are diagnosed clinically and biopsy is seldom called for. However, it may be undertaken in unusual or atypical cases or when tissue becomes readily available as, for example, when an abscess is incised.

Virus Infections

Cytomegalovirus infection in infants results from transplacental transmission of the virus. It causes premature birth, failure to thrive and haematological and other disorders. Evidence of infection is seen in a proportion of stillborn infants, variously estimated up to 30%. In adults infection may be seen in patients with terminal neoplastic or other diseases, and in other patients who have had immunosuppressive treatment. Recently, another group of adults has been found to have a very high prevalence of cytomegalovirus infection[7]. These are mainly homosexual men, and they may suffer from the acquired immune deficiency syndrome, in which there is infection by a wide variety of agents[8].

In the salivary glands, there are double contoured intranuclear and intracytoplasmic inclusion bodies in enlarged epithelial cells in the intralobular ducts (Figure 7.12).

In *mumps*, there is swelling and vacuolation of the parotid acinar cells and the lining cells of the ducts. There is oedema of the interstitial connective tissue, which is also densely infiltrated by mononuclear cells, mainly lymphocytes. Foci of fibrinoid necrosis are seen (Figure 7.13).

Sialadenitis may also be caused by a number of other viruses, usually associated with upper respiratory infections.

Bacterial Infections

Acute sialadenitis is seen most frequently in the parotid and is often the result of reduction of salivary flow, which has permitted ascending infection. The xerostomia itself may have a variety of causes, including dehydration, postoperative or in prolonged fevers, or the administration of some drugs. The usual histological picture of acute inflammation is seen – if for any reason it has been necessary to perform a biopsy. In the earlier stages the ducts contain numerous neutrophils and there is also heavy infiltration of the periductal tissues. If unarrested, the inflammation spreads to involve the acini, with abscess formation (Figure 7.14). Parotid abscess may be simulated clinically by thrombosis and infarction in an adenolymphoma, so that a biopsy may present an unexpected picture (page 90).

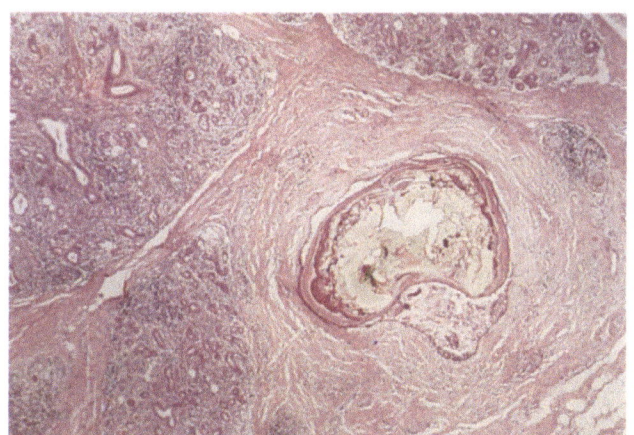

Figure 7.16 Chronic sialadenitis. A calculus is present in a dilated duct. There is surrounding fibrosis and chronic inflammatory infiltration in the adjacent acinar tissue. H & E × 40

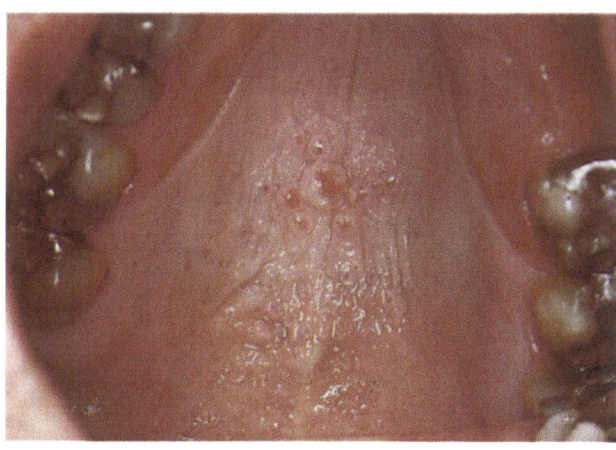

Figure 7.18 Nicotinic stomatitis. The red-centred papules on the palatal epithelium are the openings of the palatal glands

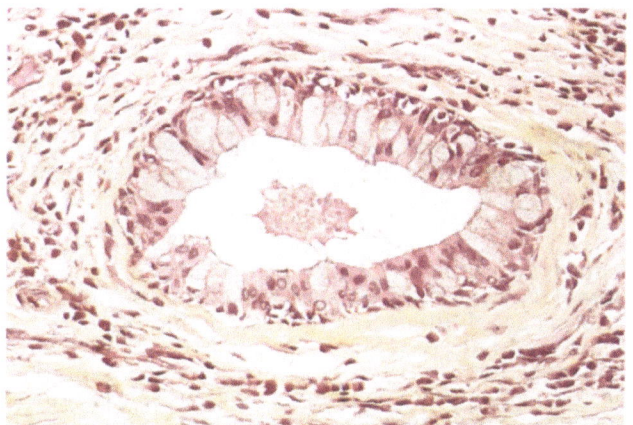

Figure 7.17 Chronic sialadenitis. The ducts in chronic sialadenitis frequently show metaplastic changes, usually squamous. Here, mucous cells have appeared. Phloxine tartrazine × 100

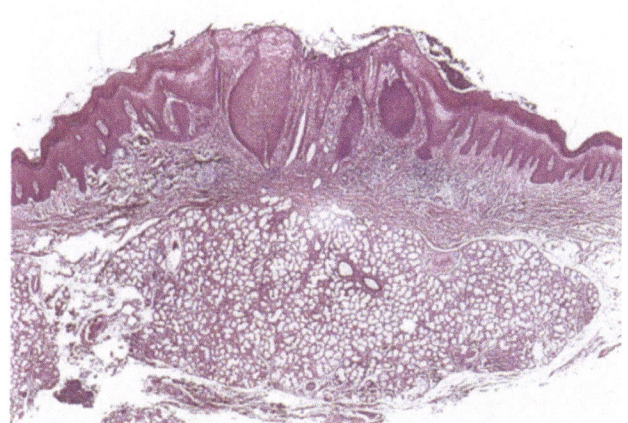

Figure 7.19 Nicotinic stomatitis. A palatal salivary gland can be seen with its excretory duct lined by metaplastic squamous epithelium. The surrounding palatal epithelium shows acanthosis and hyperkeratosis, and there is subjacent chronic inflammatory infiltration. H & E × 25

Chronic sialadenitis is very much commoner than the acute condition and is most frequent in the submandibular gland. It is often the result of duct obstruction, with impaired salivary flow. The histological picture is typical of a chronic inflammatory condition with mononuclear infiltration, mainly lymphocytic, atrophy of the parenchyma and fibrosis (Figure 7.15). Calculus formation is frequently associated with chronic sialadenitis and calculus may be seen in the dilated ducts, the epithelium of which often undergoes squamous metaplasia. Less often, mucus-secreting cells may appear, or ciliated columnar epithelium (Figures 7.16 and 7.17). If the lymphoid infiltration is pronounced, as it may be in the more severe or long-standing cases, lymphoepithelial lesion comes into the differential diagnosis (page 84).

Chronic inflammatory infiltration of minor glands is often seen when adjacent groups of these glands are included in biopsies of mucosal ulcers or other local lesions, or where there has been duct obstruction. Calculus formation in minor gland ducts is rather uncommon, and the related glandular tissue is chronically inflamed[9]. Trauma to a minor gland duct sufficient to allow secretion to escape into the surrounding tissues leads to the formation of an extravasation mucocele, with chronic inflammatory infiltration of adjacent gland lobules (page 85). Chronic inflammatory infiltration is practically always present in the labial glands in Sjögren's syndrome, and also in some other autoimmune conditions. In *cheilitis glandularis* the labial glands show chronic inflammatory infiltration, fibrosis, and dilatation of the ducts. The lip is everted and enlarged, and mucopurulent secretion can be expressed from the dilated duct openings. Here again, the inflammation may not be the primary lesion, which has been attributed to actinic damage and other causes. An important feature is dysplasia of the labial epithelium, which has been noted in most reported cases. The incidence of squamous cell carcinoma arising in *cheilitis glandularis* has been reported in up to 35% of cases.

Nicotinic stomatitis is a distinctive type of sialadenitis and epithelial hyperplasia that affects the minor glands of the palate in pipe and cigar smokers. It is also seen in those countries where reversed smoking, with the lighted end of the cigarette or cigar held in the mouth, is practised. Clinically, there is a characteristic picture, with the orifices of the palatal glands standing out as small papules with red centres against the intervening pale palatal mucosa (Figure 7.18). Microscopically, there is squamous metaplasia of the excretory duct epithelium and keratosis of the palatal epithelium which also affects the mouths of the ducts and may plug them with keratin. There is chronic inflammatory infiltration of the associated glands (Figure 7.19).

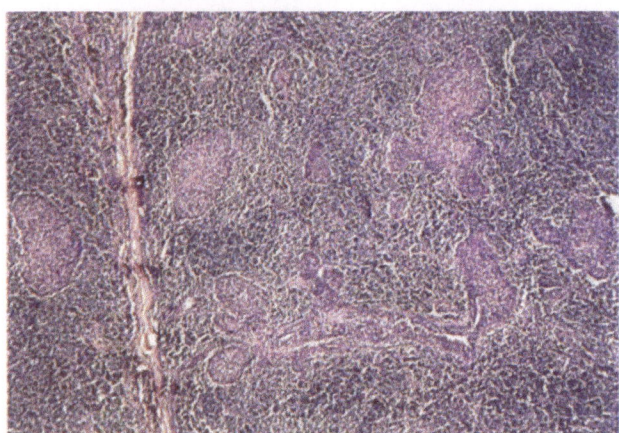

Figure 7.20 Lymphoepithelial lesion. The parotid secretory tissue has been replaced by a diffuse lymphocytic infiltration. Epimyoepithelial islands are present throughout the lymphoid background. The interlobular septa are not overrun by the cellular infiltration.   H & E × 100

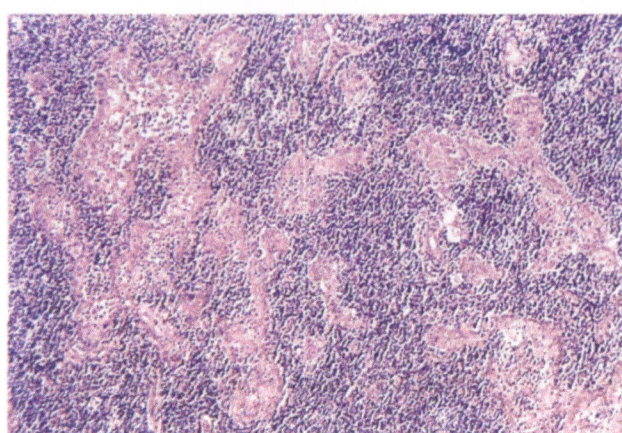

Figure 7.22 Carcinoma in lymphoepithelial lesion. Numerous epithelial islets are distributed throughout a lymphoid background.   H & E × 100

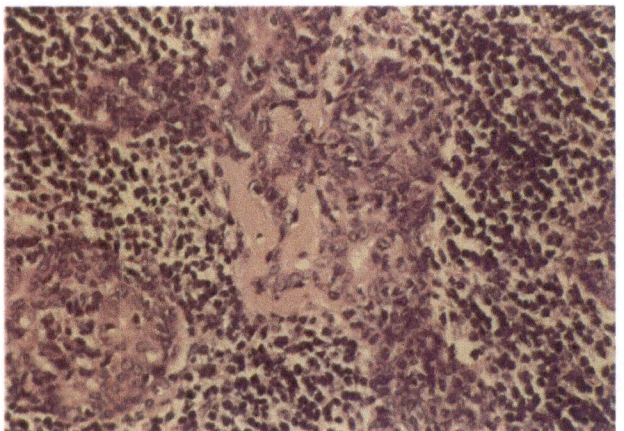

Figure 7.21 Lymphoepithelial lesion. An epimyoepithelial island, consisting of an irregularly shaped mass of epithelial cells with intermingled hyaline material. H & E × 250

The specific chronic inflammations are rare in the salivary glands. *Tuberculosis*, when it occurs, does so practically always in the parotid. The granulomas that are sometimes present in infected or infarcted adenolymphomas should not be mistaken for tubercles.

Sarcoidosis affects the parotids and less often the submandibular glands in a small number of patients. The uveal tract and lacrimal gland may also be affected (Heerfordt's syndrome). If there are symptoms from lesions in other organs such as lung, skin or lymph nodes, it is not likely that histological examination of the salivary glands will be required. However, should this eventuate, sarcoid lesions will be found in the salivary tissue and, again, they should not be confused with granulomas due to other causes.

Other specific chronic infections are very rarely seen in the salivary glands. They include actinomycosis, syphilis and deep mycoses.

AUTOIMMUNE DISEASE

Sjögren's Syndrome and Lymphoepithelial Lesion

Patients with *Sjögren's syndrome* have the triad of xerostomia, keratoconjunctivitis sicca and a connective tissue disorder, usually rheumatoid arthritis. In some patients

only the ocular and oral changes are present; this is the *sicca syndrome*. In either group there may be painless enlargement of salivary glands, usually both parotids. Less often, the submandibular glands may be affected, alone or together with the parotid glands. The lacrimal glands may also be involved. The glandular enlargement is termed *lymphoepithelial lesion* and it may be present in the absence of either Sjögren's syndrome or the sicca syndrome. There are thus a variety of combinations of symptoms, and while it is clear that Sjögren's syndrome and the sicca syndrome, with or without salivary gland enlargement, are variants of the same basic disorder, it is not yet clear whether the lymphoepithelial lesion alone may not represent a separate entity, although the histopathology of the salivary lesions is identical, whether they occur alone or as part of the syndrome. The immunological disorder in Sjögren's syndrome is evidenced by the presence of multiple organ specific and non-organ specific autoantibodies, including salivary duct antibody and rheumatoid factors[10].

Microscopically, the salivary glands show two characteristic components; lymphocytic infiltration and epimyoepithelial islands. The lymphocytes diffusely infiltrate the gland, replacing the normal architecture but not obliterating the interlobular septa. Follicles with germinal centres are sometimes seen. The epimyoepithelial islands, which develop from the ducts, are so-called because they have been thought to consist of proliferated ductal epithelium and myoepithelial cells, although the presence of the latter has not been convincingly demonstrated. The islands are scattered throughout the lymphoid infiltration and consist of rounded, ovoid or rather irregularly-shaped solid masses of spheroidal or polyhedral cells. Occasionally, a lumen is present. Homogeneous eosinophilic hyaline material is often seen in and around the islands, in variable amount. It may be entirely absent from some, others may be almost wholly replaced by it. Mitoses may be seen in cells of islands that are still enlarging, but they are infrequent (Figures 7.20 and 7.21).

The main problems in differential diagnosis are chronic sialadenitis and lymphoma. It is only when the lymphoid infiltration in sialadenitis is very heavy that difficulty may arise, since in most cases its patchy nature, with intervening remnants of ducts and acini and areas of fibrosis, differentiate it from the diffuse infiltration of lymphoepithelial lesion that obliterates all features except epimyoepithelial

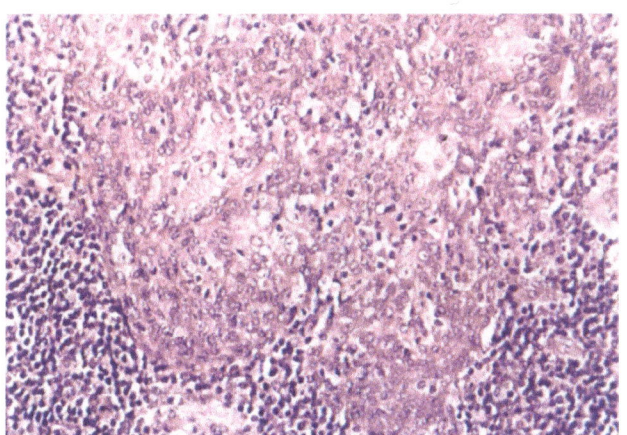

Figure 7.23 Carcinoma in lymphoepithelial lesion. The epithelial element of the lesion consists of spindle-shaped and pleomorphic cells. H & E × 250

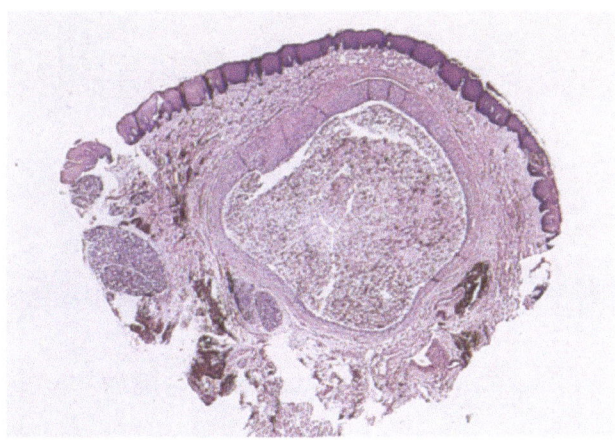

Figure 7.25 Mucous extravasation cyst of lip. The cyst is situated in the subepithelial connective tissue, adjacent to groups of mucous glands. H & E × 7·5

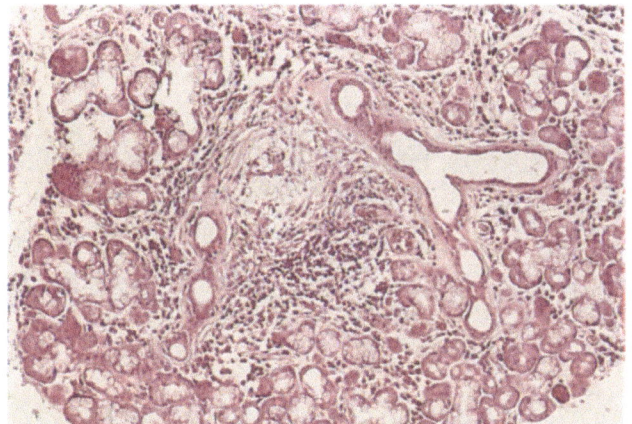

Figure 7.24 Lip biopsy in Sjögren's syndrome, showing perivascular and periductal lymphocytic infiltration in a labial salivary gland. H & E × 250

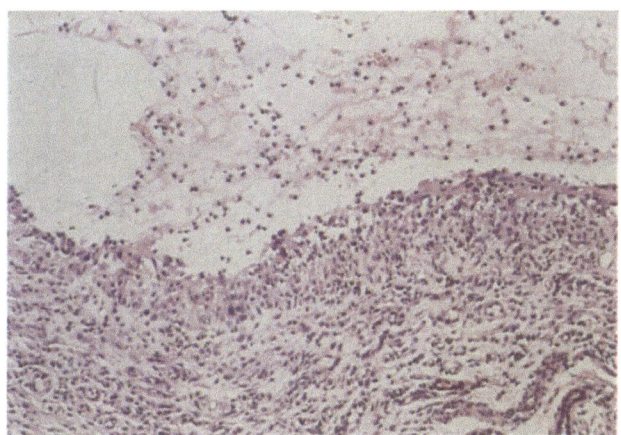

Figure 7.26 Mucous extravasation cyst. The cyst cavity is lined by macrophages and fibroblasts in varying proportions. The former usually predominate. H & E × 250

islands. In lymphoma, the diffuse infiltration effaces all other features, and passes from one lobule to another, obliterating the interlobular septa. In lymphoepithelial lesion the septa are not obliterated and epimyoepithelial islands are present. It is often a more difficult problem to decide whether an originally benign lymphoepithelial lesion has become lymphomatous, as occurs in an appreciable number of cases, since the epimyoepithelial islands and other features of lymphoepithelial lesion may still be present. Much will then depend on assessing the character of the cells of the infiltrate.

A much less common form of malignancy in lymphoepithelial lesion develops in the epithelial component. In these cases the epimyoepithelial islands proliferate and come to consist of spindle or pleomorphic cells, often with areas of squamous metaplasia. There may be numerous mitoses. Most of the reported cases have been in Eskimos and Chinese, but Europeans are also affected (Figures 7.22 and 7.23)[11,12].

Lip Biopsy in Sjögren's Syndrome

This procedure is often carried out since a positive result can be of considerable help in arriving at a clinical diagnosis. Focal lymphocytic sialadenitis has been demonstrated in the labial salivary glands of a high proportion of patients with various connective tissue disorders including Sjögren's syndrome. These lymphoid accumulations appear to be related initially to blood vessels adjacent to the ducts and the number and size of the lymphocytic foci appear to correlate with the severity of major gland involvement in the disease (Figure 7.24) Epimyoepithelial islands are seen in the minor glands only rarely.

CYSTS

Cysts of the minor salivary glands are common. They are seen much less frequently in the major glands and when they do occur the parotid is the usual site.

Minor gland cysts are seen most often in the lower lip and also frequently in the cheeks and tongue. The majority are caused by trauma to a minor salivary gland, which allows secretion to extravasate into the connective tissues (*mucous extravasation cyst*). This excavates a small cavity, the wall of which is formed by the connective tissue itself, by granulation tissue, or much less commonly and then only partially, by squamous epithelium. A group of mucous glands can usually be seen near the cyst cavity, which contains mucous and inflammatory cells. There is generally some chronic inflammatory infiltration in the tissues around the cyst and in the adjacent mucous glands. It is important to look for and report the presence or absence of minor salivary gland lobules in mucoceles as the lesion is very likely to recur if the gland related to the cyst is not removed with the lesion (Figures 7.25–7.27).

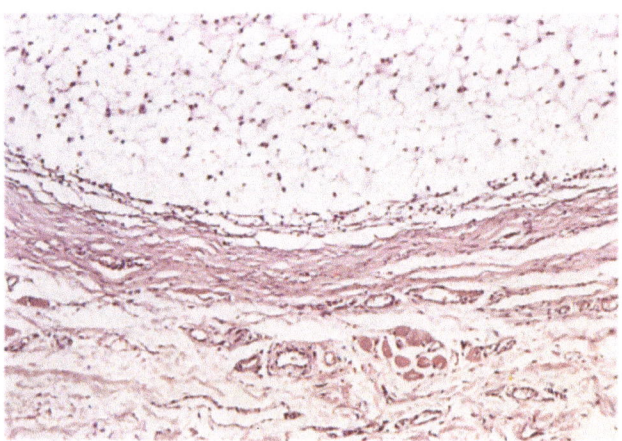

Figure 7.27 Mucous extravasation cyst. The cyst wall may be mainly fibrous. This is less common than the type of cyst lining shown in Figure 7.26, and the lesions are usually of some longstanding.   H & E × 100

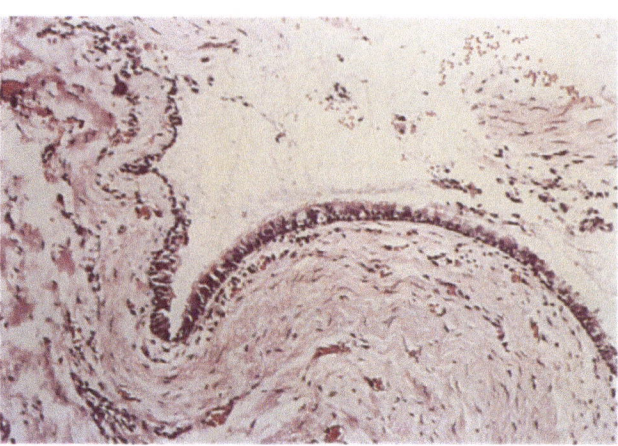

Figure 7.29 Parotid cyst. The cyst lining consists of cubical and flattened epithelium.   H & E × 250

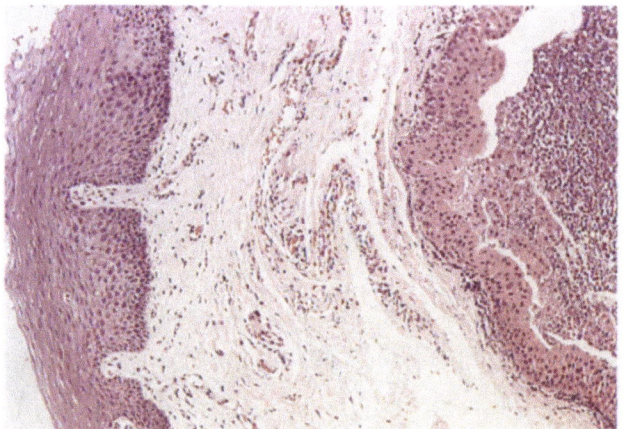

Figure 7.28 Mucous retention cyst. This cyst of the floor of the mouth is lined by cubical and colomnar epithelium.   H & E × 100

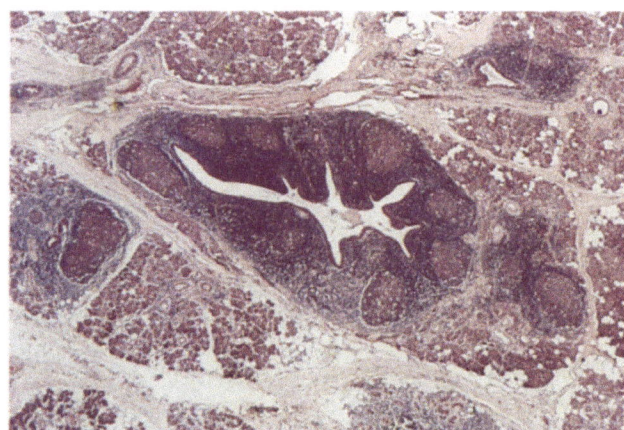

Figure 7.30 Lymphoepithelial cyst. This cyst of the parotid is lined by squamous epithelium. There is a well-defined subjacent layer of lymphoid tissue with germinal centres.   H & E × 25

Mucous cysts appear to be much less often due to obstruction of a salivary duct with consequent retention of secretion (*mucous retention cyst*). These cysts have an epithelial lining. The larger cysts of the floor of the mouth (*ranula*) are usually of the extravasation type, but occasionally they may be partly or wholly lined by epithelium (Figure 7.28).

Cysts of the parotid occur in the substance of the gland and are lined by cuboidal or squamous epithelium. They may arise as the result of duct obstruction, in which case there is likely to be associated chronic sialadenitis and the cyst, or cystically dilated duct, is simply an element of this condition. An occasional cause of cyst formation is cystic change in adenolymphoma. Most of the characteristic structure of the tumour may have disappeared, leaving only a cyst or cystic spaces lined by cubical or flattened epithelium. Very often, however, no obvious cause for cyst formation in the parotid can be found (Figure 7.29).

Some cysts arise in the intraparotid and paraparotid lymph nodes. These *lymphoepithelial cysts* are lined by squamous or cubical epithelium with subjacent lymphoid tissue (Figure 7.30).

References

1. Sicher, H. (1980). *Orban's Oral Histology and Embryology*. 9th Edn. (St. Louis: C. V. Mosby Company)
2. Pesavento, G. and Ferlito, A. (1980). Benign mixed tumour of heterotopic salivary gland tissue in upper neck. Report of a case with a review of the literature on heterotopic salivary gland tissue. *J. Larngol. Otol.*, **90**, 577
3. Arafat, A., Brannon, R. B. and Ellis, G. L. (1981). Adenomatoid hyperplasia of mucous salivary glands. *Oral Surg.*, **52**, 51
4. Mason, D. K. and Chisholm, D. M. (1975). *Salivary Glands in Health and Disease*. (London, Philadelphia, Toronto: W. B. Saunders Co. Ltd)
5. Doggett, R. G., Bentinck, B. and Harrison, G. M. (1971). Structure and ultrastructure of the labial salivary glands in patients with cystic fibrosis. *J. Clin. Pathol.*, **34**, 270
6. Grillon, G. L. and Lally, E. T. (1981). Necrotizing sialometaplasia: literature review and presentation of five cases. *J. Oral Surg.*, **39**, 747
7. Drew, W. I., Mintz, L., Miner, R. C., Sands, M., and Ketterer, B. (1981) Prevalence of cytomegalovirus infection in homosexual men. *J. Infect. Dis.*, **143**, 188
8. Waterson, A. P. (1983). Acquired immune deficiency syndrome. *Brit. Med. J.*, **286**, 743
9. Jensen, J. L., Howell, F. U., Rick, G. M. and Correll, R. W. (1979). Minor salivary gland calculi. A clinicopathologic study of forty-seven new cases. *Oral Surg.*, **47**, 44
10. Hughes, G. R. V. (1977). *Connective Tissue Diseases*. (Oxford: Blackwell Scientific)
11. Redondo, C., Garcia, A. and Vazquez, F. (1981). Malignant lymphoepithelial lesion of the parotid gland: poorly differentiated squamous cell carcinoma with lymphoid stroma. *Cancer*, **48**, 289
12. Hanji, D. and Gohao, L. (1983). Malignant lymphoepithelial lesions of the salivary glands with anaplastic carcinomatous change. Report of nine cases and review of literature. *Cancer*, **52**, 2245

The Salivary Glands
2. Tumours

8

Classification

Tumours of the salivary glands may be classified as follows[1]:

Epithelial Tumours
    Adenomas
        Pleomorphic adenoma
        Monomorphic adenoma
            Adenolymphoma
            Oxyphilic adenoma
            Other types
    Mucoepidermoid tumour
    Acinic cell tumour
    Carcinomas
        Adenoid cystic carcinoma
        Adenocarcinoma
        Epidermoid carcinoma
        Undifferentiated carcinoma
        Carcinoma in pleomorphic adenoma

Non-epithelial Tumours
    The non-epithelial tumours of the salivary glands have the same classification and terminology as comparable tumours elsewhere in the body.

The minor glands are less often the site of neoplasms than the major glands, but practically all the varieties of salivary gland tumours can affect both groups of glands, although the proportions are rather different. In the minor glands there are relatively more carcinomas and fewer adenomas than in the major glands, and some of the less common tumours of the major glands are distinctly uncommon or rare in the minor glands. However, the differences are not such as to allow the pathologist to neglect the possibility of any of the tumour types arising in any of the glands.

Pleomorphic Adenoma

This is the commonest tumour of both major and minor glands and has its most frequent location in the parotid and in the glands of the palate respectively[2]. If the tumour has been removed entire with a margin of normal tissue it will be seen to have a complete fibrous capsule, although this may be quite thin in some areas, and may readily separate from the tumour. The frequency with which this artefact of histological preparation is seen reflects the ease with which the capsule may separate from the tumour during surgical removal if suitable procedures are not adopted (Figures 8.1 and 8.2). The capsule may also contain apparently separate islets or nodules of tumour,

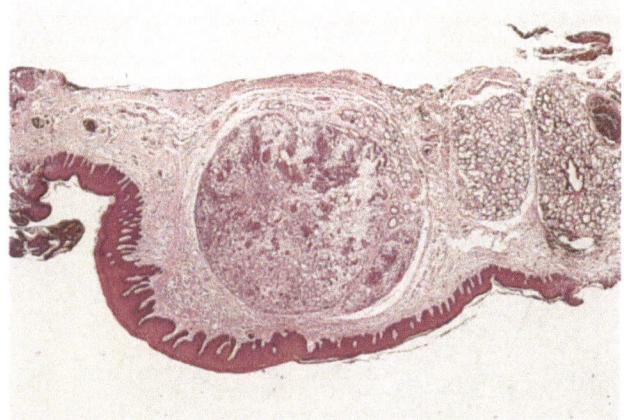

Figure 8.1 Pleomorphic adenoma of palate. The tumour is well circumscribed, but the capsule has separated from it in one area (lower right). Also in the same area there is an apparently separate island of tumour. H & E × 10

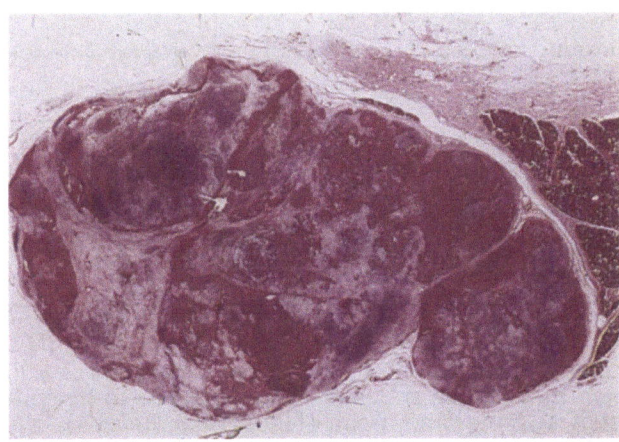

Figure 8.2 This parotid pleomorphic adenoma shows the characteristic mixture of epithelial cells (eosinophilic areas) and myxochondroid tissue (basophilic). As in Figure 8.1 the capsule has separated from the tumour. H & E × 2·5

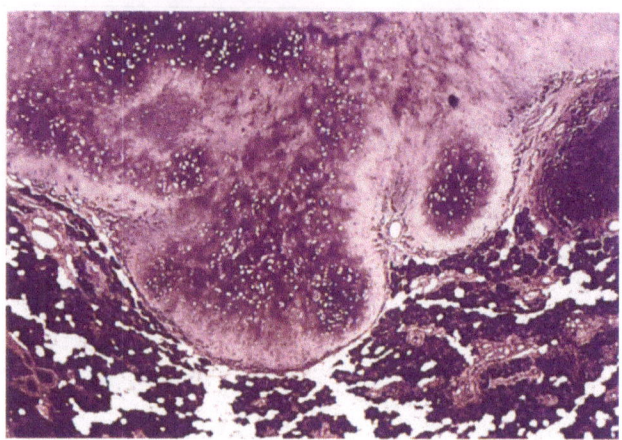

Figure 8.3 A parotid pleomorphic adenoma showing a nodular protrusion. At other levels an outgrowth like this might appear to be a separate nodule. This tumour consisted largely of chondroid tissue, but ducts and strands of cells can be seen around the edge, where the tumour abuts on the normal parotid tissue. H & E × 25

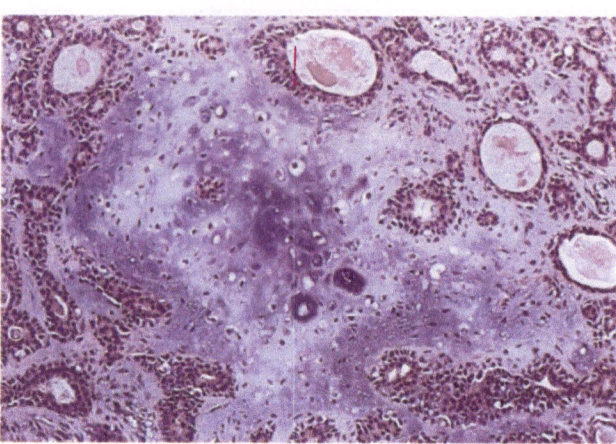

Figure 8.5 This field from a parotid pleomorphic adenoma shows the characteristic mixture of epithelial cells and myxochondroid elements. The epithelium forms ducts lined by an inner layer of flattened or cubical cells and an outer layer or layers of smaller often vacuolated cells. Small clumps and single cells are scattered throughout the chondroid tissue. H & E × 250

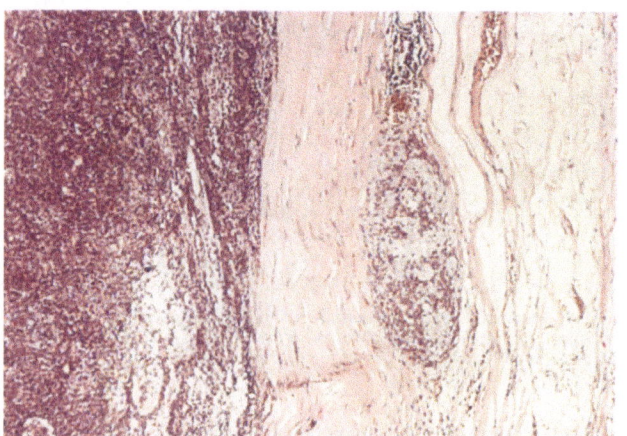

Figure 8.4 Pleomorphic adenoma of parotid. There is an apparently separate islet of tumour in the capsule. H & E × 20

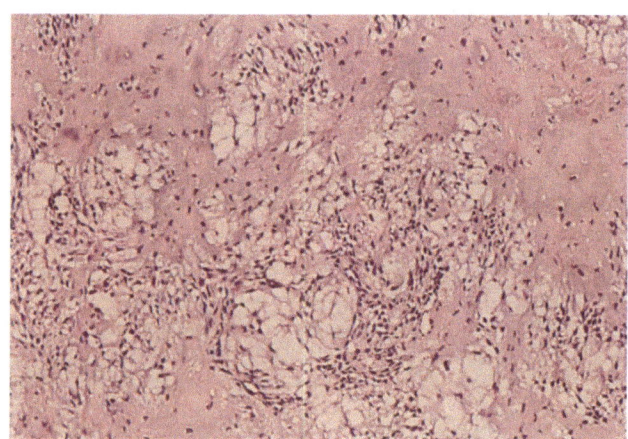

Figure 8.6 A common pattern in pleomorphic adenoma, in which the cells form interlacing strands in a myxoid background. H & E × 250

but these are outgrowths from the main tumour mass with which they can be shown by serial sections to be connected at some other point (Figures 8.3 and 8.4). The presence of a capsule is an important diagnostic feature, since a growth that is unencapsulated or only partially capsulated will be something other than a primary (that is, previously untreated) pleomorphic adenoma, although the general cellular pattern may have suggested that diagnosis on preliminary microscopical examination. If the tumour has been removed piecemeal or has been sent to the laboratory in that state, then the capsular feature is unlikely to be discernible and the cellular appearances alone will have to be relied upon.

Microscopically, a typical pleomorphic adenoma consists of epithelial cells arranged in strands, sheets and duct-like structures in a mucoid or myxochondroid background, but there are many variations of this pattern with differing proportions of the cellular and the mucoid or myxochondroid elements (Figure 8.5)[3]. When all or most

of these elements are present in a tumour diagnosis is not difficult, but when one element preponderates this may be less easily accomplished. The ducts are often similar to those of normal salivary gland, with an inner layer of flattened or cubical cells and an outer layer or layers of smaller cells that are often vacuolated. These are thought to be derived from myoepithelium and they frequently proliferate extensively. They may form interlacing strands that are intimately intermingled with myxoid tissue, or they may be arranged in more solid-appearing masses (Figure 8.6). It is probably the same cells that can appear as the so-called hyaline or plasmacytoid cells (Figures 8.7 and 8.8). These cells are seen only in pleomorphic adenoma and, uncommonly, a type of monomorphic adenoma (Figure 8.25). They have not been found in other types of salivary tumour[4].

Squamous epithelium, often with keratinization, is frequently seen in pleomorphic adenoma (Figure 8.9). It is not usually extensive, but in the very occasional tumour a

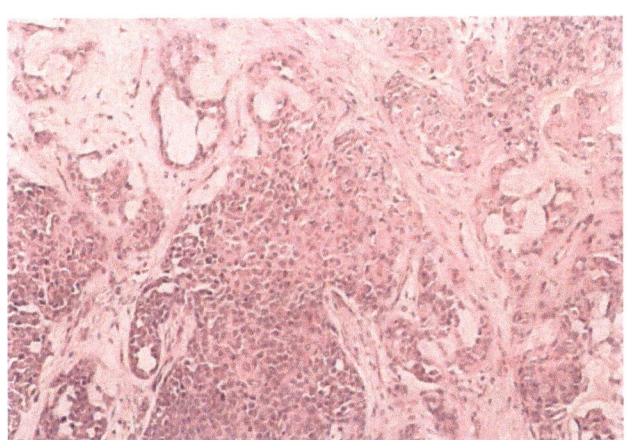

Figure 8.7 Hyaline cells in pleomorphic adenoma. The cells form groups of varying size. In the tumour shown here, appreciable areas were occupied by these cells. H & E × 100

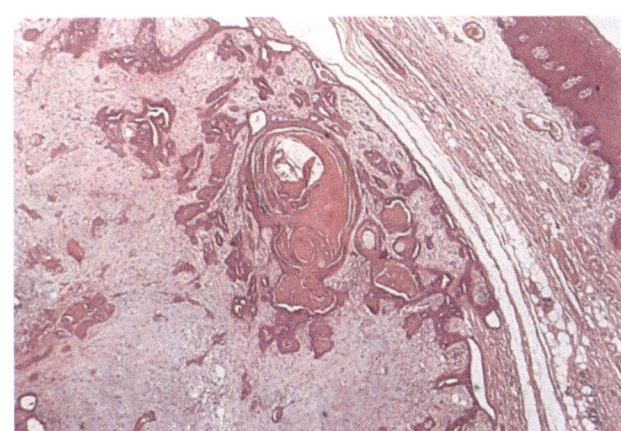

Figure 8.9 Keratinization in a palatal pleomorphic adenoma. H & E × 65

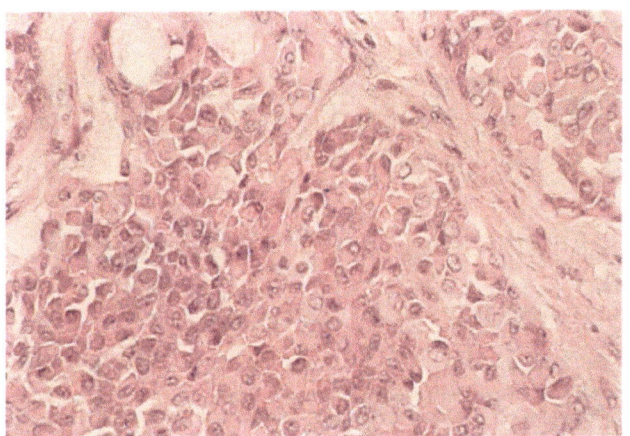

Figure 8.8 Higher magnification from Figure 8.7. The hyaline cells have some resemblance to plasma cells. The cytoplasm is eosinophilic and hyaline. H & E × 250

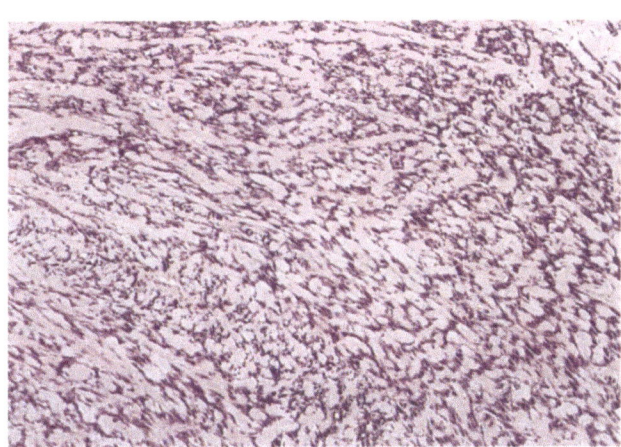

Figure 8.10 Pleomorphic adenoma of palate consisting largely of spindle cells. H & E × 100

well differentiated squamous cell carcinoma may be simulated. Mucoepidermoid tumour might also come into the differential diagnosis, but tubules and duct structures are nearly always to be found somewhere in pleomorphic adenoma if sufficient material is examined. The presence of myxochondroid tissue, again possibly present in only a small amount, will exclude mucoepidermoid tumour. Less common variants of pleomorphic adenoma include tumours that have a large spindle cell component. They can closely resemble smooth muscle or neural tumours (Figure 8.10). Here again, the presence of ducts or tubules, which may be extremely scanty, aids diagnosis.

The intercellular components of pleomorphic adenoma can be as variable as the cellular elements. Hyaline material, sometimes of homogeneous appearance but often with a fibrillar structure, may be present between the cells. This is a distinctive feature, not seen in other salivary tumours (Figure 8.11). Crystals of tyrosine may be present,

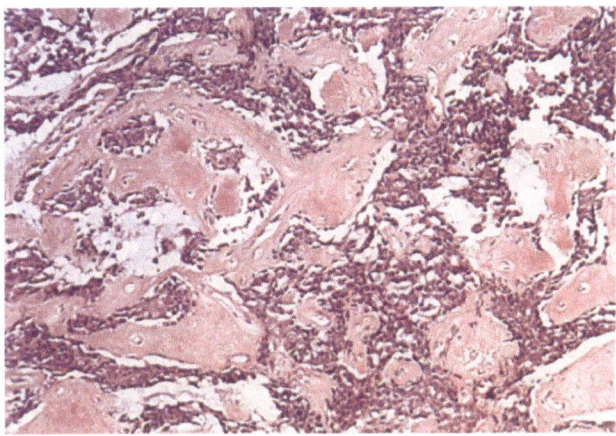

Figure 8.11 Intercellular fibrillar material in pleomorphic adenoma. H & E × 250

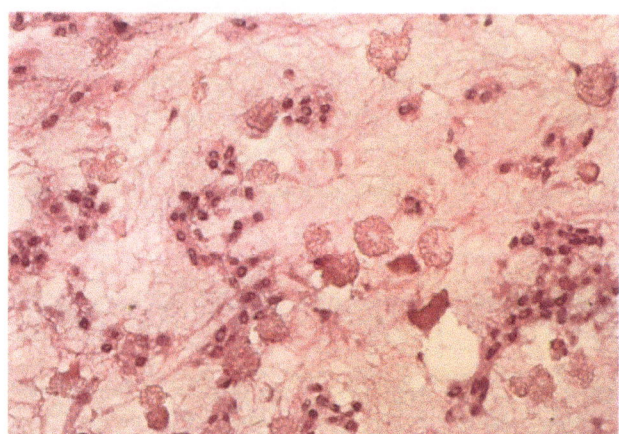

Figure 8.12 Tyrosine crystals in pleomorphic adenoma.   H & E × 250

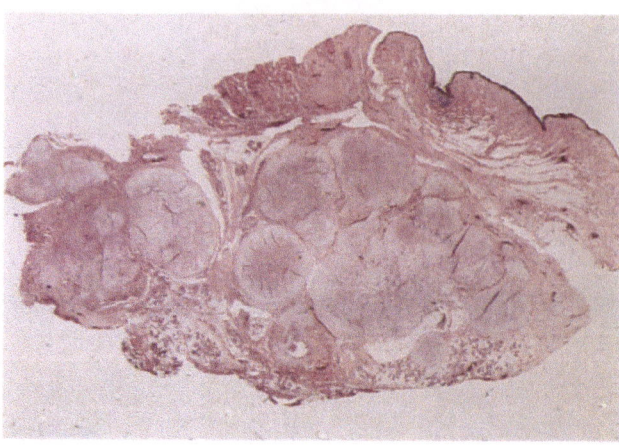

Figure 8.14 Recurrent pleomorphic adenoma. The foci of recurrent tumour extend into the skin and scar of the previous excision.   H & E × 5

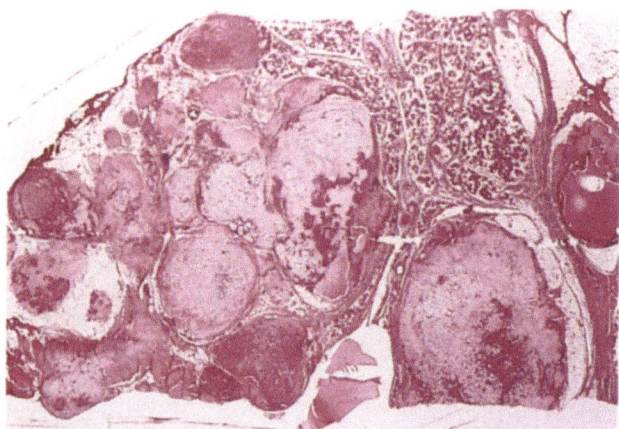

Figure 8.13 Recurrent pleomorphic adenoma. Multiple nodules of tumour are present.   H & E × 4·5

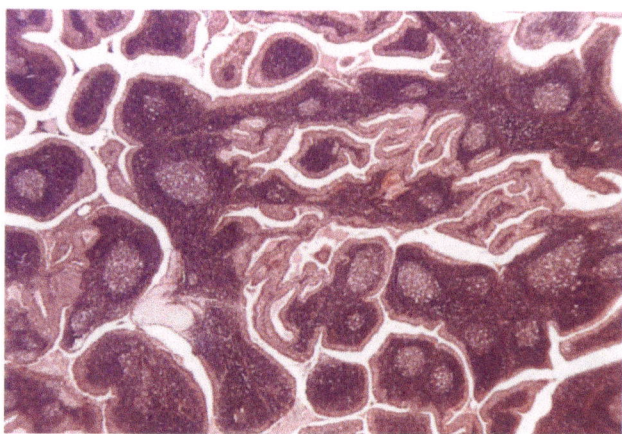

Figure 8.15 Adenolymphoma. The tumour consists of double-layered columns of epithelial cells lining cystic spaces, with intervening lymphoid tissue.   H & E × 25

very infrequently, in the matrix (Figure 8.12). This again appears to be a finding peculiar to pleomorphic adenoma. When chondroid tissue is present it is usually interspersed with obviously epithelial cellular elements, but very occasionally this type of tissue may be so preponderant that, especially with palatal or maxillary tumours, the question of chondroma or even chondrosarcoma arises. A thorough search will then be necessary to find tubules or ducts or other obviously epithelial formations, the presence of which will settle the diagnosis.

Recurrent Pleomorphic Adenoma

Recurrent tumours can result when enucleation has been used as a method of treatment instead of excision. They are likely to follow incomplete excision, or rupture during removal of a tumour that is of the type containing much myxoid tissue. Characteristically, recurrence is in the form of multiple nodules of tumour scattered over the field of the previous operation (Figures 8.13 and 8.14). Recurrent growth may take a long time, sometimes many years, before becoming apparent clinically.

Monomorphic Adenomas

These tumours, in contradistinction to the varied and often complex histological patterns of pleomorphic adenoma,

have a much more uniform appearance and they lack the myxochondroid element which is so common a component of the pleomorphic tumour.

Adenolymphoma occurs almost exclusively in the parotid, although rare examples have been reported from the other glands. It has a very characteristic structure consisting of double-layered columns of cells with intervening lymphoid tissue, often with prominent germinal follicles. The inner layer of the cell columns consists of columnar cells with finely granular eosinophilic cytoplasm. The cells of the outer layer are smaller and polygonal. Typical tumours are readily recognized (Figures 8.15 and 8.16). Variants are uncommon[5]. They include infection, which may lead to a clinical diagnosis of parotid abscess and also considerably obscure the histological picture. Local thrombosis and resulting infarction may also render a growth largely necrotic, with squamous metaplasia of the surviving epithelium, which should not be mistaken for squamous cell carcinoma (Figure 8.17). Nor should the granulomas that may be seen in these cases be mistaken for tuberculous lesions (Figures 8.18 and 8.19). Carcinoma arising in adenolymphoma is extremely rare.

Oxyphilic adenoma, like adenolymphoma, is nearly always found in the parotid, with the very occasional tumour elsewhere[6]. It is a relatively rare tumour in any situation. Again, like adenolymphoma, it has a characteristic structure, but it is more readily mimicked by other lesions. The tumour consists of large polyhedral cells with finely granular eosinophilic cytoplasm arranged in acinar

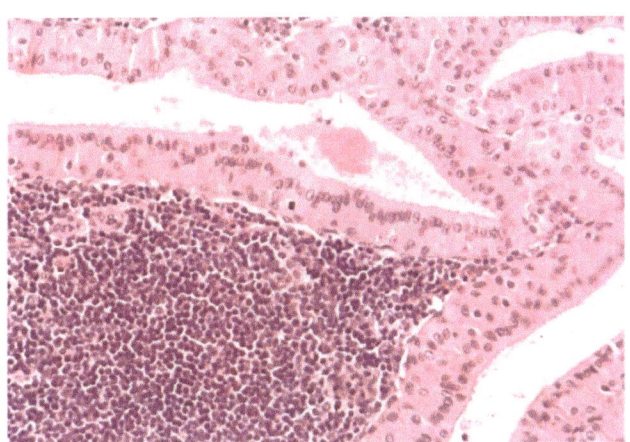

Figure 8.16 Adenolymphoma. The tumour cells are columnar and cubical, with finely granular eosinophilic cytoplasm.   H & E × 250

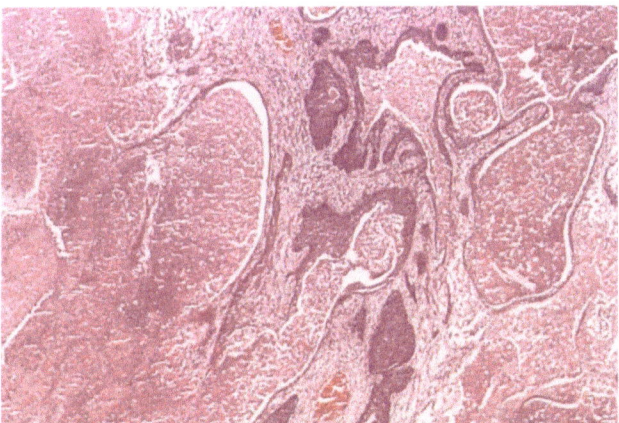

Figure 8.17 Squamous metaplasia in adenolymphoma. The cystic spaces contain necrotic material and the stroma is chronically inflamed and partially necrotic. The epithelium has undergone squamous metaplasia.   H & E × 100

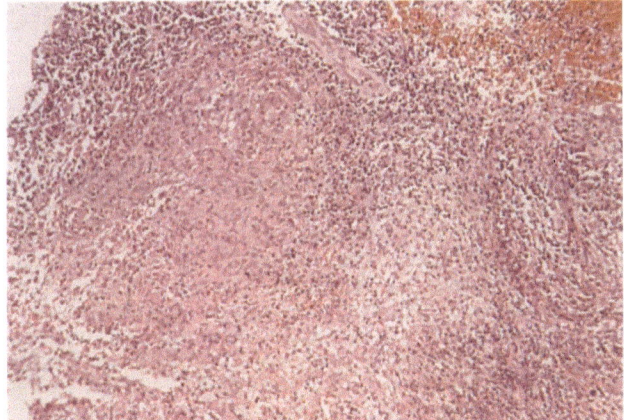

Figure 8.18 Granulomas in adenolymphoma. Follicles of large mononuclear cells may be seen in partially necrotic or infected tumours.   H & E × 100

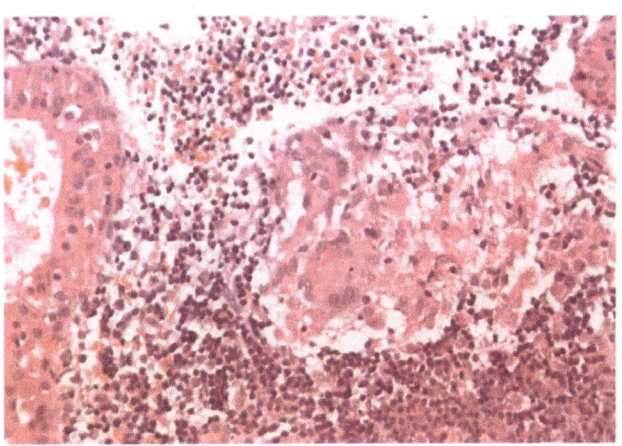

Figure 8.19 Granuloma from another adenolymphoma, showing macrophages and multinucleated giant cells.   H & E × 250

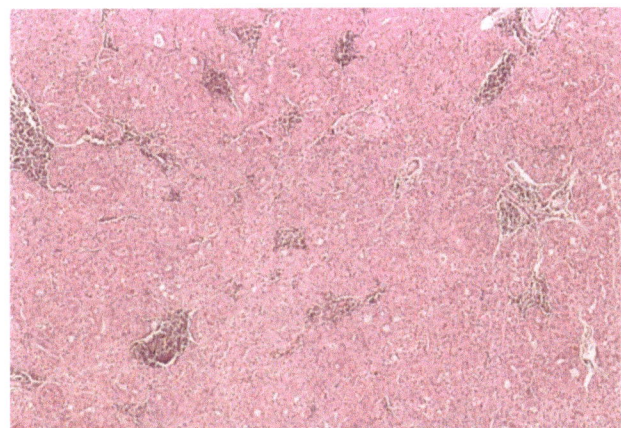

Figure 8.20 Oxyphilic adenoma. The tumour cells are arranged in a solid mass, although acinar groupings and columns can be discerned. There are some scattered foci of lymphoid tissue.   H & E × 100

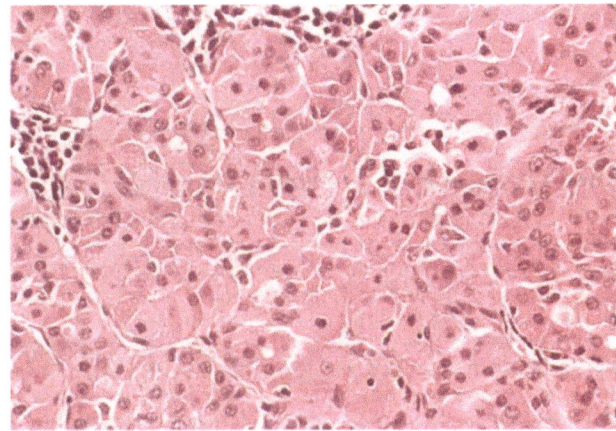

Figure 8.21 Oxyphilic adenoma. The tumour cells are rounded or polygonal, with finely granular eosinophilic cytoplasm. The acinus-like arrangement can be seen.   H & E × 250

groups or in columns. The nuclei are vesicular. Mitoses are very rarely seen. The stroma is minimal, and there may be foci of lymphoid cells here and there (Figures 8.20 and 8.21). Areas of oncocytic metaplasia in pleomorphic adenoma or other tumours may be mistaken for oxyphilic

adenoma only when extensive, which is rare. Malignant oxyphil cell tumours are extremely rare and it is highly likely that many of the tumours reported as such have really been other types of carcinoma with secondary changes of the type just mentioned.

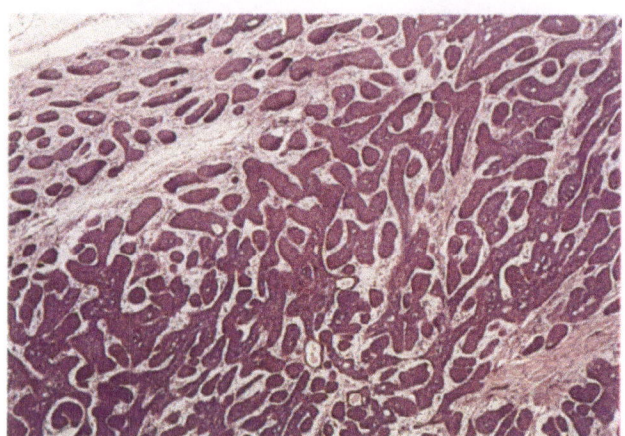

Figure 8.22 Basal cell adenoma. The well circumscribed tumour consists of strands and islets of small darkly staining cells. The pattern is uniform throughout. No myxochondroid tissue is present.   H & E × 100

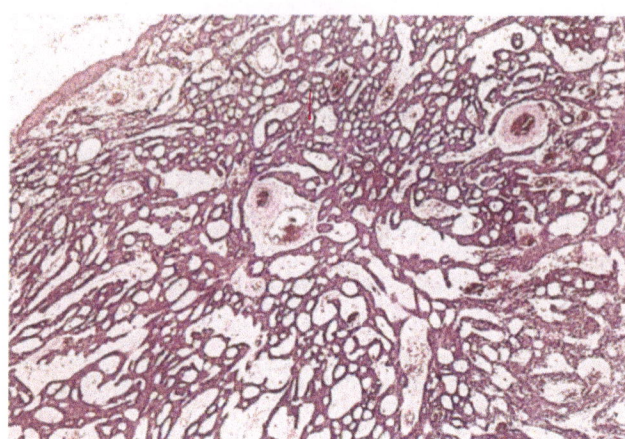

Figure 8.24 Basal cell adenoma. Stromal cyst formation is pronounced in this tumour.   H & E × 100

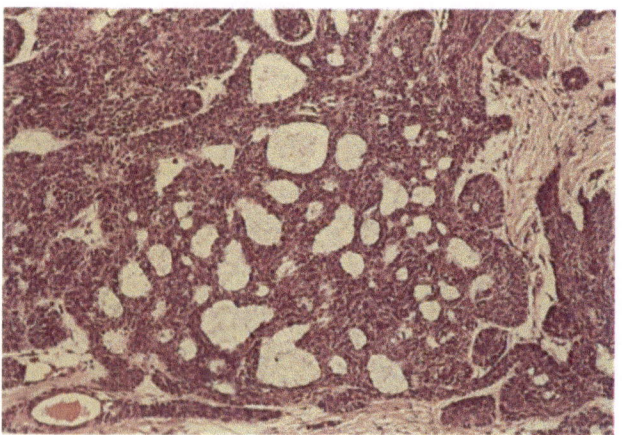

Figure 8.23 Basal cell adenoma. The strands of basal type cells are often bordered by a palisade layer. Numerous stromal cyst are present.   H & E × 250

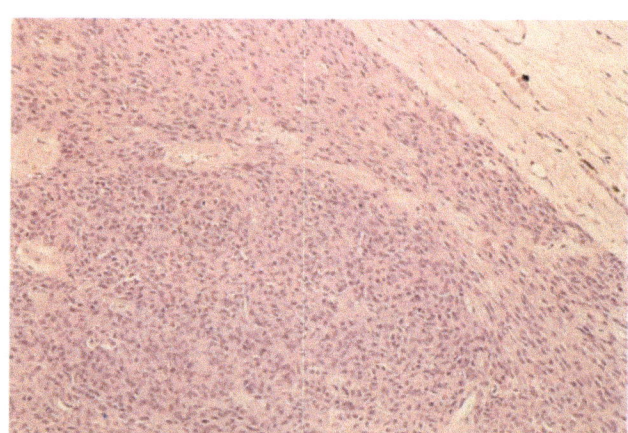

Figure 8.25 Myoepithelioma. This monomorphic adenoma consists entirely of cells of the myoepithelial type.   H & E × 250

Other Types of Monomorphic Adenoma

These comprise a number of different patterns named according to the cell type or the cell arrangement[7-9]. Like pleomorphic adenoma they are well encapsulated, but they are distinguished by their several uniform and distinctive patterns. Occasionally it is difficult to decide whether a tumour should be classified as a pleomorphic adenoma of highly homogenous pattern and having little or no myxochondroid element, or as a monomorphic adenoma. However, this is not a matter of vital importance, since the treatment and outlook for both pleomorphic and monomorphic tumours is essentially the same. Of greater importance is the differentiation between occasional monomorphic adenomas and carcinoma, usually adenoid cystic carcinoma.

Basal cell adenoma consists of small darkly staining cells arranged in islands and short columns, frequently bordered by a palisade layer and thus having a resemblance to basal cell carcinoma of the skin (Figures 8.22 and 8.23). Small cystic spaces are not uncommon. Occasionally they are quite numerous, with a resulting cribriform appearance that may suggest adenoid cystic carcinoma (Figures 8.23 and 8.24). The small darkly staining cells of the adenoma, however, can usually be distin-

guished on close examination from either of the two cell types of adenoid cystic carcinoma. Moreover, there are no ducts in the adenoma, whereas these can nearly always be found in the carcinoma. The encapsulation of the adenoma also differentiates it from adenoid cystic carcinoma, which is practically always infiltrative. However, a note of caution is necessary here. In a very small number of cases it seems probable that an adenoid cystic carcinoma has originated from a basal cell adenoma, and at an early stage of this malignant change the carcinoma may still appear to be very largely circumscribed and encapsulated. But cases of this type are rare and any errors in diagnosis are much more likely to be in the direction of over rather than under diagnosis.

Myoepithelioma has been used as the designation for adenomas that appear to consist entirely of myoepithelial cells or their derivatives. One such adenoma is composed of the hyaline cells that are often found in pleomorphic adenoma. Other monomorphic adenomas that have been described as myoepitheliomas consist of somewhat similar but smaller cells (Figure 8.25).

Clear cell adenoma is another designation that seems to embrace lesions of differing histological appearance. Some consist almost entirely of cells with much clear cytoplasm,

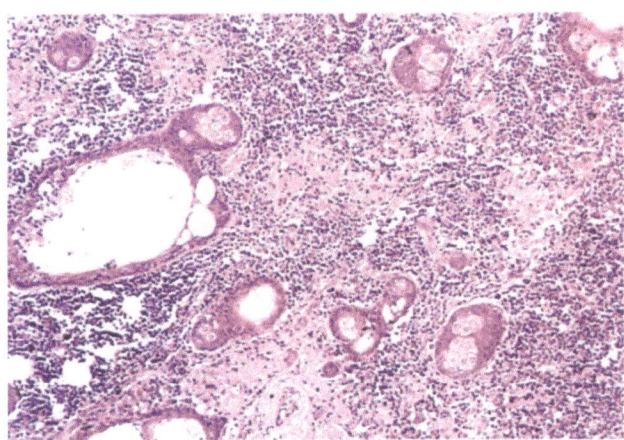

Figure 8.26 Sebaceous lymphadenoma. This tumour is characterized by sebaceous glands in a lymphoid stroma. Cysts lined by squamous epithelium are also present. H & E × 250

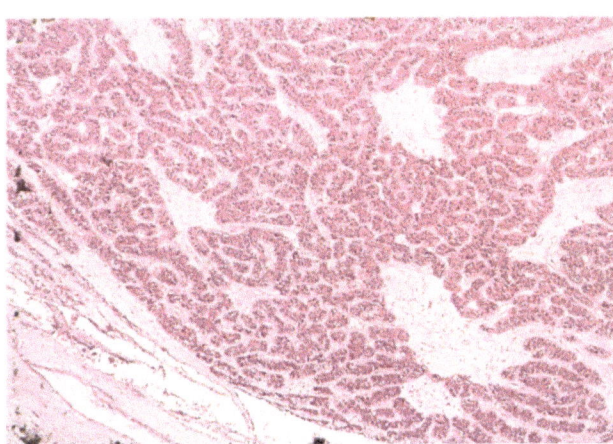

Figure 8.28 Trabecular adenoma. The tumour consists of trabeculae of small cells, often with vacuolated cytoplasm. H & E × 100

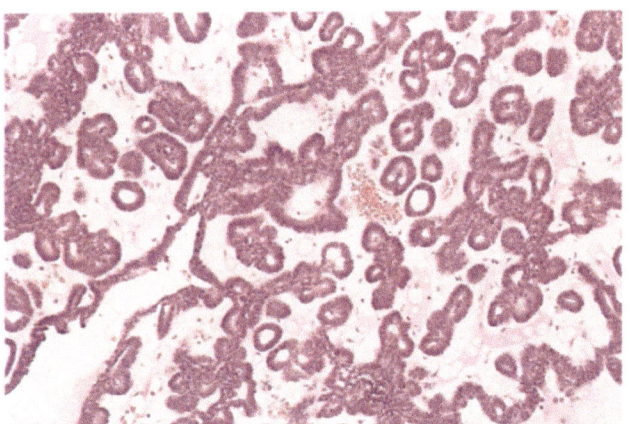

Figure 8.27 Canalicular adenoma. The tumour epithelium forms ducts lined by columnar cells. H & E × 250

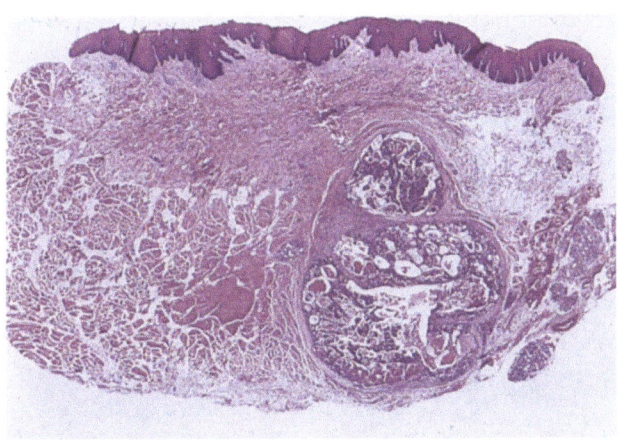

Figure 8.29 Cystadenoma. This adenoma of the lip is partly cystic, with papillary and interlacing ingrowths of epithelium. Labial mucous glands are seen adjacent to the tumour. H & E × 7·5

in which glycogen is present. Other clear cell adenomas are characterized by duct-like structures with bordering cells that have a markedly clear cytoplasm. These latter lesions should probably be considered as a very well differentiated type of adenocarcinoma (page 98).

Sebaceous adenoma is a rare tumour, consisting of sebaceous epithelium in a fibrous stroma. In the sebaceous lymphadenoma, sebaceous glands and squamous cysts are present in a fibrous stroma containing lymphoid tissue (Figure 8.26).

Tubular adenoma consists of small tubules or ducts with an inner lining layer of ductal epithelium and an outer layer or layers of smaller myoepithelial-type cells. In the *canalicular adenoma* there is only one type of cell, forming convoluted duct-like structures (Figure 8.27). In the *trabecular adenoma* the cells, mainly of the myoepithelial type, form strands or trabeculae (Figure 8.28).

Papillary cystadenoma is seen particularly in the minor glands of the lip and palate. It consists of interlacing strands of cells in and around a cystic space of variable size. The arrangement of the cells is frequently in a cribriform pattern, with a consequent superficial resemblance to adenoid cystic carcinoma (Figures 8.29 and 8.30). Differentiation from that tumour depends on recognition

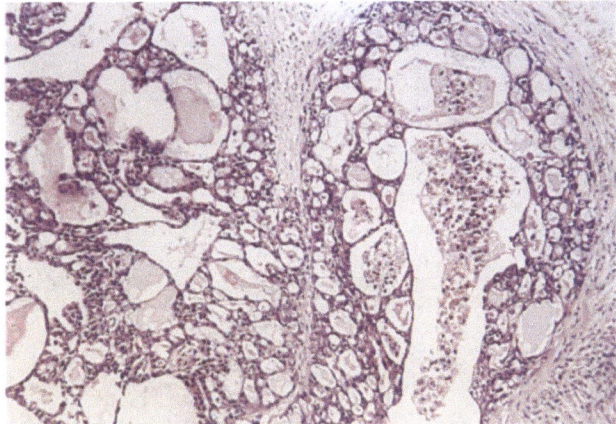

Figure 8.30 Detail from Figure 8.29, showing the cribriform pattern of the epithelium. H & E × 100

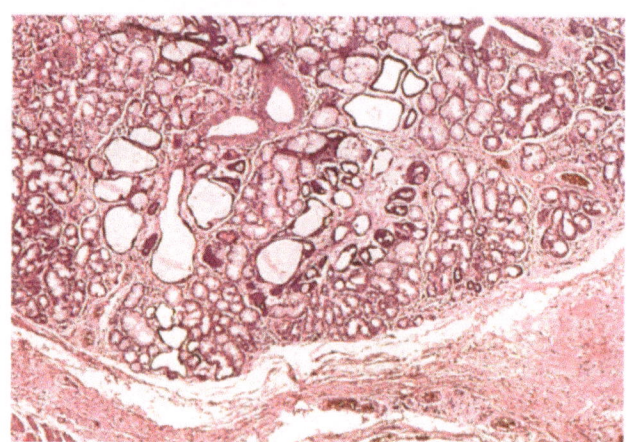

Figure 8.31 Mucous glands adjacent to a papillary cystadenoma. The darkly staining areas are foci of commencing adenomatous proliferation.   H & E × 100

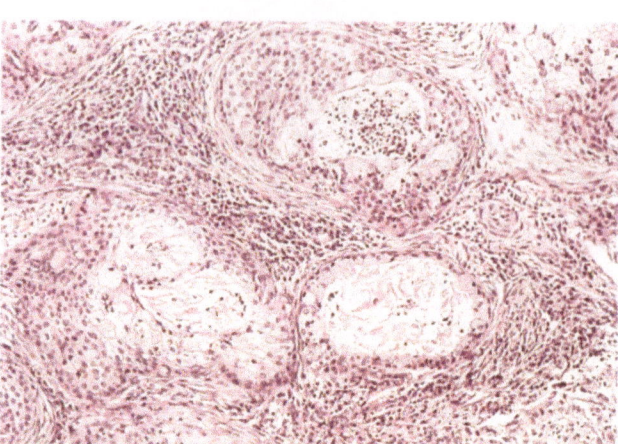

Figure 8.34 Mucoepidermoid tumour of the parotid. A well differentiated tumour with numerous mucous cells lining small cysts. Epidermoid cells are also present. There is chronic inflammatory infiltration in the stroma.   H & E × 250

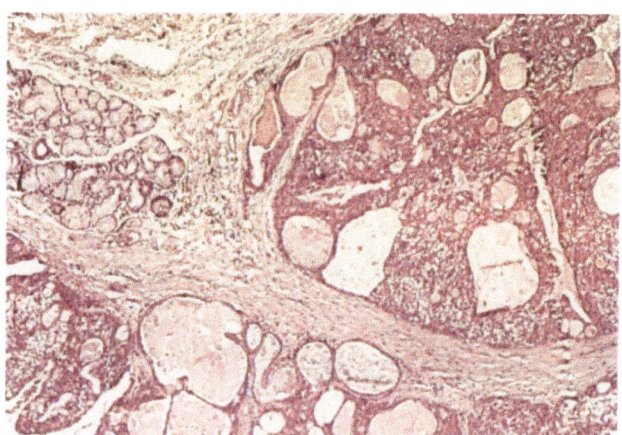

Figure 8.32 Mucoepidermoid tumour of the palate. The tumour islets are set in a fibrous stroma. There is no capsule. This is a well differentiated tumour, with cyst formation and both mucous and epidermoid cells. Clear cells are prominent. H & E × 100

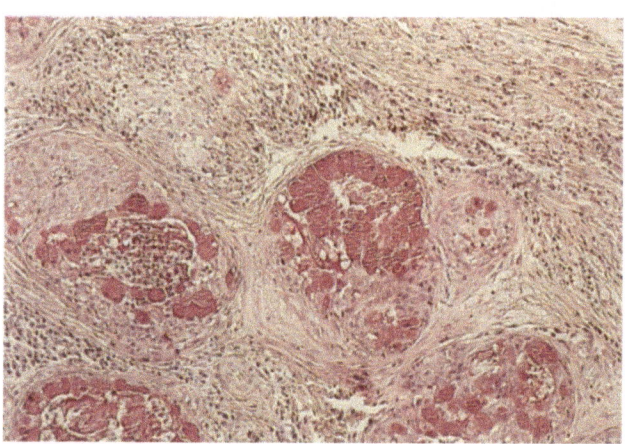

Figure 8.35 A nearby section to that shown in Figure 8.34, showing copious mucus production.   Mucicarmine × 250

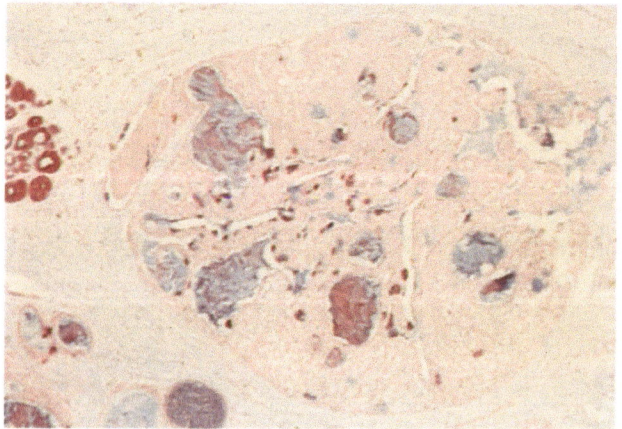

Figure 8.33 An adjacent section to that shown in Figure 8.32, showing abundant mucus formation.   Alcian Blue × 100

of similar features to those that distinguish basal cell adenoma from adenoid cystic carcinoma. Proliferative changes or microtumours can sometimes be seen in the ducts of adjacent mucous glands (Figure 8.31). This field change in the ducts accounts in at least some cases for apparent recurrence after excision and for those infrequent cases where multiple tumours have been present.

Mucoepidermoid Tumour

This tumour is seen rather more frequently in the minor glands, especially in the palate, than in the major glands[10,11]. Most mucoepidermoid tumours are not encapsulated or are only partly so, this being a distinctive difference from the adenomas. The tumour tissue is arranged in islets and sheets in a fibrous stroma, and in those tumours of low-grade malignancy, which are much the commonest, cyst formation is often seen (Figures 8.32–8.35). The two chief components of the mucoepidermoid tumour, mucus-secreting cells and epidermoid cells, are readily seen in these low-grade tumours, but the less common tumours that are of greater invasiveness and that are more likely to metastasize are generally mainly

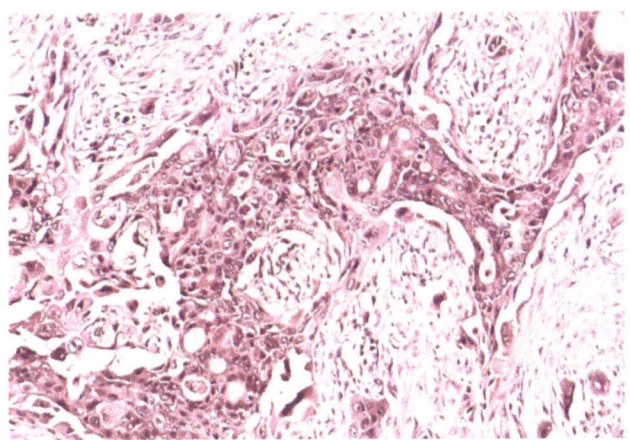

Figure 8.36 A less well differentiated mucoepidermoid than those shown in the preceding figures. The tumour consists mainly of epidermoid cells, with some interspersed mucus-secreting cells. There is pleomorphism and hyperchromatism. H & E × 250

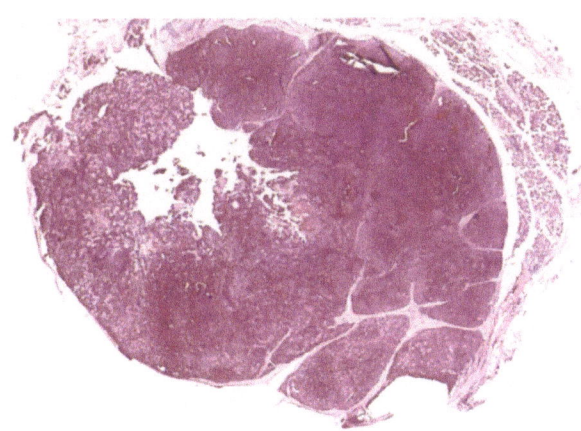

Figure 8.38 Acinic cell tumour. This parotid tumour is well circumscribed, although there are one or two small extensions into and beyond the capsule. The violaceous colour in H & E preparations is characteristic of many of these tumours. H & E × 2·5

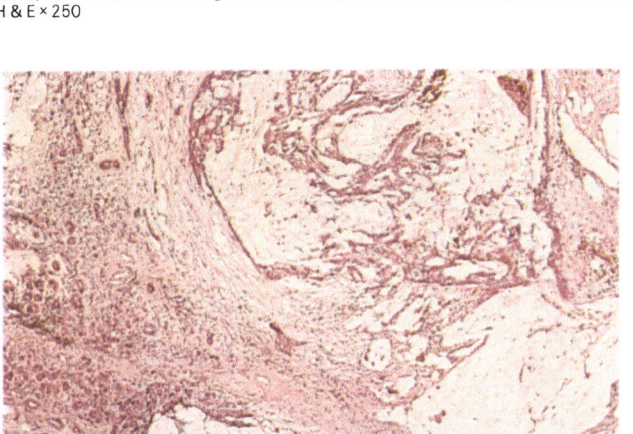

Figure 8.37 The cysts in mucoepidermoid tumour often rupture, to liberate mucus into the stroma with an ensuing chronic inflammatory reaction.   H & E × 100

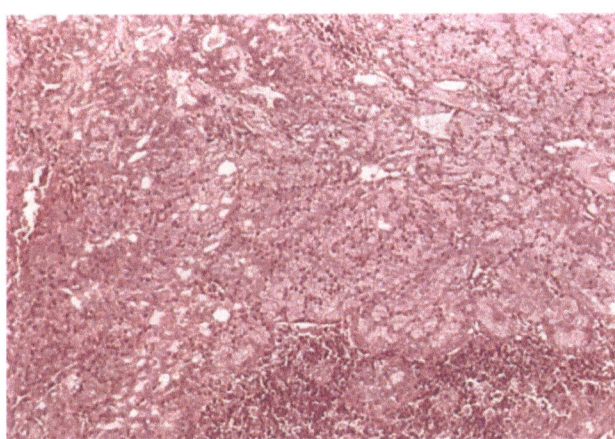

Figure 8.39 Acinic cell tumour. The tumour is composed of finely granular cells in a solid arrangement with occasional acinus-like groupings. Small intercellular spaces are present throughout.   H & E × 250

epidermoid, and cysts are infrequent (Figure 8.36). In some tumours some or many of the epidermoid cells have clear cytoplasm. Keratin formation is occasionally seen. The stroma in mucoepidermoid tumours may show areas of lymphocytic infiltration. There is not infrequently chronic inflammatory infiltration and a foreign body reaction due to the escape of mucus from ruptured microcysts into the stroma (Figure 8.37).

From the point of view of differential histological diagnosis, other mucus-secreting tumours have to be considered. Mucus secretion in pleomorphic adenoma can often be abundant, but the mucus is seen mainly in duct-like structures, which are not a constituent of mucoepidermoid tumours. In addition, there is the lack of, or deficient, encapsulation already mentioned. Salivary adenocarcinomas are not infrequently mucus-secreting but the cells are of glandular type and not epidermoid. In tumours with a predominance of the epidermoid element the possibility of squamous cell carcinoma has to be considered, especially where there is also cellular atypia. In fact, sometimes the distinction cannot be made, but in such cases this is probably of little practical importance. The more a mucoepidermoid tumour resembles squamous cell carcinoma the more it is likely to behave like one.

Acinic Cell Tumour

This relatively uncommon tumour, which occurs mainly in the parotid and rather rarely in the other glands, is composed of cells resembling those of normal serous acini[12]. Although many tumours are encapsulated, some have ill-defined borders. Small infiltrations of the capsule are common (Figure 8.38). These features account for the fact that recurrences of acinic cell tumour are often in the form of multiple nodules. The tumour cells are arranged in solid masses, although acinar groupings can often be detected, or the cells may have a tendency to form columns. A feature of the tumour is the absence of ducts, which results in the accumulation of secretion in spaces (Figure 8.39). Usually these spaces are small or inconspicuous, but occasionally they are extensive. The round or polyhedral tumour cells have a finely granular basophilic cytoplasm. The granules are PAS-positive and sometimes they are coarse and chunky. In occasional tumours some or many of the cells may have a vacuolated or partially clear cytoplasm, or it may be entirely clear. Pleomorphism and mitotic activity are generally absent (Figures 8.40–8.43). The stroma in acinic cell tumour is usually inconspicuous. Lymphoid tissue is quite often present, and calcospheroids are not uncommonly seen (Figure 8.42).

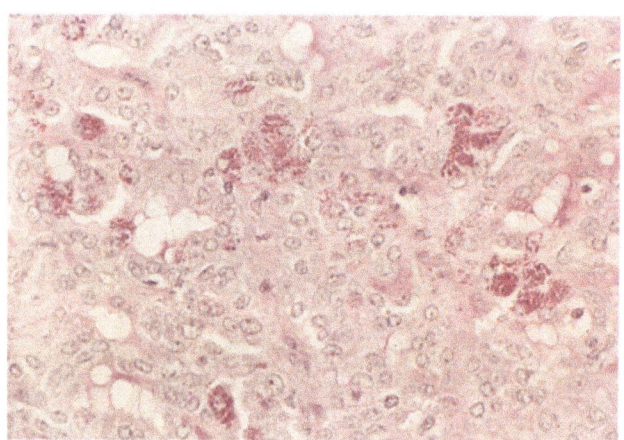

Figure 8.40 Acinic cell tumour, showing coarse cytoplasmic granules. PAS × 250

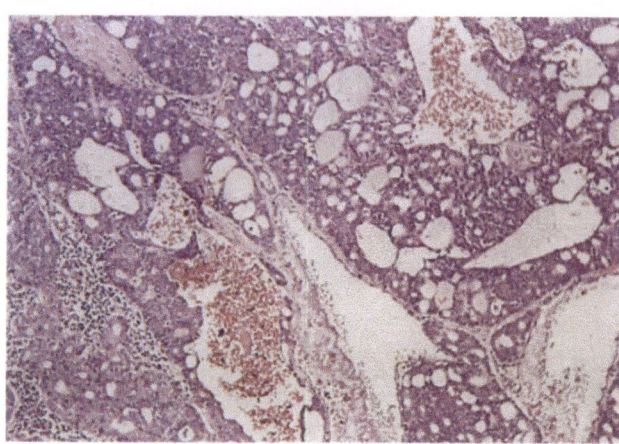

Figure 8.43 The intercellular spaces in acinic cell tumour may become large enough to produce a cribriform pattern in some areas, or larger cysts.   H & E × 100

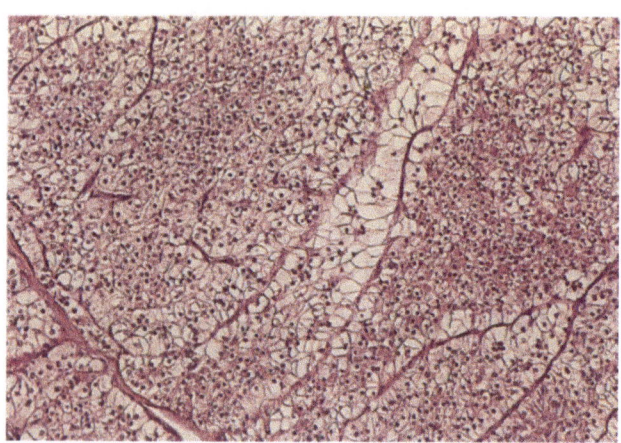

Figure 8.41 Acinic cell tumour, in which many of the cells are vacuolated. In some the cytoplasm has become completely clear.   H & E × 250

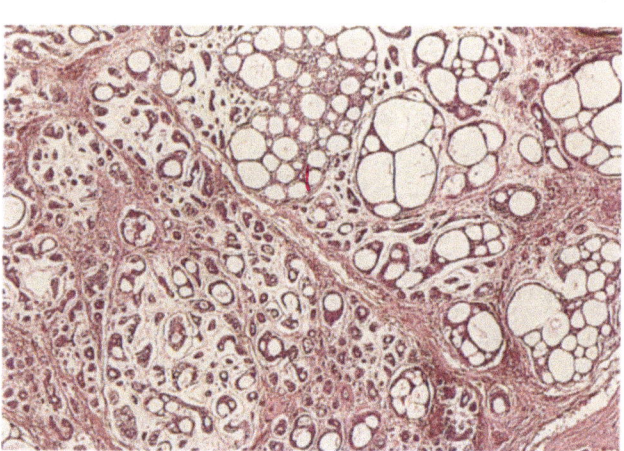

Figure 8.44 Adenoid cystic carcinoma, showing the typical cribriform pattern. Most of the cystic spaces are stromal cysts, but much smaller spaces, representing duct lumens, are also present.   H & E × 50

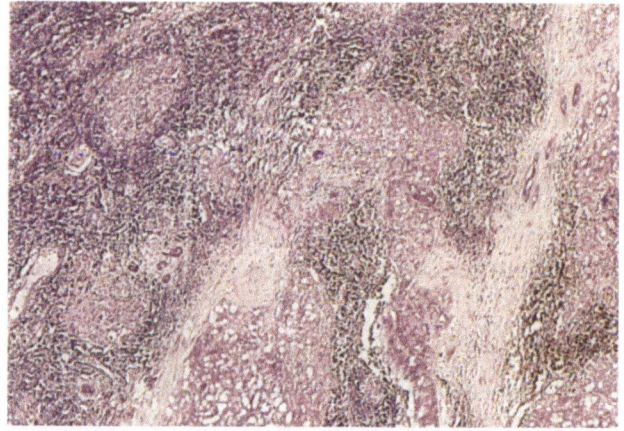

Figure 8.42 Acinic cell tumour with prominent intercellular spaces in some areas. Lymphoid tissue is present in the stroma.   H & E × 100

Typical tumours, consisting of a uniform mass of characteristically basophilic cells, are readily recognizable. Variants, with large cystic spaces and often with cells with eosinophilic rather than basophilic cytoplasm, may suggest adenocarcinoma or adenoid cystic carcinoma. The presence of PAS-positive granules, copious in some tumours, scanty in others, is an aid to differentiation (Figure 8.40).

Adenoid Cystic Carcinoma

This tumour is seen relatively much more often in the minor glands, especially of the palate, than in the major glands. The parotid is the commonest site for major gland tumours, but the submandibular gland is nearly as frequently affected[13,14]

The typical adenoid cystic carcinoma, with its cribriform pattern and pronounced invasive activity, including perineural infiltration, presents a characteristic picture (Figures 8.44 and 8.45). However, there are many variations, although it is usually possible to find areas of more typical

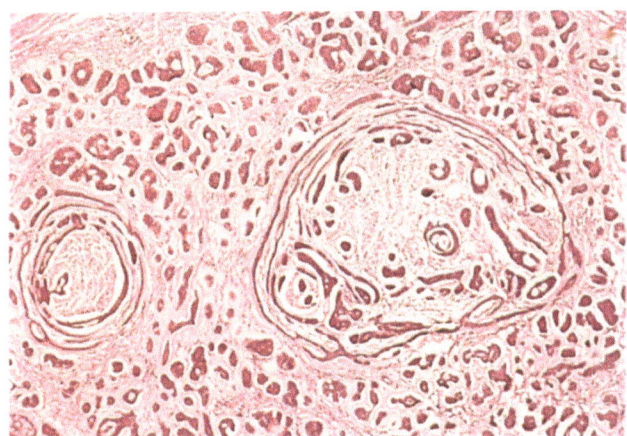

Figure 8.45 Perineural infiltration in adenoid cystic carcinoma. H & E × 50

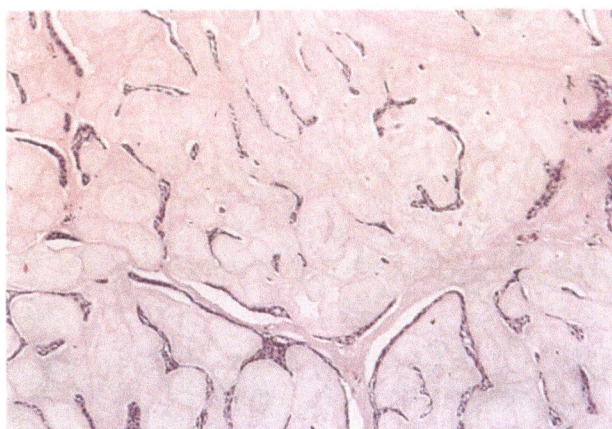

Figure 8.47 Adenoid cystic carcinoma. A tumour with prominent hyalinized stroma. H & E × 100

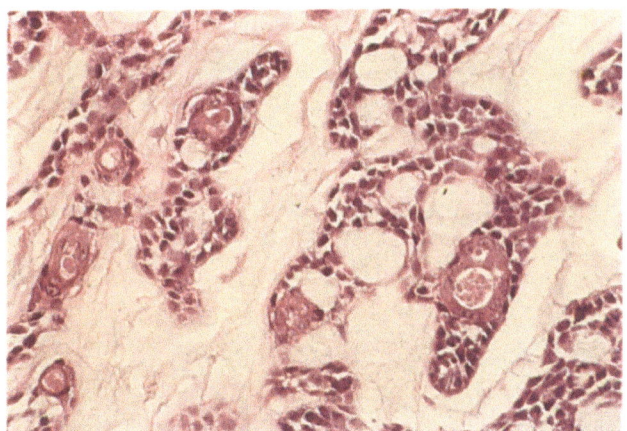

Figure 8.46 Detail from the tumour shown in Figure 8.44. The stromal cysts are lined by vacuolated cells with deeply staining nuclei, the duct formations by cells with vesicular nuclei and eosinophilic cytoplasm. H & E × 250

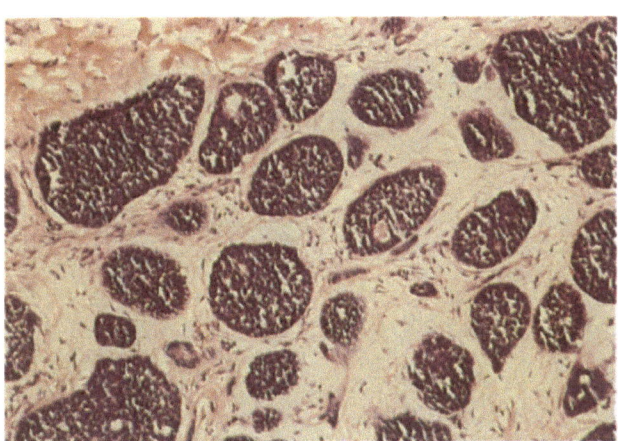

Figure 8.48 Adenoid cystic carcinoma. A solid variant, in which the tumour consists of islets of cells in solid formations. Ducts can be seen in some of the islets. H & E × 100

growth in these less common configurations that lead to the correct diagnosis.

The characteristic cribriform pattern is largely due to the encirclement of areas of stroma by proliferating strands of cells of the vacuolated duct lining type. The enclaved stroma then degenerates to form cysts. Some spaces, however, are the lumens of ducts. These spaces are much smaller than the stromal cysts, and they are lined by cells with eosinophilic cytoplasm (Figure 8.46). In tumours with prominent stromal changes, such as hyalinization or mucoid change, the epithelial structures may tend to be separated, but the basic features can usually be readily recognized (Figure 8.47). An important variant is the solid type of growth, in which the cells form masses of apparently uniform structure. However, closer examination will reveal the presence of small ducts, although they may be few in number (Figures 8.48 and 8.49). Much of a tumour may consist of this solid type of growth, but more typical areas may be found on examination of further material. Tumours with this pattern in whole or part are more aggressive than the usual type of adenoid cystic carcinoma, and have a worse prognosis.

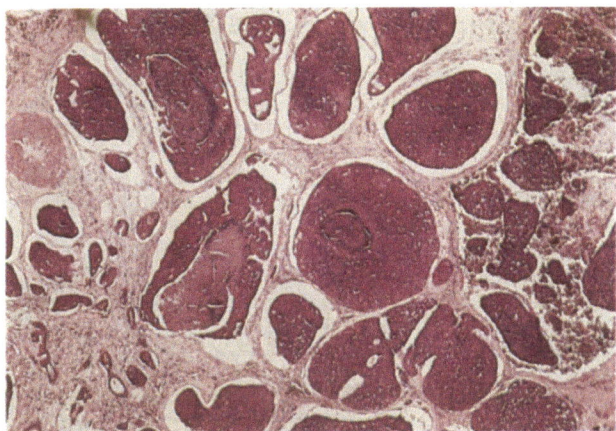

Figure 8.49 Another example of the solid variant in adenoid cystic carcinoma. The cell masses frequently show central necrosis. H & E × 100

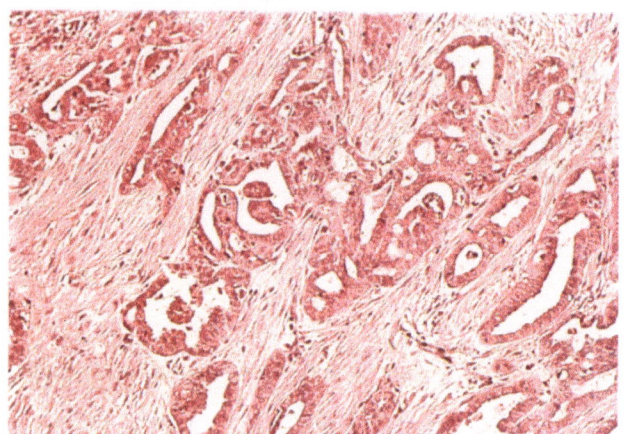

Figure 8.50 Adenocarcinoma of palate. The neoplastic ducts are lined by columnar and cubical cells.   H & E × 100

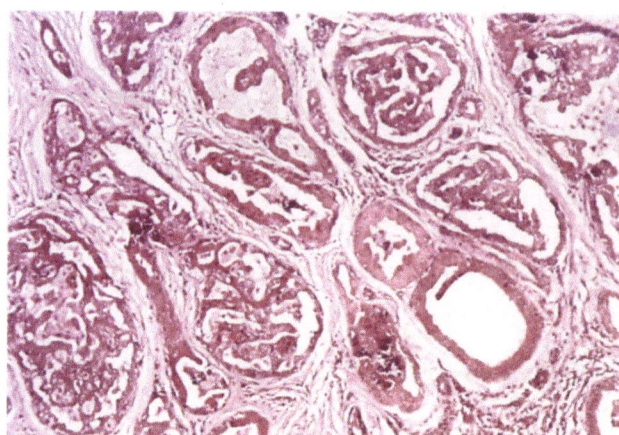

Figure 8.52 Adenocarcinoma of parotid, showing oncocytic metaplasia. The oncocytic cells have a markedly eosinophilic cytoplasm.   H & E × 100

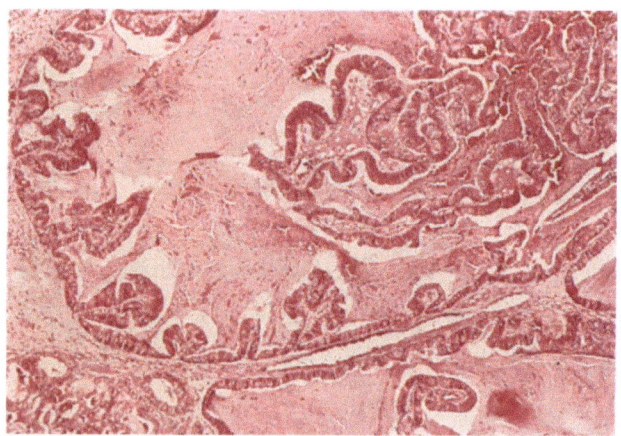

Figure 8.51 Adenocarcinoma of parotid, showing a papillary pattern.   H & E × 100

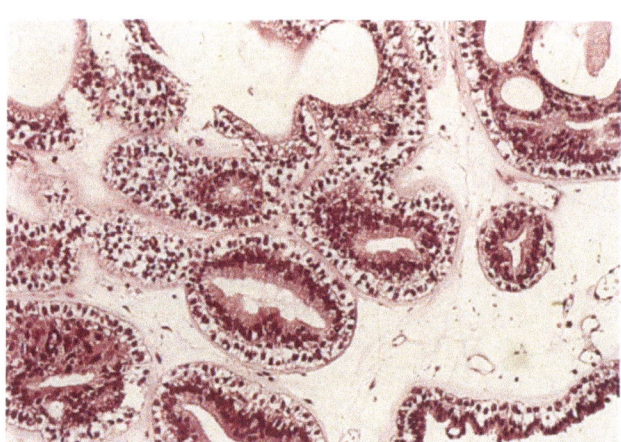

Figure 8.53 Intercalated duct carcinoma. A well differentiated example, with ducts lined by an inner layer of columnar cells with eosinophilic cytoplasm and an outer layer of cells with clear cytoplasm.   H & E × 150

It is the cribriform pattern of adenoid cystic carcinoma that generally causes most difficulty in differential diagnosis, since a somewhat similar pattern can be seen in a number of other tumours. These include other salivary tumours, some odontogenic tumours and even on occasion metastatic deposits in or near the salivary glands. Among salivary tumours monomorphic adenomas have already been mentioned. Adenocarcinoma may also sometimes have a pattern suggestive of adenoid cystic carcinoma. An important distinguishing feature in most of these tumours is, in general, their monocellular structure. The cysts or spaces that may give them a cribriform appearance occur within one type of cell only, whereas in adenoid cystic carcinoma the spaces are ductal as well as stromal.

Adenocarcinoma and Other Carcinomas

Adenocarcinomas are relatively more frequent in the minor than in the major glands, and very often they are well differentiated, low-grade growths. Occasionally they secrete much mucus and sometimes they have a papillary configuration (Figures 8.50 and 8.51). They resemble in general adenocarcinomas in many other tissues[15,16].

Occasionally, as in some other salivary tumours, oncocytic metaplasia may be seen (Figure 8.52). This is a helpful feature in assigning provenance to a tumour that might otherwise have no special appearances to point to its tissue of origin.

A distinctive although uncommon type of adenocarcinoma, the intercalated duct carcinoma, consists of ducts lined by an inner layer of cubical or columnar cells with eosinophilic cytoplasm and an outer layer or layers of cells with clear cytoplasm. Well differentiated tumours of this type tend to be circumscribed and have been described as clear cell adenomas, but the less well differentiated tumours show increasing irregularity of pattern, pleomorphism and mitotic activity, and infiltrative growth (Figures 8.53 and 8.54).

Other types of carcinoma include squamous cell and undifferentiated growths (Figures 8.55 and 8.56). These resemble tumours of the same type elsewhere, and although when encountered in a salivary gland it is likely that this is where they have originated, the possibility of their being metastatic deposits should be considered. Metastatic tumours in the salivary glands are rare, relative to the numbers of primary tumours of salivary tissue, but should be kept in mind as a possibility in unusual cases.

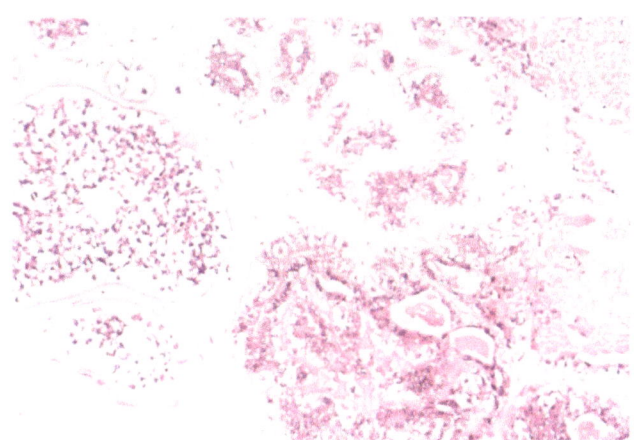

Figure 8.54   This duct carcinoma has a more irregular pattern than the tumour shown in Figure 8.53, and areas of necrosis are present.   H & E × 100

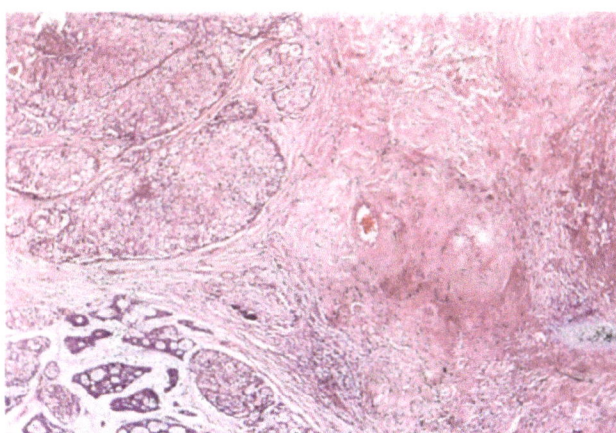

Figure 8.57   Carcinoma in pleomorphic adenoma. Differing histological patterns are present.   H & E × 100

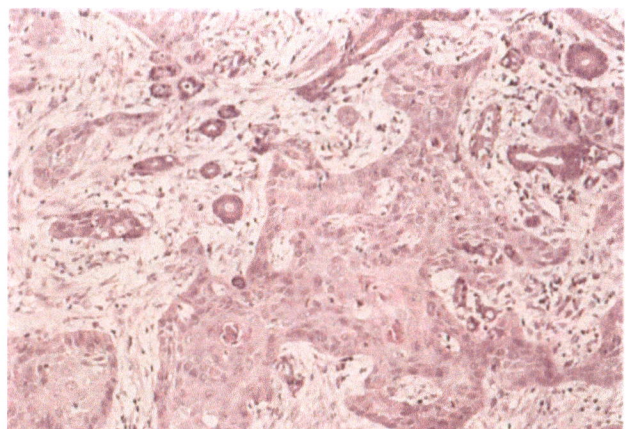

Figure 8.55   Squamous cell carcinoma of submandibular gland. Persisting submandibular ducts can be seen.   H & E × 250

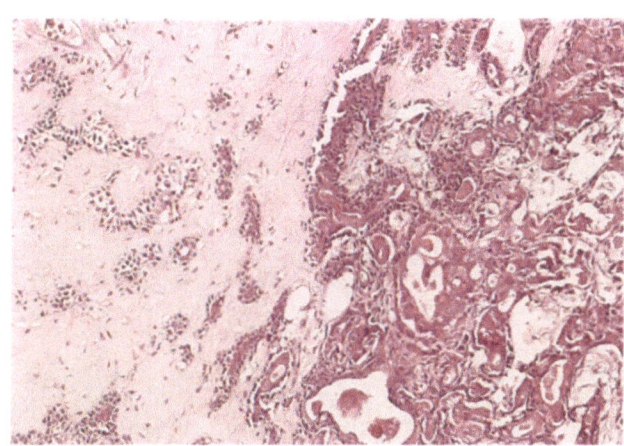

Figure 8.58   Carcinoma in pleomorphic adenoma. Recognizable elements of pleomorphic adenoma are seen on the left. On the right, there is adenocarcinoma. H & E × 100

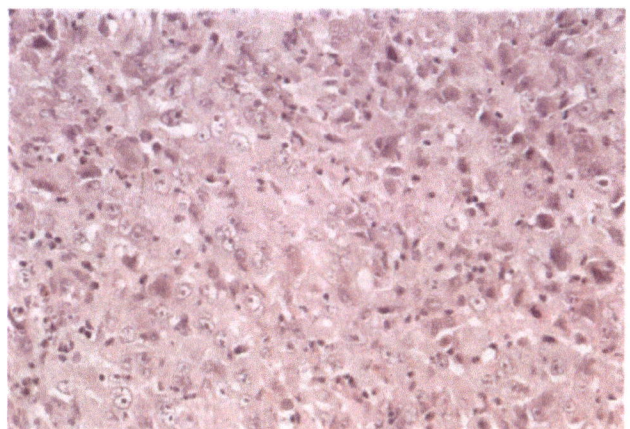

Figure 8.56   Undifferentiated carcinoma of parotid. Pleomorphism and hyperchromatism are marked.   H & E × 250

Most metastases come from primary tumours elsewhere in the head and neck, but they may derive from distant and as yet undiscovered primaries. Some metastases are sufficiently like primary salivary tumours as to be readily taken for them, for example, metastatic renal clear cell carcinoma may mimic a clear cell salivary adenoma, or a metastatic mucus-secreting adenocarcinoma from the gastrointestinal tract may simulate a primary salivary adenocarcinoma or even mucoepidermoid tumour.

Carcinoma in Pleomorphic Adenoma

Malignant change in pleomorphic adenoma occurs either in a primary tumour that has practically always been present for a long time (often 10 years or more), or in one of the nodules of a recurrent pleomorphic adenoma. A third possibility is that a pleomorphic tumour may be malignant from its inception, but this appears to be comparatively rare[17,18].

The carcinoma that appears in a pre-existing pleomorphic adenoma, primary or recurrent, can be of varied histological type. It may, for example, be adenocarcinoma, squamous cell carcinoma, clear cell carcinoma or other type of growth and, a very characteristic feature, more than one of these histological types may be present in the

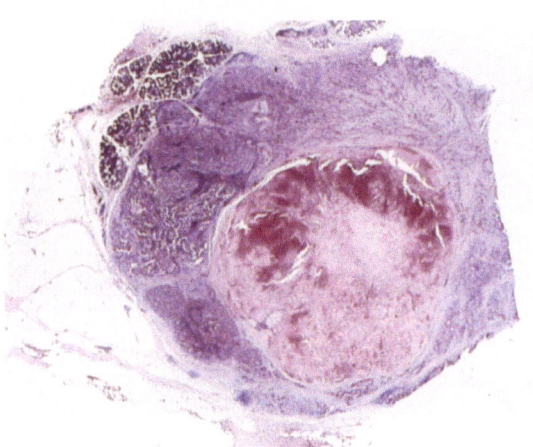

Figure 8.59 Carcinoma in pleomorphic adenoma. The old fibrosed and hyalinized pleomorphic adenoma is seen as the circular eosinophilic area. Around this is the carcinoma, with a small portion of normal parotid at top left.   H & E × 7·5

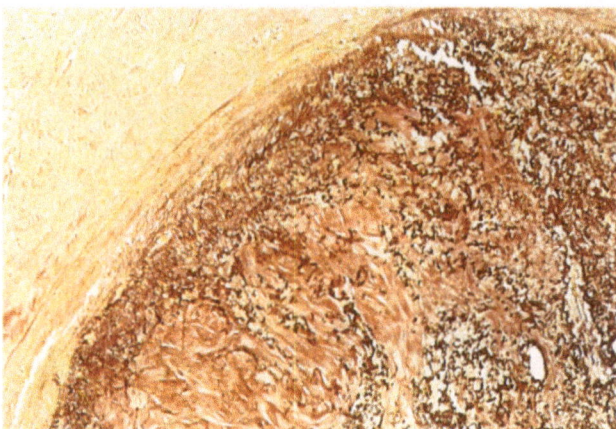

Figure 8.61 A field from the tumour in Figure 8.59, showing numerous strands of material staining positively for elastic.   Weigert × 100

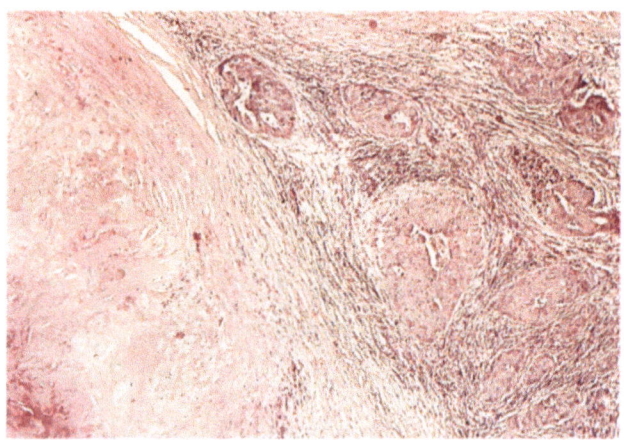

Figure 8.60 A field from the tumour shown in Figure 8.59. The fibrous and hyaline area to the left contains more deeply eosinophilic strands which stain positively with elastic strains. To the right, the carcinoma is seen.   H & E × 100

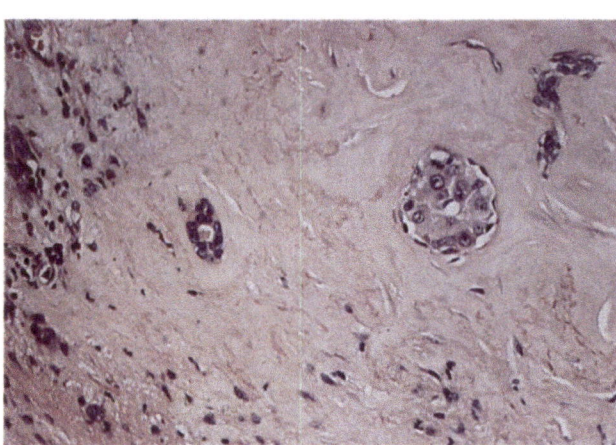

Figure 8.62 Islets of carcinoma in the hyalinized area of a longstanding pleomorphic adenoma.   H & E × 250

same tumour (Figure 8.57). Parts of the original pleomorphic adenoma may still be apparent, but not infrequently these may be difficult to find (Figure 8.58). In this event the diagnosis is presumptive, depending on a combination of the histological features, especially if two or more types of carcinoma are present, and the long history, possibly with one or more previous attempts at removal. When there are extensive areas of scarring in a salivary carcinoma, and especially when significant amounts of elastic tissue can be demonstrated, origin from a pleomorphic adenoma should always be considered (Figures 8.59–8.63).

Non-epithelial Tumours

Mesenchymal and other non-epithelial tumours of the salivary glands are rare. Haemangioma, usually in the parotid, is found in infants as a locally infiltrative growth and is probably the best known. Fibrosarcoma, neural tumours, lymphomas and others have all been noted, less commonly.

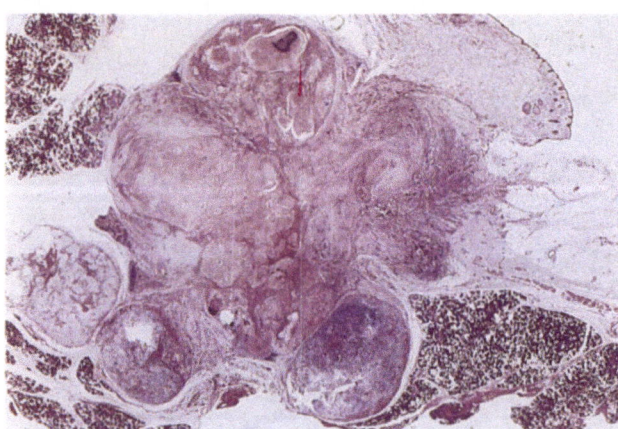

Figure 8.63 Carcinoma arising in recurrent pleomorphic adenoma. Three nodules of recurrent tumour with the usual appearances of pleomorphic adenoma are seen at the lower edge of the section, with some normal parotid tissue at each side. Above these nodules there is a large area of relatively homogeneous appearance representing an islet of recurrent tumour that has become carcinomatous.   H & E × 2·5

References

1. Thackray, A. C. and Sobin, L. (1972). *International Histological Classification of Tumours. Histological Typing of Salivary Gland Tumours.* (Geneva: World Health Organization)

2. Thackray, A. C. and Lucas, R. B. (1974). *Tumors of the Major Salivary Glands.* Atlas of Tumor Pathology—Second Series—Fascicle 10. (Washington, D.C.: Armed Forces Institute of Pathology)

3. Evans, R. W. and Cruickshank, A. H. (1970). *Epithelial Tumours of the Salivary Glands.* (Philadelphia: W. B. Saunders Company)

4. Lomax-Smith, J. D. and Azzopardi, J. G. (1978). The hyaline cell: a distinctive feature of 'mixed' salivary tumours. *Histopathology,* **2**, 77

5. Seifert, G., Bull, H. G. and Donath, K. (1980). Histologic sub-classification of the cystadenolymphoma of the parotid gland. *Virchows Arch. (Path. Anat.),* **388**, 13

6. Gray, S. R., Cornog, J. L. and Seo, I. S. (1976). Oncocytic neo-plasms of salivary glands. A report of fifteen cases including two malignant oncocytomas. *Cancer,* **38**, 1306

7. Crumpler, C., Scharfenberg, J. C. and Reed, R. J. (1976). Mono-morphic adenomas of salivary glands. Trabecular–tubular, canal-icular, and basaloid varieties. *Cancer,* **38**, 193

8. Fantasia, J. E. and Neville, B. W. (1980). Basal cell adenomas of the minor salivary glands. A clinicopathologic study of seventeen new cases and a review of the literature. *Oral Surg.,* **50**, 433

9. Sciubba, J. J. and Brannon, R. B. (1982). Myoepithelioma of salivary glands: report of twenty-three cases. *Cancer,* **49**, 562

10. Healey, W. V., Perzin, K. H. and Smith, L. (1970). Mucoepidermoid carcinoma of salivary gland origin. Classification, clinical–patho-logic correlation, and results of treatment. *Cancer,* **26**, 368

11. Melrose, R. J., Abrams, A. M. and Howell, F. V. (1973). Muco-epidermoid tumors of the intraoral minor salivary glands: a clinico-pathologic study of fifty-four cases. *J. Oral Path.,* **2**, 314

12. Spiro, R. H., Huvos, A. G. and Strong, E. W. (1978). Acinic cell carcinoma of salivary origin. *Cancer,* **41**, 924

13. Perzin, K. H., Gullane, P. and Clairmont, A. C. (1978). Adenoid cystic carcinomas arising in salivary glands. A correlation of histo-logic features and clinical course. *Cancer,* **42**, 265

14. Tarpley, T. M. and Giansanti, J. S. (1976). Adenoid cystic carci-noma. Analysis of fifty oral cases. *Oral Surg.,* **41**, 484

15. Blanck, C., Eneroth, C.-M. and Jakobsson, P. A. (1971). Mucus-producing adenopapillary (non-epidermoid) carcinoma of the parotid gland. *Cancer,* **28**, 676

16. Allen, M. S., Fitz-Hugh, G. S. and Marsh, W. L. (1974). Low-grade papillary adenocarcinoma of the palate. *Cancer,* **33**, 153

17. LiVolsi, V. A. and Perzin, K. H. (1977). Malignant mixed tumors arising in salivary glands. 1. Carcinomas arising in benign mixed tumors: a clinicopathologic study. *Cancer,* **39**, 2209

18. Spiro, R. H., Huvos, A. G. and Strong, E. W. (1975). Cancer of the parotid gland. A clinicopathologic study of 288 primary cases. *Am. J. Surg.,* **130**, 452

Cysts of the Oral Tissues

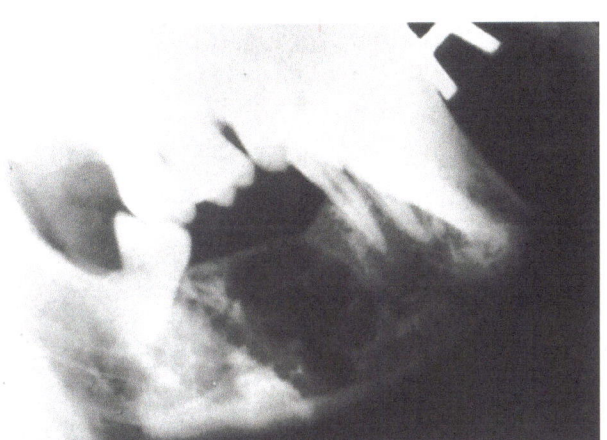

Figure 9.1   Odontogenic keratocyst. The radiograph shows a well defined area of radiolucency with irregular outline and multilocular appearance.

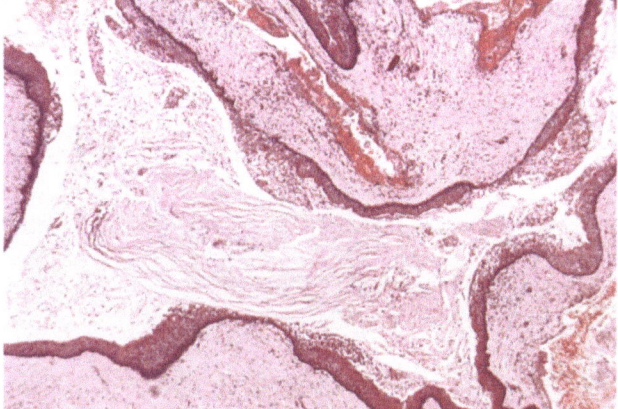

Figure 9.2   The keratocyst extends and ramifies extensively. The epithelial lining is thin and tends to separate in places from the underlying connective tissue. H & E × 70

Cysts in the oral tissues fall into two main groups: odontogenic cysts associated with the dental tissues, and non-odontogenic cysts[1].

ODONTOGENIC CYSTS

These cysts are of developmental origin, or they are inflammatory.

Developmental Cysts

Odontogenic Keratocyst (primordial cyst)

This type of cyst originates in odontogenic epithelium, possibly in some cases before a tooth has formed and thus replacing it, or in odontogenic rests. In either case, there need be no close relationship between the cyst and a tooth such as occurs with dentigerous or radicular cysts. There may be extensive involvement of the jaw before there is any expansion, and these cysts may thus be very large at the time of discovery. They are usually detected in young adults, but because of the symptomless growth they may be seen in older patients also. Radiographs show a well defined radiolucency that may appear to be multilocular or unilocular with a scalloped margin and that may ramify extensively in the jaw (Figure 9.1). Unless there has been superadded infection with consequent inflammatory infiltration and thickening, the cyst wall which is otherwise very thin almost invariably ruptures during removal, when it has the macroscopic appearance of a collapsed balloon.

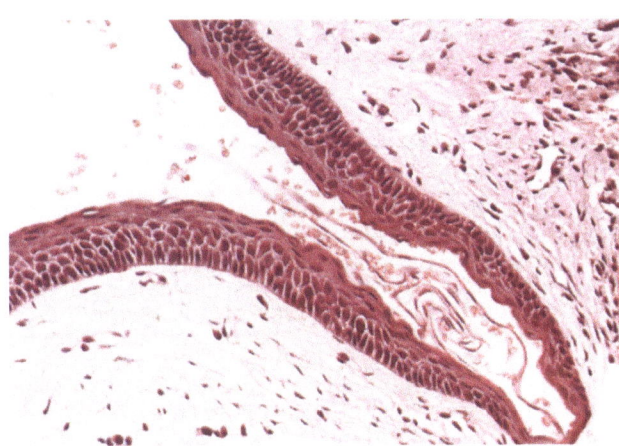

Figure 9.3   Higher magnification, showing the regularity of the keratocyst lining, with its prominent basal layer and parakeratosis in the superficial layers.   H & E × 250

Microscopically, the cyst wall consists of fibrous tissue with a regular lining of squamous epithelium without the downgrowths and variations in thickness that are so commonly seen in radicular cysts (Figures 9.2 and 9.3). The lining is quite narrow, a few cells only in depth, with keratinization at the surface adjacent to the lumen. Sometimes there is a definite but narrow layer of keratin, or there may be parakeratosis only. Keratin scales may be present

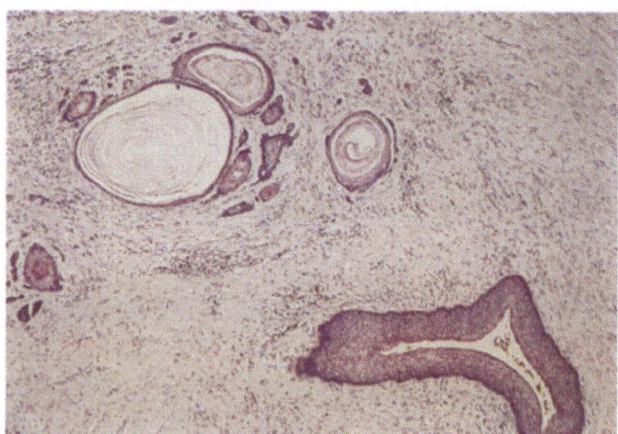

Figure 9.4 Small apparently isolated islands of epithelium in the wall of a keratocyst, and microcysts containing keratin scales.   H & E × 100

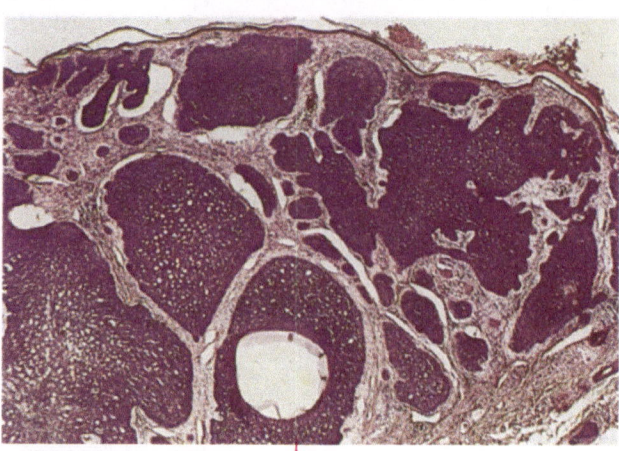

Figure 9.6 A basal cell carcinoma from a case of the naevoid carcinoma and multiple jaw cyst syndrome.   H & E × 70

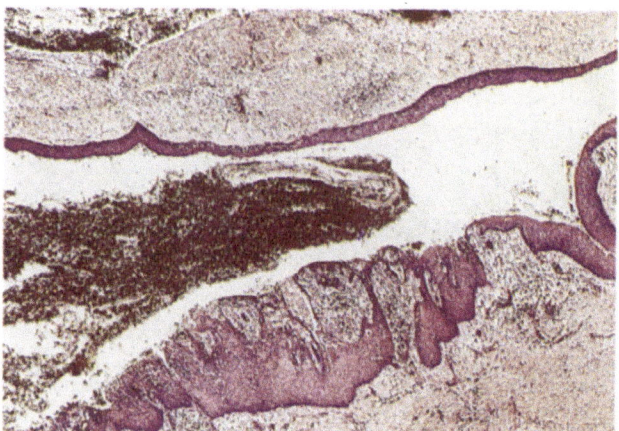

Figure 9.5 Infected keratocyst. There is chronic inflammatory infiltration throughout the cyst wall. Where this is relatively light, as in the upper part of the field, the lining epithelium preserves its usual characteristics, but elsewhere, where the infiltration is more pronounced, the epithelium has proliferated.   H & E × 100

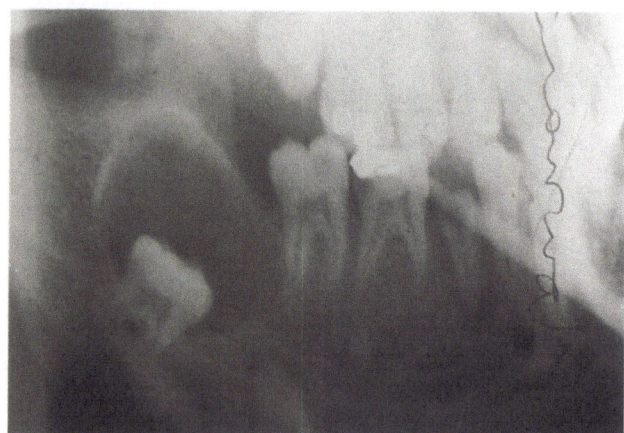

Figure 9.7 Dentigerous cyst. The crown of an unerupted tooth is surrounded by a well defined radiolucency.

in the lumen. The lining is very regular and without rete processes, although occasionally there may be bud-like protuberances. The basal layer, composed of low columnar or cuboidal cells with well stained nuclei stands out distinctly (Figure 9.3). Small groups of odontogenic type epithelial cells may be seen in the subepithelial fibrous tissue. These cell groups, when present, help to confirm that the lesion is developmental. They may also be seen in the dentigerous cyst but not in inflammatory or nonodontogenic cysts. Some of these groups of cells can develop into microcysts (Figure 9.4).

The cyst wall is frequently convoluted and the attachment between epithelium and connective tissue appears to be rather weak, since in the course of histological preparation partial separation is often seen. No doubt this weakness accounts for some of the difficulty experienced in enucleating these cysts completely, and the consequent high rate of recurrence. Inflammation is generally absent unless the cyst has eroded the cortex of the bone and thus communicates with the oral cavity. Chronic inflammatory infiltration of varying degree is then seen. The epithelium in inflamed areas tends to lose its specific character and becomes much more like the epithelium of a radicular cyst (Figure 9.5). This should be borne in mind when dealing with small biopsy specimens[2].

Naevoid Carcinoma and Multiple Jaw Cyst Syndrome

The multiple jaw cysts present in this syndrome are keratocysts similar to those that arise as solitary lesions in otherwise normal persons. They are first seen in childhood, and may continue to appear for many years. The basal cell carcinomas are also multiple. They usually appear about puberty and, as do the cysts, may continue to occur throughout the patient's lifetime. They may appear in any area of skin, but the face, trunk and arms are especially common sites of involvement (Figure 9.6). There are also many other abnormalities that may be present in the syndrome, including skeletal abnormalities, skin cysts and tumours and neurological conditions[3].

Dentigerous Cyst

If cyst formation takes place in the remaining layers of the enamel organ that cover the crown of a tooth when it has been fully formed, a dentigerous cyst results. The tooth remains embedded in the jaw with its crown protruding into the cyst, which is attached to the tooth at the cementum-enamel junction. Whether it is the cyst formation that prevents eruption of the affected tooth, or whether teeth that fail to erupt for other reasons are especially liable to form dentigerous cysts, is not certain[1].

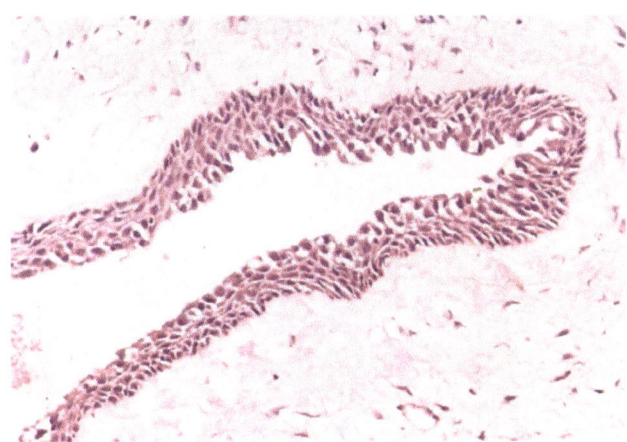

Figure 9.8 Dentigerous cyst. The wall consists of fibrous tissue with a lining of squamous epithelium.   H & E × 250

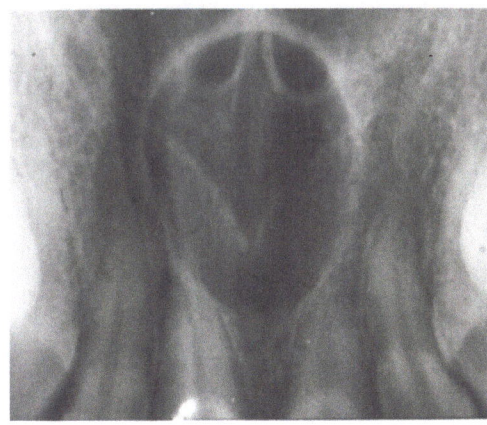

Figure 9.9 Nasopalatine duct cyst. The cyst appears as a radiolucency in the midline of the palate, displacing the roots of the central incisor teeth.

Dentigerous cysts can enlarge to a considerable size and replace much bone. They are usually detected in children or adolescents and they can cause appreciable expansion of the jaw. They are associated only with permanent teeth. Radiographs show a well defined radiolucency around the crown of an unerupted tooth (Figure 9.7).

The cyst is lined by a regular layer of stratified squamous epithelium, a few cells in depth (Figure 9.8). Occasional mucous cells may be present. Small islets of odontogenic epithelium like those that are sometimes seen in keratocysts may also be seen in dentigerous cysts, situated in the connective tissue some little distance beneath the epithelial lining. Again, like keratocysts, dentigerous cysts may open into the mouth. Where this has happened infection, usually low-grade, ensues, with chronic inflammatory infiltration. The epithelium proliferates and the microscopic appearances are then very similar to those of the radicular cyst.

Figure 9.10 Nasopalatine duct cyst. The cyst is lined by squamous epithelium with occasional mucous cells. Small blood vessels and nerves are seen in the fibrous tissue of the cyst wall.   H & E × 50

Inflammatory Cysts

Radicular Cyst (dental cyst, apical cyst, periapical cyst)

This is the commonest cyst of the oral region. It is inflammatory in origin and usually results from dental caries (page 33).

NON-ODONTOGENIC CYSTS
Developmental Cysts

There are a number of cysts in the oral region which are unrelated to the dental tissues and are collectively described as developmental, since they form in situations where it has been postulated that there are epithelial residues in the areas of contiguity of the embryonic facial processes. Although the precise nature and origin of some of them is a matter of dispute these cysts are recognizable clinicopathological entities. They include the following lesions, which may be asymptomatic and discovered incidentally, but which may give rise to pain and swelling if they become infected.

Nasopalatine Duct Cyst

This cyst is situated in the nasopalatine (incisive) canal, where it produces a clearly demarcated radiolucency that is heart-shaped, ovoid or round, situated between or above the maxillary central incisor teeth (Figure 9.9). It is lined by stratified squamous epithelium, ciliated columnar epithelium, or both types of epithelium may be present (Figure 9.10). Small blood vessels, nerve bundles and mucous glands are often seen in the subepithelial connective tissue[4].

Median Palatal Cyst

Situated in the midline of the palate, this cyst is probably a variety of nasopalatine duct cyst.

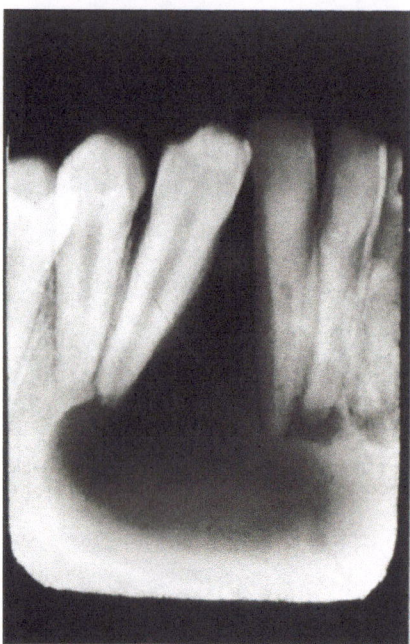

Figure 9.11 Median mandibular cyst. A well defined radiolucency is seen in the symphysis area.

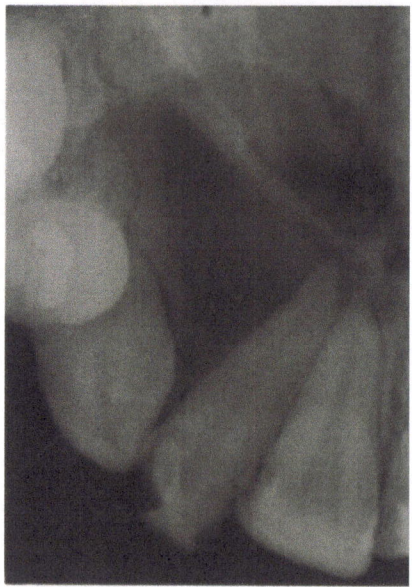

Figure 9.13 Globulomaxillary cyst. There is a radiolucency between the roots of the lateral incisor and canine teeth, which are diverged.

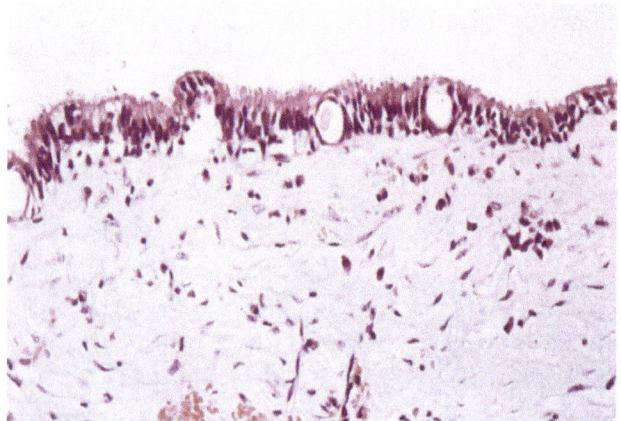

Figure 9.12 Median mandibular cyst. This cyst was lined by squamous and by ciliated columnar epithelium. An area with the latter is shown here. H & E × 250

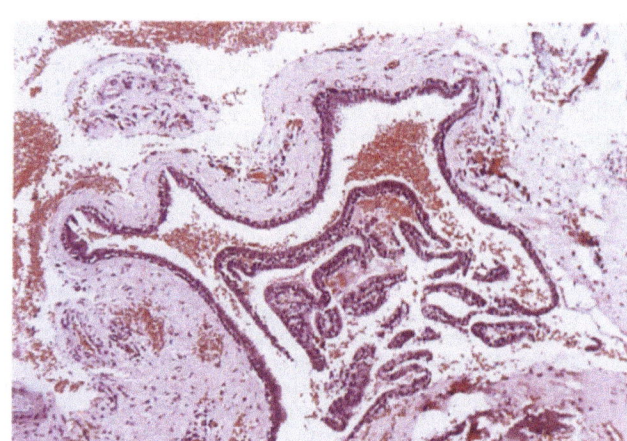

Figure 9.14 Globulomaxillary cyst. The cyst wall is lined by columnar and cubical epithelium. H & E × 100

Median Mandibular Cyst

This cyst is situated in the midline of the mandible. Radiographs show a radiolucency near the central incisor teeth (Figure 9.11). The cyst is lined by stratified squamous epithelium, possibly with areas of columnar epithelium (Figure 9.12). There should be no evidence of inflammatory changes, otherwise the lesion may be a radicular cyst associated with an adjacent tooth[5].

Globulomaxillary Cyst

The globulomaxillary cyst is situated between the roots of the maxillary lateral incisor and canine teeth, where it produces a radiolucency resembling an inverted pear (Figure 9.13). The cyst is lined by stratified squamous or ciliated columnar epithelium[6] (Figure 9.14).

Nasolabial Cyst

This is a soft tissue cyst, arising in the tissues subjacent to the nasolabial fold below the alae nasi. It is lined by stratified squamous or columnar epithelium[7] (Figure 9.15).

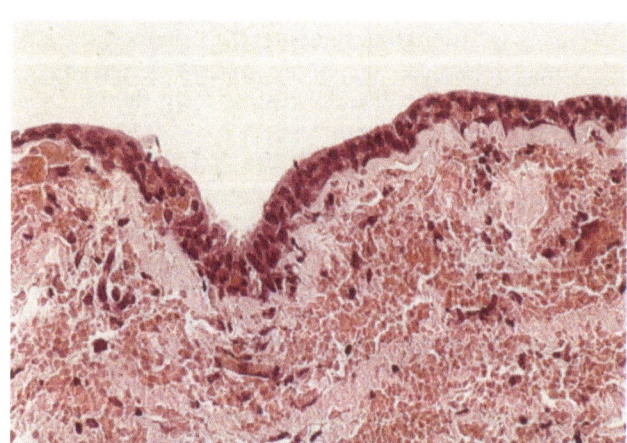

Figure 9.15 Nasolabial cyst. The lining consists of flattened squamous and low cubical epithelium. H & E × 250

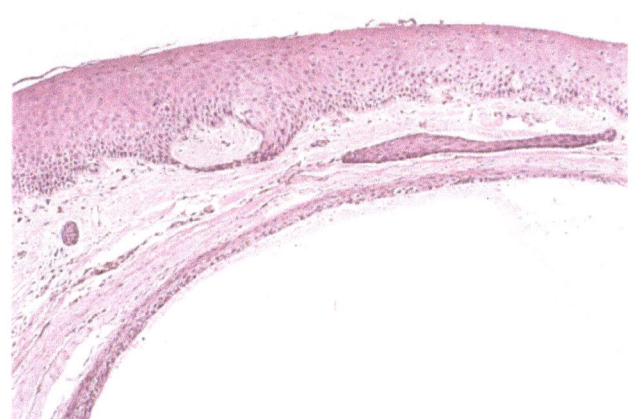

Figure 9.16 Gingival cyst. The cyst is situated in the gingiva a short distance from the oral epithelium. The lining consists of flattened squamous epithelium. H & E × 100

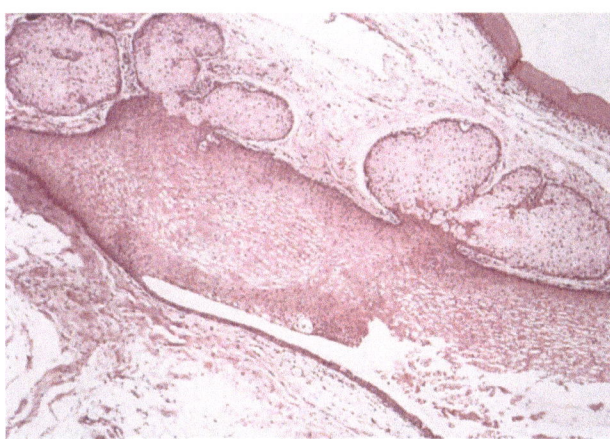

Figure 9.18 Dermoid cyst of cheek. The lining consists of squamous epithelium with sebaceous differentiation. H & E × 60

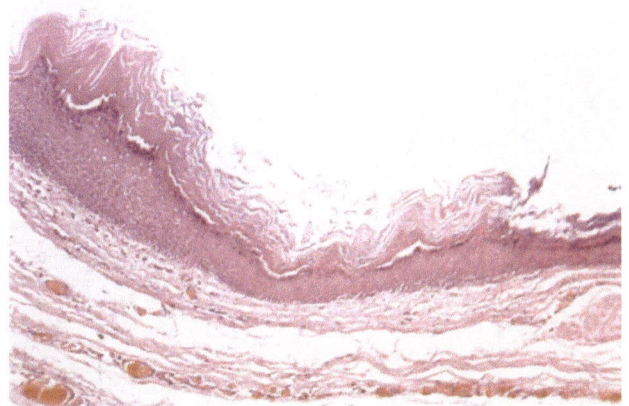

Figure 9.17 Implantation cyst of lip, lined by squamous epithelium and containing keratin scales. H & E × 100

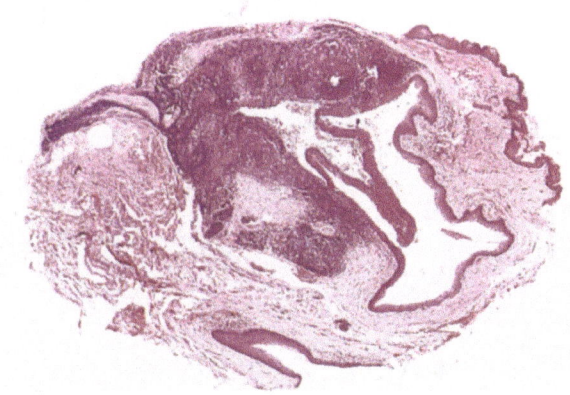

Figure 9.19 Lymphoepithelial cyst of floor of mouth. The cyst is lined mainly by squamous epithelium, with lymphoid tissue in the subepithelial fibrous tissue. H & E × 15

Soft Tissue Cysts

Nasolabial Cyst

This cyst has already been mentioned with the developmental cysts.

Salivary Cyst (Mucocele)

See page 85.

Gingival Cyst

Small cysts in the gingivae are occasionally found in infants. They probably arise in epithelial residues from the dental lamina and it seems likely that most of them involute and disappear, since they are seldom found after the age of 3 months. In adults, cysts in the gingivae may be found at any age and probably have a varied etiology, including an origin from epithelial rests or from implantation of surface epithelium[8].

Gingival cysts are lined by squamous or occasionally cuboidal epithelium (Figure 9.16).

Epidermoid and Dermoid Cysts

These designations are used for a variety of cysts. Epidermoid cysts are lined simply by squamous epithelium, and may contain keratin scales (Figure 9.17). Dermoid cysts may have sebaceous glands, sweat glands and hair follicles in the cyst wall, and rarely other tissues such as muscle, bone and respiratory or alimentary epithelium (Figure 9.18). These cysts are most often seen in the floor of the mouth and the tongue[9].

Lymphoepithelial Cyst

These cysts have the same structure as the branchial cysts of the neck (Figure 9.19). In the oral tissues they are seen, as not very common lesions, in those areas where lymphoid tissue is normally present[10].

Thyroglossal Cyst

In the oral tissues thyroglossal cysts may arise at the foramen caecum in the posterior part of the tongue and in the floor of the mouth. In this area the cyst lining is usually squamous epithelium, but occasionally ciliated respiratory type epithelium may be present, although this is much more often found in those cysts that are situated below the level of the hyoid bone[11].

Aberrant thyroid tissue may be found in the tongue, where it can form a tumour-like mass if cervical thyroid insufficiency has induced its hyperplasia.

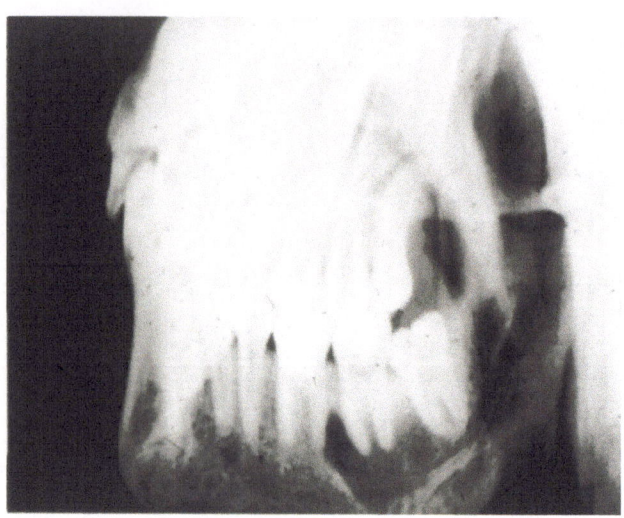

Figure 9.20   Solitary bone cyst. The radiograph shows a well defined radio-lucency in the body of the mandible near the angle.

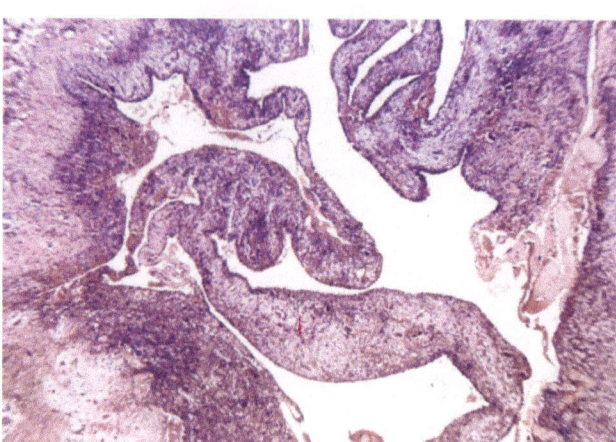

Figure 9.22   Aneurysmal bone cyst. Intercommunicating spaces are lined by connective tissue in which there are areas of osteoid.   H & E × 40

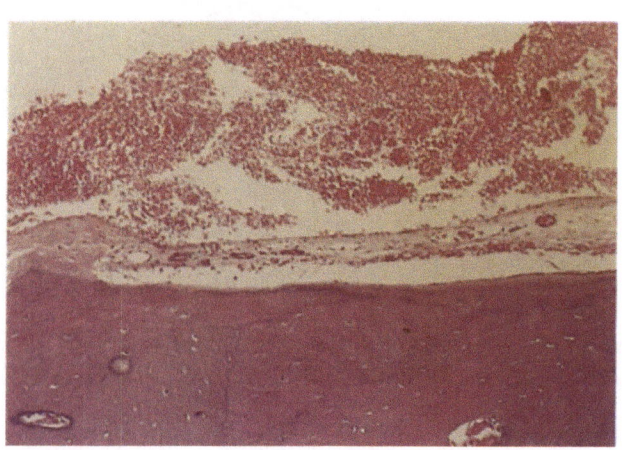

Figure 9.21   Solitary bone cyst. The cyst wall consists of connective tissue only.
H & E × 100

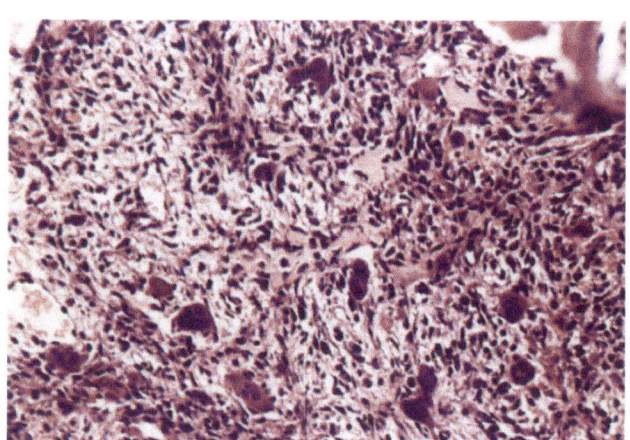

Figure 9.23   A field showing numerous giant cells.   H & E × 250

Bone Cysts

Simple Bone Cyst
(solitary bone cyst; haemorrhagic bone cyst)

This lesion of children and young adults is seen occasionally in the jaws, mainly the mandible and much less often the maxilla. Since it is generally painless it is usually discovered during routine examination. The posterior part of the mandible is the common location, where the lesion presents as a well defined radiolucency (Figure 9.20). When biopsy is carried out the cyst is found to have only a thin connective tissue lining, with perhaps some small accumulations of granulation tissue (Figure 9.21). Otherwise; the contents comprise only a little clear or blood-stained fluid[12]. Minimal surgical intervention, even biopsy, almost invariably leads to resolution of the lesion.

Aneurysmal Bone Cyst

This lesion is rare in the jaws. When it does occur the appearances are the same as in other bones, but in the jaws there may be some local diagnostic difficulties. Microscopically, the lesion consists of numerous capillaries and blood-filled spaces in a connective tissue matrix. Areas of old and recent haemorrhage are seen, and there are usually numerous multinucleated giant cells, especially around areas of haemorrhage. Osteoid is also often present (Figures 9.22–9.24). Some areas of giant cell granuloma of the jaws can closely resemble aneurysmal bone cyst and in fact a relationship between the two conditions has been postulated. There also appears to be a relationship between aneurysmal bone cyst and other bone lesions such as fibrous dysplasia and ossifying fibroma, since appearances typical of aneurysmal bone cyst and these other bone conditions can sometimes be found in the same lesion[13].

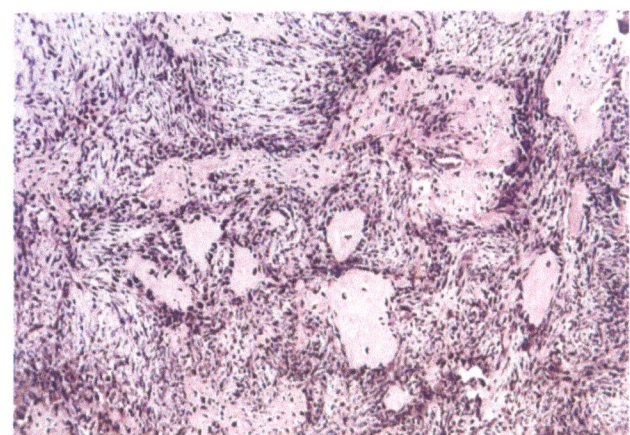

Figure 9.24 A field showing florid osteoid formation. H & E × 100

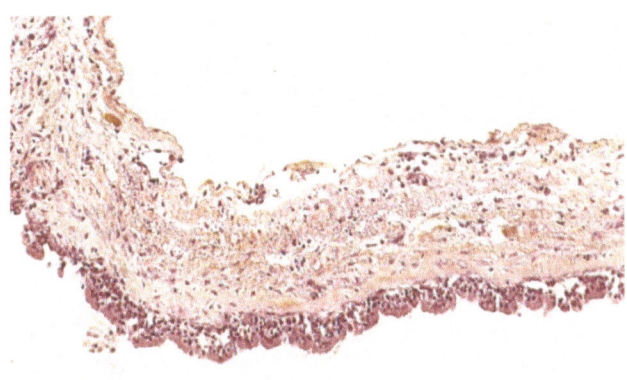

Figure 9.25 Maxillary antral cyst. A post-operative cyst, lined by columnar epithelium. H & E × 250

References

1. Shear, M. (1983). *Cysts of the Oral Regions*. 2nd Edn. (London, Boston: Wright PSG)
2. Hodgkinson, D. J., Woods, J. E., Dahlin, D. C. and Tolman, D. E. (1978). Keratocysts of the jaw. Clinicopathologic study of 79 patients. *Cancer*, **41**, 803
3. Donatsky, O., Hjørting-Hansen, E., Philipsen, H. P. and Fejerskov, O. (1976). Clinical, radiologic, and histopathologic aspects of 13 cases of nevoid basal cell carcinoma syndrome. *Int. J. Oral Surg.*, **5**, 19
4. Courage, G. R., North, A. F. and Hansen, L. S. (1974). Median palatine cysts. Review of the literature and report of a case. *Oral Surg.*, **37**, 745
5. White, D. K., Lucas, R. M. and Miller, A. S. (1975). Median mandibular cyst: review of the literature and report of two cases. *J. Oral Surg.*, **33**, 372
6. Hollinshead, M. B. and Schneider, L. C. (1980). A histologic and embryologic analysis of so-called globulomaxillary cysts. *Int. J. Oral Surg.*, **9**, 281
7. Roed-Petersen, B. (1969). Nasolabial cysts. A presentation of five patients with a review of the literature. *Brit. J. Oral Surg.*, **7**, 84
8. Moskow, B. S., Siegel, K., Zegarelli, E. V., Kutscher, A. H. and Rothenberg, F. (1970). Gingival and lateral periodontal cysts. *J. Periodont.*, **41**, 249
9. Kelln, E. E. (1965). Oral epidermal cysts and probable histogenesis. Report of a case. *Oral Surg.*, **19**, 359
10. Buchner, A. and Hansen, L. S. (1980). Lymphoepithelial cysts of the oral cavity. A clinicopathologic study of 38 cases. *Oral Surg.*, **50**, 441
11. Wampler, H. W., Krolls, S. O. and Johnson, R. P. (1978). Thyroglossal-tract cyst. *Oral Surg.*, **45**, 32
12. Hansen, L. S., Sapone, J. and Sproat, R. C. (1974). Traumatic bone cysts of jaws. Report of 66 cases. *Oral Surg.*, **37**, 899
13. Steidler, N. E., Cook, R. M. and Reade, P. C. (1979). Aneurysmal bone cysts of the jaws: a case report and review of the literature. *Brit. J. Oral Surg.*, **16**, 254
14. Kaneshiro, S., Nakajima, T., Yoshikawa, Y., Iwasaki, H. and Tokiwa, N. (1980). The postoperative maxillary cyst: report of 71 cases. *J. Oral Surg.*, **39**, 191

Maxillary Antral Cysts

Cysts lined by fibrous or granulation tissue and very seldom by epithelium may be found in the maxillary antrum. These *mucosal cysts* resemble the common mucous extravasation cysts of the lip and elsewhere in the oral mucosa, and they probably arise from mucous glands in the antral lining. They grow very slowly, are frequently asymptomatic and are usually detected on routine radiographic examination.

Postoperative or *surgical maxillary cysts* are seen in patients who have a history of sinus infections and surgical treatment. When the cyst appears, characteristically many years after the original surgery, it gives rise to swelling in the maxillary region which may be accompanied by pain and purulent discharge. Cysts of this type are thought to arise in epithelium implanted in the wound of the original surgical operation. They have a thin fibrous tissue wall with a lining of ciliated columnar epithelium (Figure 9.25). There may also be areas of cubical or squamous epithelium[14].

Tumours of the Oral Tissues
1. Odontogenic Tumours

10

The odontogenic tumours arise from the dental tissues either during the period of active development of the teeth or after tooth formation has been completed. In the former case the tumours arise in the developing tissues and they are in this sense embryonic tumours. In the latter, they develop from the remnants of the odontogenic tissues in the jaws after the teeth have been fully formed. Odontogenic tumours are therefore often seen in children and adolescents, but they also occur in adults of all age groups since the odontogenic tissue remnants, or rests, persist throughout life. Moreover, since most of the odontogenic tumours are benign and grow relatively slowly, often with few symptoms, they may have been present for a long time before being detected.

Most odontogenic tumours are intraosseous, although occasional examples are confined to the soft tissues. The information accompanying the biopsy specimen should tell the pathologist if there is a swelling of the mandible or maxilla, and it should also inform him of the radiological appearances, as this investigation will almost certainly have been done. It is, in fact, advantageous for the pathologist to see the films himself, as they will give a good idea of the site and extent of the lesion. Microscopic examination will show a tumour that in most cases has a variable degree of resemblance to normal developing dental tissues[1,2]. The developing tooth consists at first of epithelium only, then of epithelium and mesenchyme, followed by the appearance of dentine, enamel and cementum, so similarly odontogenic tumours show varying degrees of differentiation. A morphological classification can be made on this basis and this is of practical value in arriving at a histological diagnosis.

Morphological Classification of Odontogenic Tumours

1. *Tumours consisting principally of odontogenic epithelium*

Although the tumours in this group are essentially cellular lesions, they may contain calcified material:

Ameloblastoma
   Small amorphous calcifications may be present but are very rare.
Adenomatoid odontogenic tumour
   Small scattered amorphous calcifications are common. Tubular dentine may rarely form.

Calcifying epithelial odontogenic tumour
   Calcification is an abundant and distinctive feature.
Calcifying odontogenic cyst
   Dentine and enamel may be seen.

2. *Tumours consisting of odontogenic epithelium and mesenchyme*

These tumours consist of two neoplastic elements:
Ameloblastic fibroma.
Ameloblastic sarcoma.

3. *Tumours consisting of odontogenic epithelium and calcified dental tissues*

Odontoameloblastoma
   The epithelium is similar to that in ameloblastoma, but mature dentine and enamel are also present.

4. *Tumours consisting of calcified dental tissues, but without odontogenic epithelium (except that directly associated with the formation of the calcified tissue)*

Complex odontome
   An irregular mass of enamel, dentine and cementum.
Compound odontome
   The calcified tissues are organized into recognizable tooth-like structures. Many such teeth may be present, in a fibrous capsule.
Enameloma
   A lesion consisting of small ectopic deposits of enamel on a tooth.
Dentinoma
   A lesion in which the only calcified tissue is dentine.
Cementoma
   A basically fibrous lesion in which cementum or cementum-like tissue is also present.

5. *Tumours consisting of odontogenic mesenchyme*

These lesions are basically fibrous, but they may also contain small groups of odontogenic epithelial cells:
Odontogenic fibroma.
Odontogenic myxoma.

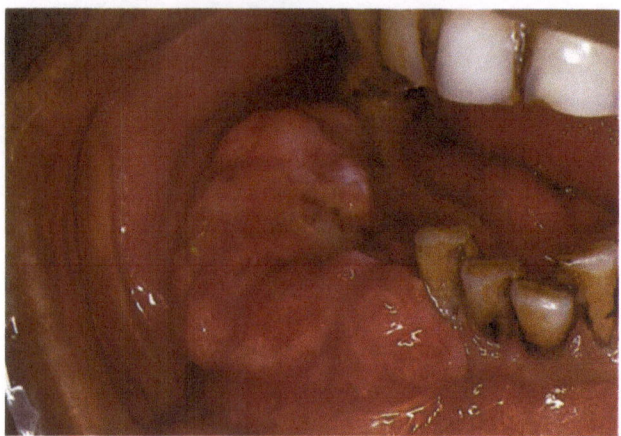

Figure 10.1 Ameloblastoma. A tumour of some years duration, appearing as an irregular expansion of the mandible, buccally and lingually. There is ulceration of the overlying mucosa

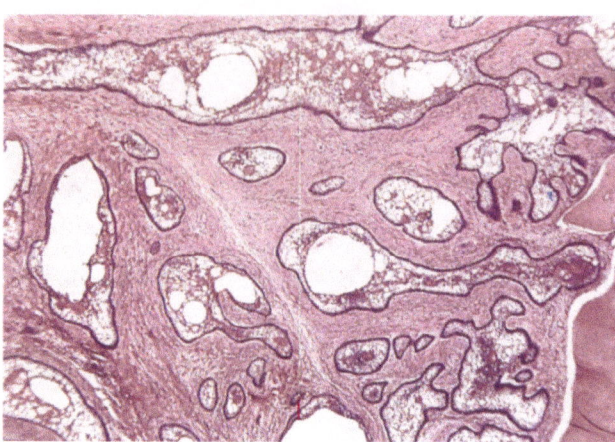

Figure 10.4 The follicular type of ameloblastoma. The tumour consists of islets of follicles of epithelium in a fibrous stroma. Microcyst formation in the follicles is common.   H & E × 50

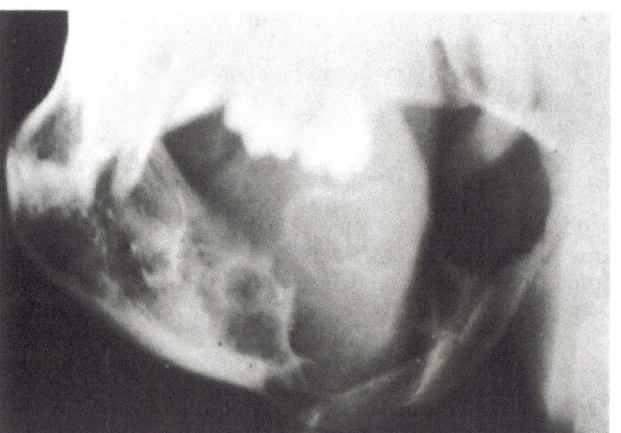

Figure 10.2 Ameloblastoma. The radiograph shows a large multilocular radiolucency extending from the body of the mandible into the ramus

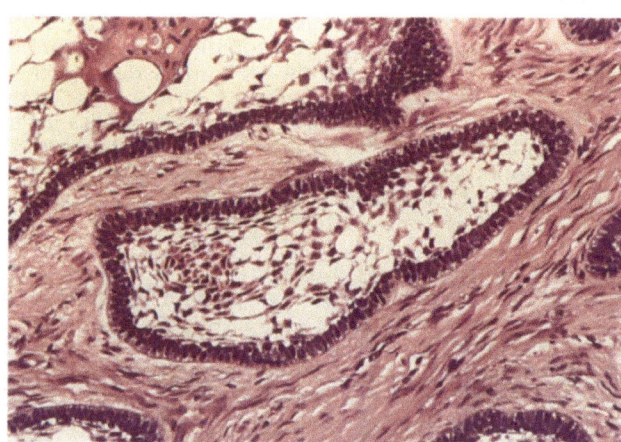

Figure 10.5 Higher magnification of an islet, showing it to consist of stellate cells similar to those of the stellate reticulum of the developing tooth germ surrounded by a peripheral layer of cubical or columnar cells.   H & E × 250

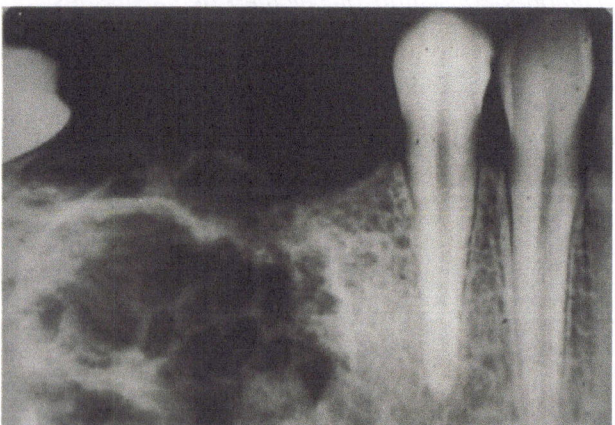

Figure 10.3 Ameloblastoma. This intraoral radiograph shows a multilocular radiolucency

Ameloblastoma

This tumour arises mainly in the mandible (80%), at any age[2]. Most patients are in the third and fourth decades. It grows very slowly and is usually symptomless, apart from gradually increasing facial asymmetry (Figure 10.1). There are two main modes of growth: as a solid or semisolid tumour with or without cystic spaces of variable size, and as a unilocular cystic lesion. Correspondingly, the radiographic appearances are a multilocular radiolucency expanding the jaw (Figures 10.2 and 10.3), or a unilocular radiolucency frequently associated with an unerupted tooth, and thus resembling a dentigerous cyst (page 104).

Microscopically, the tumour consists of odontogenic epithelium in a fibrous stroma. The epithelium is arranged either in discrete islets (follicular type) or in continuous interconnected strands (plexiform type). Both arrangements may be found in different parts of the same tumour. The islets of epithelium resemble the enamel organ of the developing tooth germ, consisting of a central area of

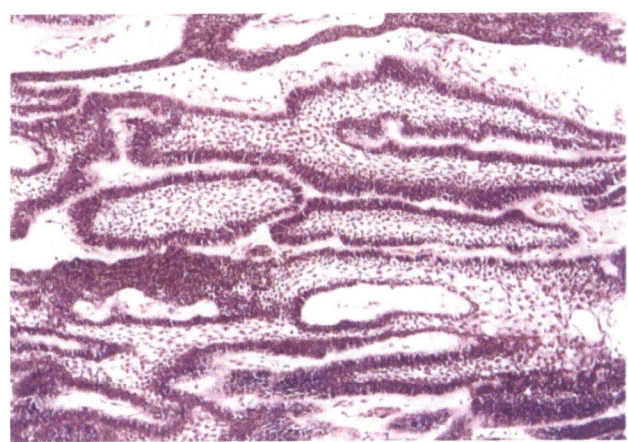

Figure 10.6 The plexiform pattern in ameloblastoma. The tumour epithelium forms continuous interconnected strands. As in the follicular type of tumour, cysts are present in the epithelium. They are also present in the stroma. H & E × 75

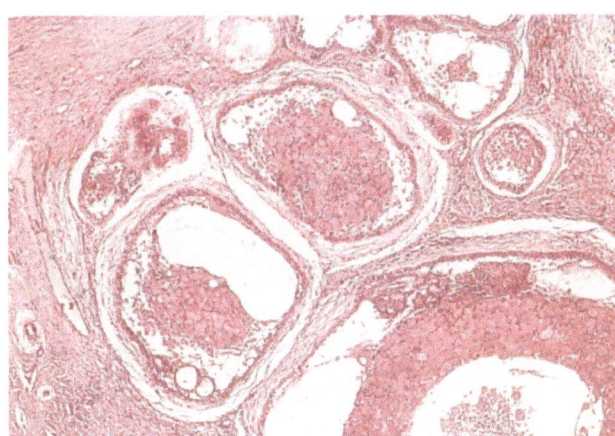

Figure 10.8 Granular cells in ameloblastoma. The stellate cells of the tumour follicles have been largely replaced by granular cells. H & E × 100

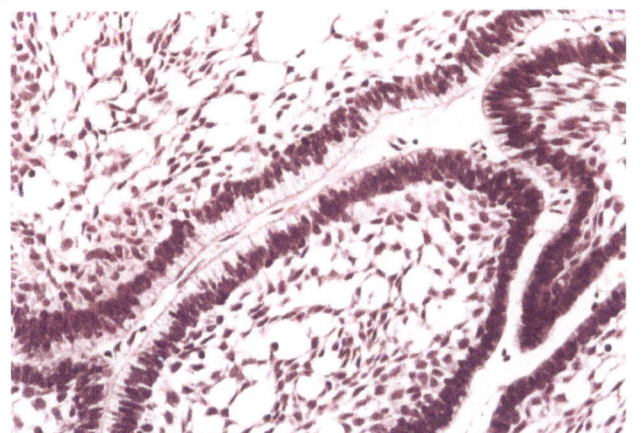

Figure 10.7 A field from the tumour in Figure 10.6, showing the stellate cells of the epithelial strands bordered by columnar cells. H & E × 250

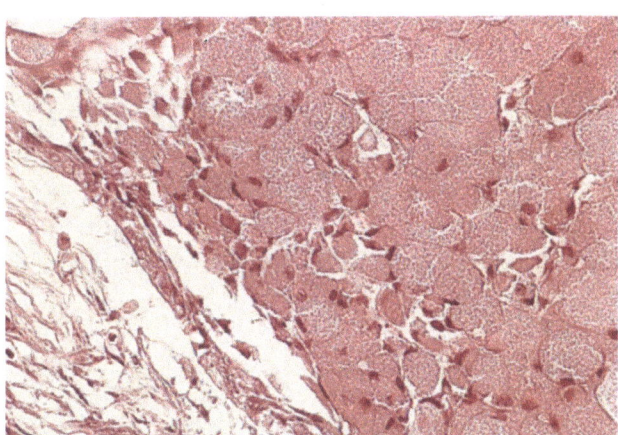

Figure 10.9 The large granular cells contain numerous eosinophilic cytoplasmic granules. H & E × 250

stellate cells similar to stellate reticulum, bordered by a peripheral layer of columnar or cubical cells resembling ameloblasts. In the plexiform type the continuous strands of epithelium show a similar appearance (Figures 10.4–10.7).

Cyst formation is common, both in the epithelium and in the stroma. Other changes that may be present in the epithelium include a type of colloid degeneration that resembles squamification, squamous metaplasia itself, and the presence of granular cells rather like those of granular cell myoblastoma (Figures 10.8 and 10.9).

Metastasis of ameloblastoma is rare[3]. When it does occur, it is usually in patients with recurrent tumours who have had repeated surgery over many years, and the metastases are pulmonary, almost certainly the result of aspiration. The histology of the primary tumour and the metastatic deposits in these cases is often unremarkable. In addition, tumours have been described as malignant ameloblastoma because of an unusual degree of local aggressiveness and possibly metastases, together with histological evidence of malignancy such as pleomorphism, mitotic activity and the like. Tumours of this type are very rare.

Differential Diagnosis

The following possibilities should be considered:

Other odontogenic tumours. Some other odontogenic tumours contain areas of epithelium that may be very similar to ameloblastoma, but there will also be calcified dental tissues, as in the odontomes, or some other additional feature such as the ghost cells in calcifying odontogenic cyst or the fibroblastic element in ameloblastic fibroma.

Other odontogenic tumours that can have some resemblance to ameloblastoma may appear as peripheral, extra-osseous lesions. Tumours of this type, which are rather ill-defined at present because they are relatively uncommon, include lesions that resemble the usual intra-osseous ameloblastoma in most respects except for their

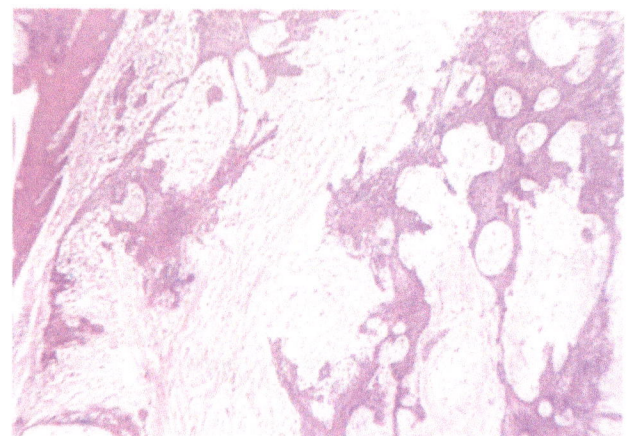

Figure 10.10 Extraosseous ameloblastoma. This lesion consists of strands and islets of epithelium situated in the gingival connective tissue. H & E × 40

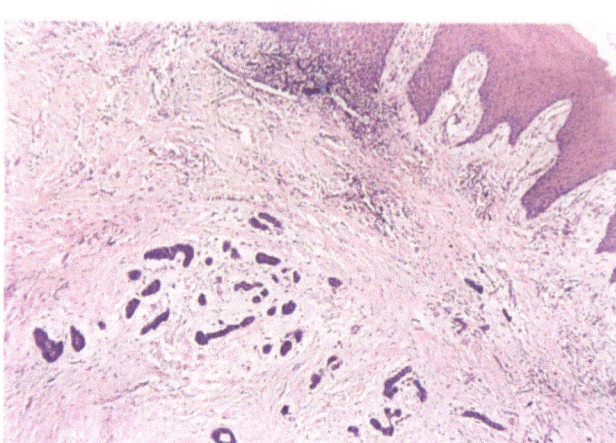

Figure 10.12 Groups of odontogenic epithelial cells in the gingiva. H & E × 100

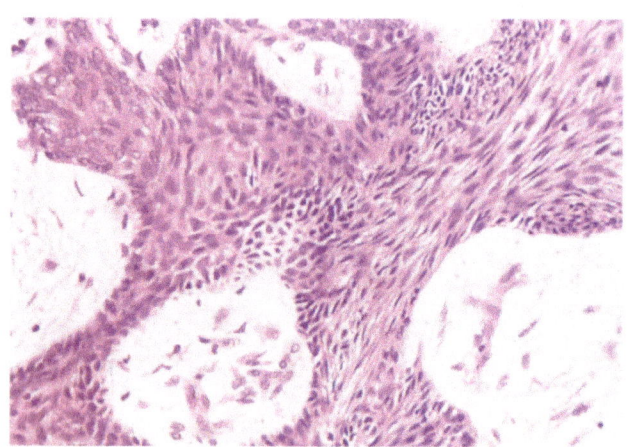

Figure 10.11 Higher magnification from Figure 10.10, showing squamous metaplasia in the tumour epithelium. H & E × 250

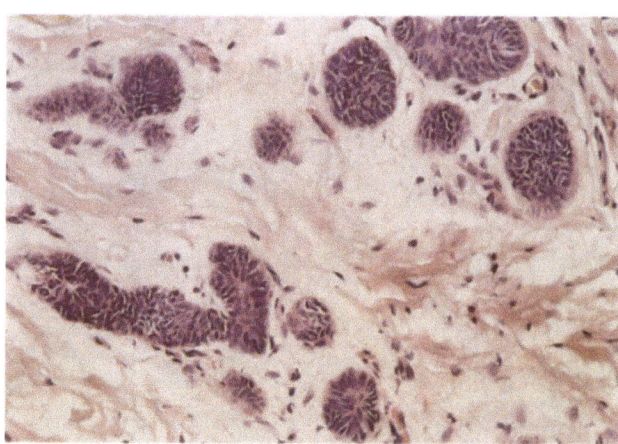

Figure 10.13 Detail from Figure 10.12. The strands of cells are somewhat reminiscent of the dental lamina. They probably represent hyperplastic rests. H & E × 250

soft tissue location[4] (Figures 10.10 and 10.11). Another tumour that can appear as an extraosseous or intraosseous growth is the recently described squamous odontogenic tumour[5]. This tumour is composed of strands and islets of well differentiated squamous epithelium, and seems previously to have been described as ameloblastoma with extensive squamous metaplasia. Rarely, odontogenic epithelium may be seen in the gingiva forming unusually large strands and groups of cells (Figures 10.12 and 10.13). This localized collection of odontogenic epithelium has been termed gingival epithelial hamartoma. The lesion seems to be of little significance other than in differentiating it from some more serious condition.

Salivary tumours. Adenoid cystic carcinoma is the salivary tumour most likely to be mistaken for ameloblastoma. Careful study of the cell types should help to avoid this error.

Squamous cell carcinoma. Some squamous cell carcinomas which have invaded the jaws from their origin in the overlying mucosa may be mistaken for ameloblastoma with extensive squamous metaplasia. Alternatively, some squamous cell carcinomas may develop hydropic or similar changes and resemble stellate reticulum.

Metastatic carcinoma. Metastatic deposits in the jaws may arise from many primary sites, the most common of which are the breast and bronchus. Microscopy may show discrete islets of tumour, sometimes with central necrosis, suggestive of ameloblastoma. The resemblance is superficial, however, and the characteristic cell types of ameloblastoma are lacking.

Odontogenic cysts. Ameloblastoma may present as a unilocular radiolucency, and resemble an odontogenic cyst[6]. In such circumstances the lining epithelium is frequently compressed and the ameloblastomatous nature of the lesion may not be immediately apparent (Figure 10.14). Careful examination of different areas usually reveals places where the epithelium is less compressed and its true nature thus more obvious (Figure 10.15). It is sometimes possible to find small islets of ameloblastoma in areas of the connective tissue of the cyst wall. Conversely, islets of non-neoplastic epithelium in the wall of a dentigerous or other odontogenic cyst should not be mistaken for ameloblastomatous follicles (Figures 10.16–10.19).

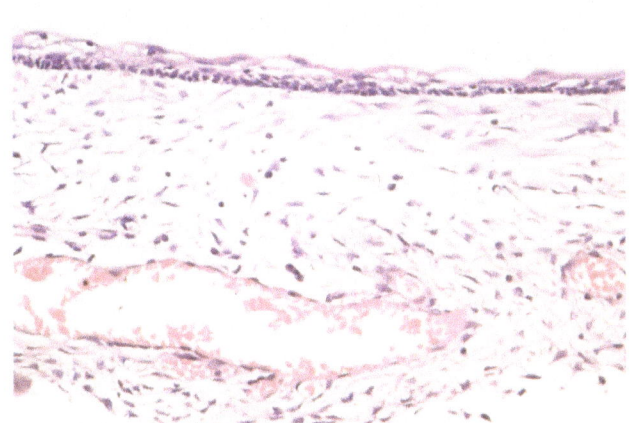

Figure 10.14 Monocystic ameloblastoma. This tumour presented as a uni-cameral cystic lesion, resembling a dentigerous cyst. Most of the lining consisted of flattened cells.   H & E × 250

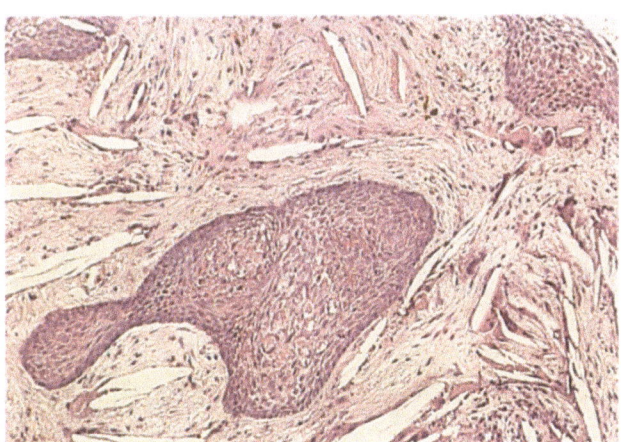

Figure 10.17 Islets of epithelium in the wall of a dentigerous cyst. Like those in Figure 10.16 they might be taken for ameloblastoma.   H & E × 250

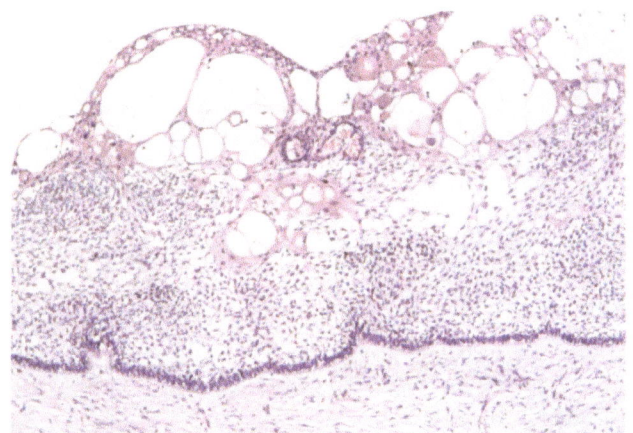

Figure 10.15 An area from the cystic lesion shown in Figure 10.14, where the lining is less compressed and can be seen to consist of typical ameloblastomatous epithelium.   H & E × 100

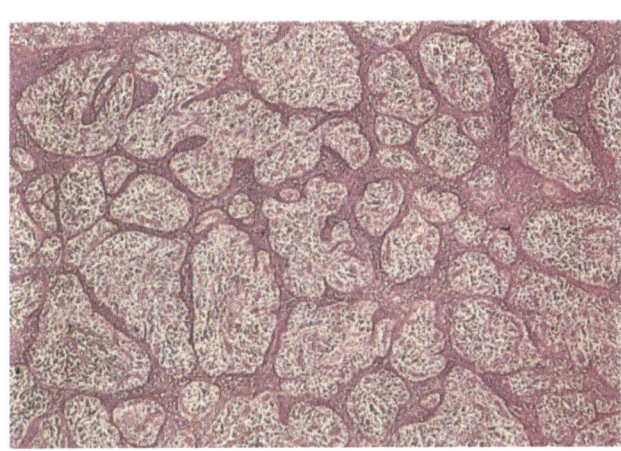

Figure 10.18 Periapical granuloma. Granulomas at the apices of infected teeth often become permeated by strands of epithelium. Some ameloblastomas can show a somewhat similar pattern, but note that the epitheliated granuloma shows heavy inflammatory infiltration.   H & E × 50

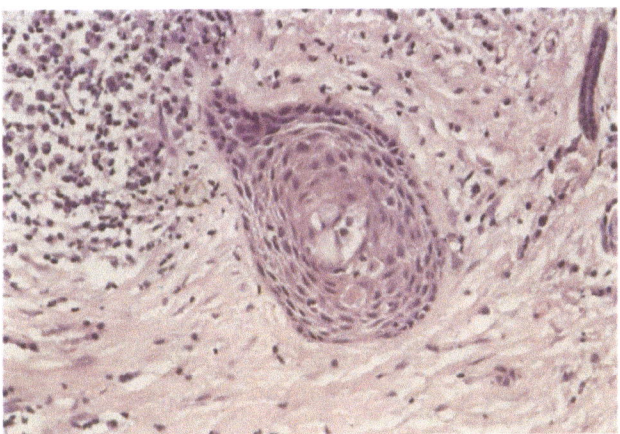

Figure 10.16 Islets of epithelium in the wall of a keratocyst, showing a resem-blance to ameloblastoma.   H & E × 250

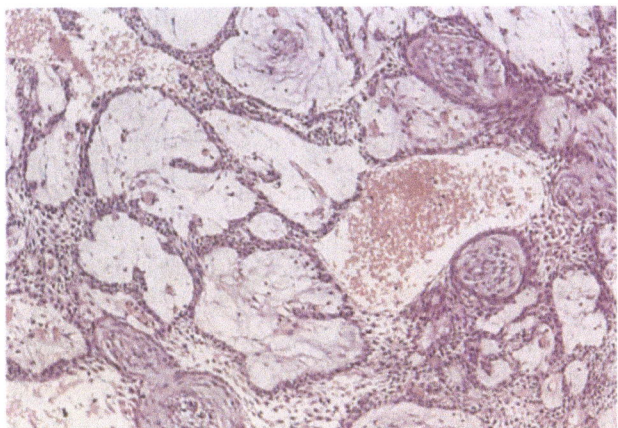

Figure 10.19 A plexiform ameloblastoma showing a similar appearance to an epitheliated granuloma. Inflammatory infiltration, however, is absent.   H & E × 100

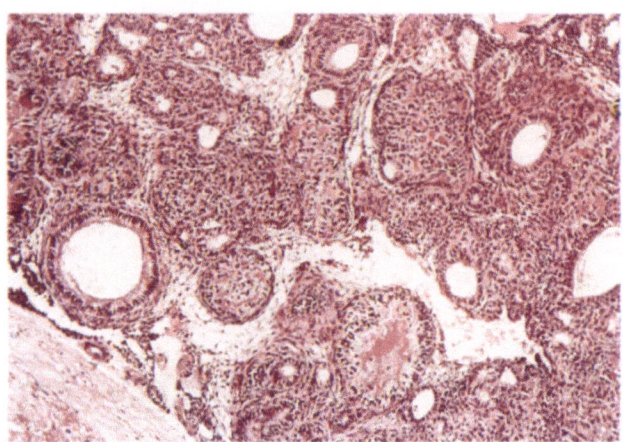

Figure 10.20   Adenomatoid odontogenic tumour. The well-formed capsule, a part of which is seen at bottom left, surrounds a tumour in which tubule-like structures are prominent.   H & E × 65

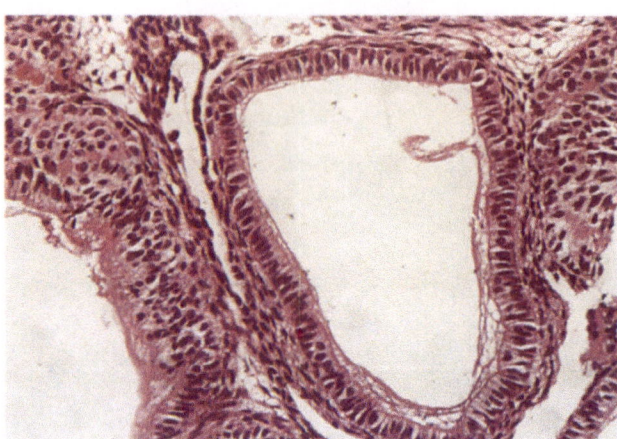

Figure 10.22   Higher magnification of tubule-like structures.   H & E × 250

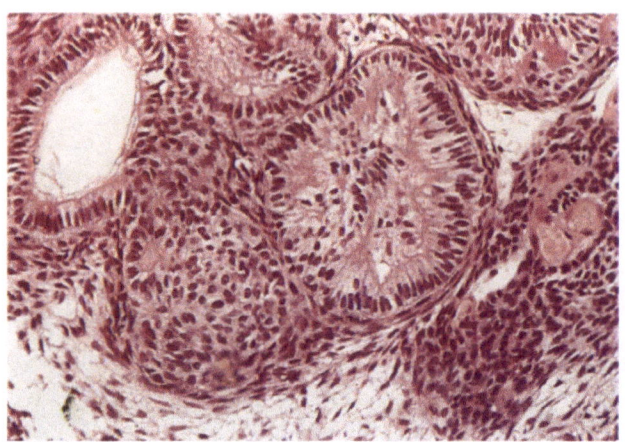

Figure 10.21   The tubule-like structures in adenomatoid odontogenic tumour consist of columnar cells resembling ameloblasts arranged around a central space. H & E × 250

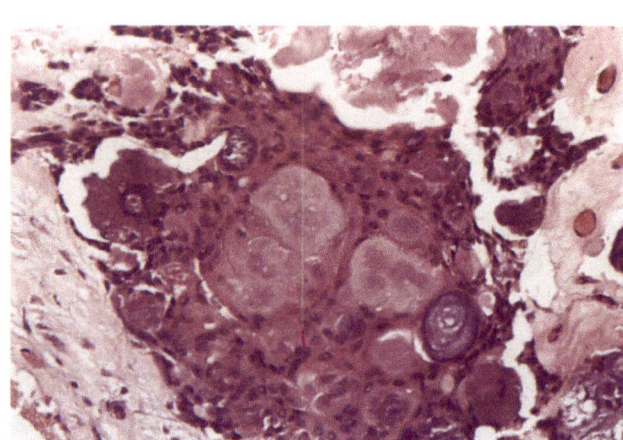

Figure 10.23   An area of calcification.   H & E × 250

Adenomatoid Odontogenic Tumour

Like ameloblastoma, this tumour is essentially epithelial. It presents in a younger age group than ameloblastoma, usually adolescents or young adults, although it can appear up to quite a late age[7]. The lesion is commoner in the maxilla than in the mandible and is often associated with an unerupted tooth. Very occasionally, it may be situated entirely in the gingiva. Radiographically, the typical finding is a well defined cyst-like radiolucency, possibly associated with an unerupted tooth. Sometimes the foci of calcification that are frequently present in the tumour can be detected in the radiograph, and give a clue to the diagnosis. The tumour has a well formed fibrous capsule. It may be solid, but not infrequently it is cystic, with a central fluid-filled cavity and solid tumour tissue forming a lining of variable thickness inside the capsule.

Microscopically, the striking feature is the presence of structures that superficially resemble glandular tubules but which are really abortive enamel organs (Figure 10.20). They consist of columnar cells resembling ameloblasts, arranged as a single layer around a central space. These spaces contain homogeneous eosinophilic material, which forms a layer over the free ends of the cells (Figures 10.21 and 10.22). Between the tubule-like structures the tumour consists of small cells with oval nuclei forming sheets of tissue. In some areas the cells surround cystic spaces that have formed in the scanty fibrous stroma. This arrangement can result in a lace-like or cribriform appearance. Although the tubule-like structures are the characteristic feature of the tumour, they may not be numerous. Moreover, the columnar cells that form these structures can form convoluted bands that do not enclose a central space.

Small areas of calcification can be found throughout the tumour and probably represent attempted enamel or dentine formation (Figure 10.23).

Differential Diagnosis

Although the adenomatoid odontogenic tumour has a very characteristic appearance, the tubule-like structures might suggest a salivary gland tumour, as might the cribriform areas, when these are present. Other possible diagnoses are as listed under ameloblastoma.

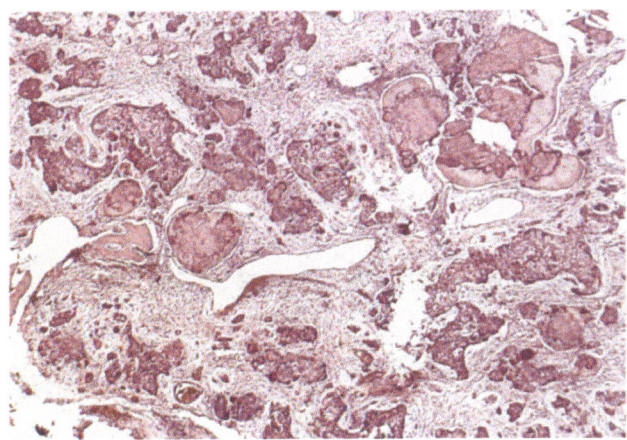

Figure 10.24 Calcifying epithelial odontogenic tumour. The tumour consists of sheets of epithelial cells in a fibrous stroma. There is extensive calcification in the epithelial cells and in the stroma. H & E × 65

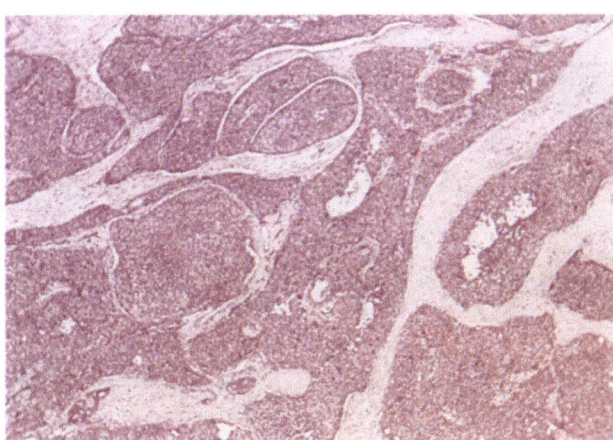

Figure 10.26 In the non-calcifying variant of calcifying epithelial odontogenic tumour, calcification is either absent or only a few small deposits are seen. The epithelial element is similar to that of the usual type of tumour. H & E × 40

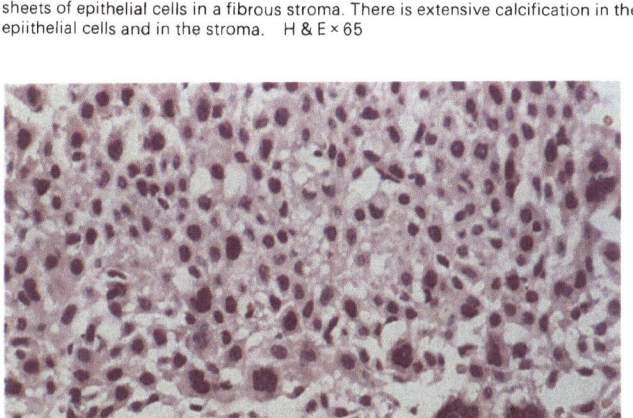

Figure 10.25 Higher magnification from the tumour shown in Figure 10.24. The tumour cells have intercellular bridges, the cytoplasm is eosinophilic and the nuclei vesicular. Pleomorphic cells with bizarre and multiple nuclei are often seen. H & E × 250

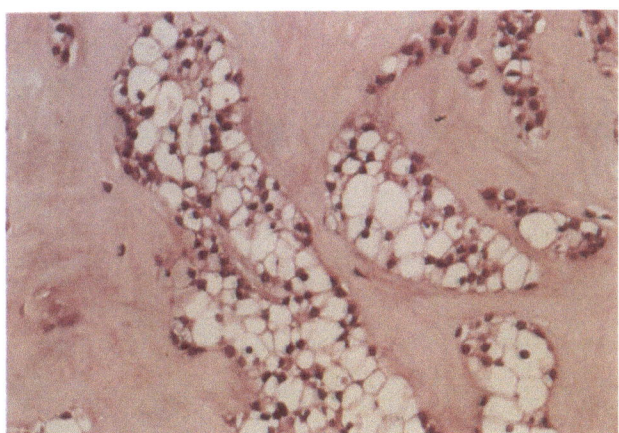

Figure 10.27 The clear cell variant of calcifying epithelial odontogenic tumour. H & E × 250

Calcifying Epithelial Odontogenic Tumour

The clinical features of this tumour closely resemble those of ameloblastoma and radiographically the appearances might also be compatible, since there is frequently a multi-locular radiolucency. In an appreciable number of cases the tumour is associated with an unerupted tooth. If the tumour presents as a unilocular radiolucency in association with an unerupted tooth, the clinical diagnosis may be dentigerous cyst. If the calcification which is so characteristic of the tumour is evident radiographically, this is of considerable help in the clinical diagnosis[8].

Microscopically, the tumour consists of sheets of epithelial cells in a fibrous stroma (Figure 10.24). Prominent intercellular bridges are often seen, and the cytoplasm is eosinophilic and homogeneous. The nucleus is vesicular, with distinct nucleoli. A characteristic feature is the presence of bizarre cells with giant nuclei and of cells with two or more nuclei (Figure 10.25). Mitoses, however, are rare. The sheets and strands of epithelium alternate with areas of acellular hyaline appearance which have many of the staining characteristics of amyloid. Calcification takes place in the hyaline-appearing material and in and around the epithelial elements. It occurs in concentric layers, which can build up to form large, confluent, irregular masses.

Variants of this tumour are not infrequent. There may be very little or no calcification, when diagnosis depends on recognizing the epithelial element and perhaps demonstrating the presence of amyloid-like material (Figure 10.26). Some tumours consist in part or almost entirely of clear cells (Figure 10.27).

Differential Diagnosis

Typical examples of the calcifying epithelial odontogenic tumour are readily recognized; the variants with little calcification may cause difficulty. The multinucleated and giant cells, when present, may suggest a primary or metastatic malignant tumour, a view that may be reinforced by the indefinite edge of the tumour. Some calcifying epithelial odontogenic tumours are reasonably well defined and encapsulated but many are not.

The epithelial cells in some poorly calcified variants tend to have clear cytoplasm and the general appearance suggests a mucoepidermoid tumour, in which clear cells are sometimes seen. Mucus, however, cannot be demonstrated in the odontogenic tumour. Some types of salivary monomorphic adenomas are composed partly or wholly of clear cells which may contain glycogen but not mucus. However, these tumours have other distinctive features.

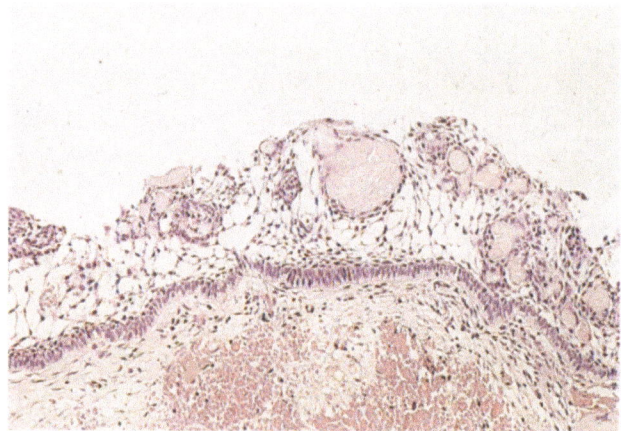

Figure 10.28   Calcifying odontogenic cyst. The epithelium is similar to that of ameloblastoma, but in addition there are areas of keratinization.   H & E × 100

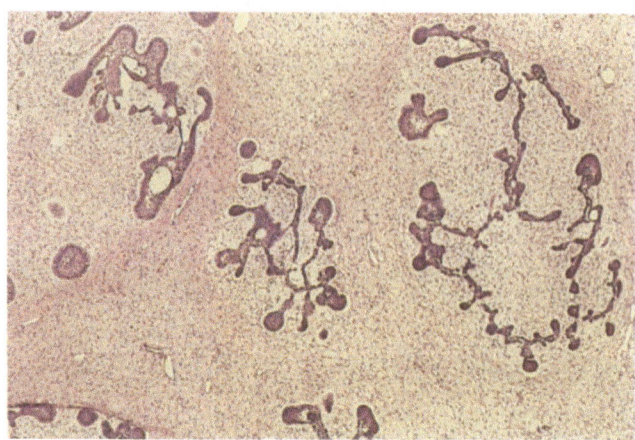

Figure 10.31   Ameloblastic fibroma. Strands of odontogenic epithelium are present in a cellular fibroblastic background.   H & E × 65

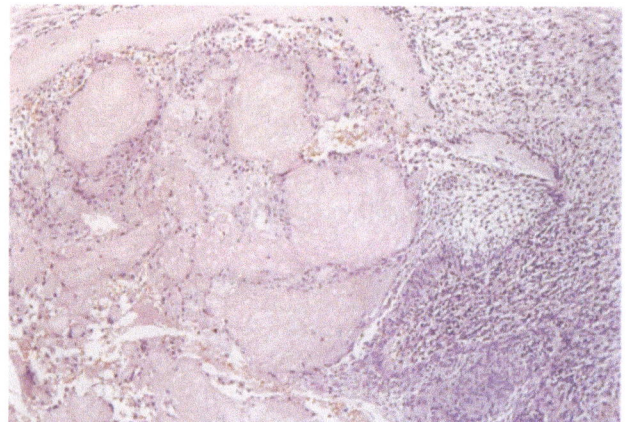

Figure 10.29   The typical ghost cells of calcifying odontogenic cyst are seen in the epithelium.   H & E × 100

Calcifying Odontogenic Cyst

Although this lesion is often cystic it can present as a solid mass. It usually arises within the bone of the mandible, but not infrequently it appears as a soft tissue growth in the gingiva. When in bone, the lesion usually presents radiographically as a well defined unilocular or multilocular radiolucency and may be associated with an unerupted tooth[9].

Microscopically, the cyst is lined by epithelium that is similar to that of ameloblastoma, consisting of a basal layer of well stained cubical or columnar cells with an overlying zone of cells that resemble stellate reticulum (Figure 10.28). The characteristic feature of the lesion, however, is the presence of ghost cells. These are epithelial cells that are undergoing an aberrant type of keratinization in which the cell enlarges and the keratin does not stain as deeply as normal keratin. The outlines of the affected cells become indistinct, so that large masses of keratin accumulate. These can excite a florid foreign body reaction, with the presence of numerous giant cells (Figures 10.29 and 10.30). Calcification is not uncommon.

Differential Diagnosis

The tumour epithelium is very similar to that of ameloblastoma but the ghost cells are the distinctive feature. These cells have been noted in other odontogenic tumours, but never with the prominence that they assume in calcifying odontogenic cyst.

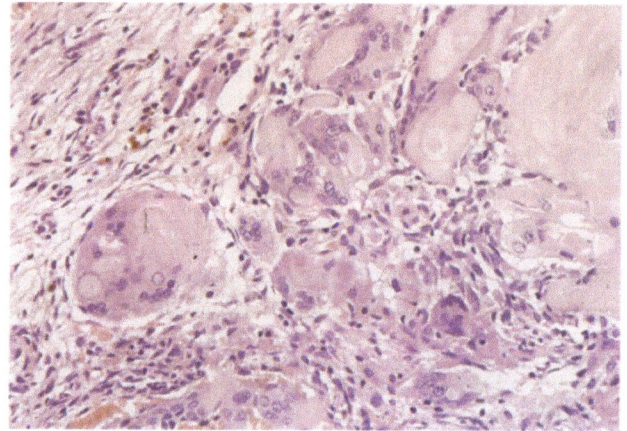

Figure 10.30   Ghost cells and keratin in the connective tissue in calcifying odontogenic cyst, with accompanying foreign body reaction.   H & E × 250

Ameloblastic Fibroma

This tumour is seen more often in the maxilla than the mandible and presents as a slowly growing painless mass expanding the jaw. It generally develops in patients of a rather younger age group than ameloblastoma. Radiographically, there is a unilocular radiolucency[10], generally well defined and possibly associated with an unerupted tooth or teeth. Sometimes the radiolucency is multilocular.

Microscopically, the tumour consists of strands and islets of epithelial cells somewhat resembling the arrangement seen in ameloblastoma. The intervening tissue, however, is a richly cellular connective tissue that resembles the dental papilla of the developing tooth (Figures 10.31 and 10.32). Dentine may occasionally be present; tumours of this type have been termed ameloblastic fibro-odontoma.

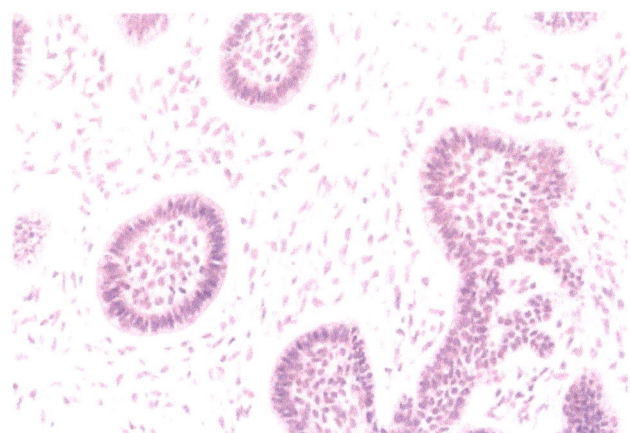

Figure 10.32 The epithelial component of ameloblastic fibroma consists of irregularly branching strands that resemble the epithelium in ameloblastoma. The mesenchymal component is a richly cellular tissue similar to the developing dental pulp. H & E × 250

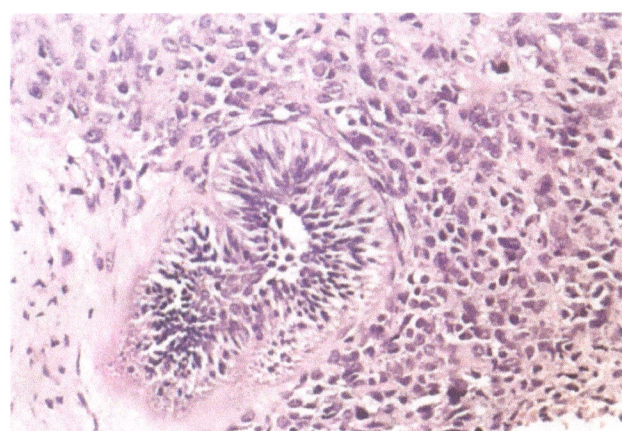

Figure 10.33 Ameloblastic sarcoma. The mesenchymal cells are pleomorphic, the epithelial component appears as in ameloblastic fibroma. H & E × 250

Very rarely, the cellular connective tissue may show pleomorphism and there may be numerous mitoses, associated with an aggressive course (Figure 10.33). This is the ameloblastic sarcoma. Some of these sarcomas have apparently originated as ameloblastic fibromas, but recurrences have shown progressively sarcomatous changes.

Differential Diagnosis

The characteristic feature of the ameloblastic fibroma is the double neoplastic element. It might be confused with odontogenic fibroma or myxoma, in which strands of odontogenic epithelium may be present. These strands, however, do not form the ameloblastoma-like islets that are seen in ameloblastic fibroma. They tend, instead, to remain as rather narrow columns or small groups.

Odontomes

Odontomes are essentially hamartomas consisting of fully formed dental tissues which are more or less normal qualitatively but are present in abnormal quantity and arrangement. When fully mature, odontomes consist principally of enamel and dentine, but during the period of active growth ameloblastic epithelium and odontoblastic tissue are present.

Most of these lesions are detected in children and adolescents, and more often in the mandible than the maxilla. There are frequently no symptoms and the lesion may be discovered in the course of routine radiographic examination. In most cases the lesion is associated with the permanent dentition and is solitary. Multiple odontomes are rare.

There are two main types of odontome, the complex and the compound. The former consists of a circumscribed tumour-like mass of dental tissues laid down in a quite irregular manner. The latter is a collection of small teeth or tooth-like structures in a fibrous capsule[11]. However, all gradations of organization between the two extremes can be encountered (Figures 10.34–10.37).

Complex odontome. The lesion forms a circumscribed mass that is frequently about the size of a normal tooth, or perhaps larger, when it may expand the jaw. Microscopically, it consists of a mass of irregularly disposed enamel, dentine and cementum, together with connective tissue similar to normal dental pulp. Since most of the enamel is

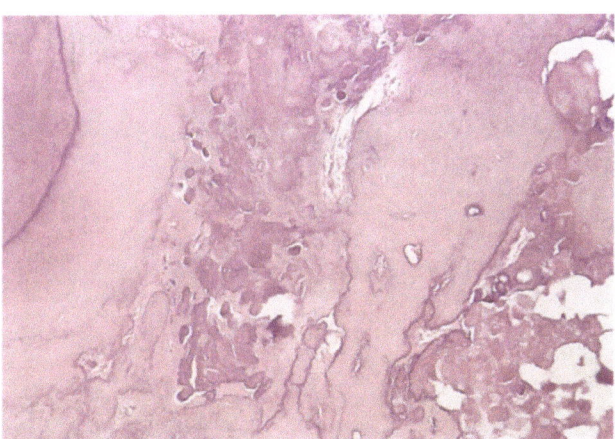

Figure 10.34 Complex odontome, consisting of an irregularly disposed mass of calcified dental tissues. The clear space at top left, and smaller ones elsewhere, were occupied by enamel before decalcification. H & E × 100

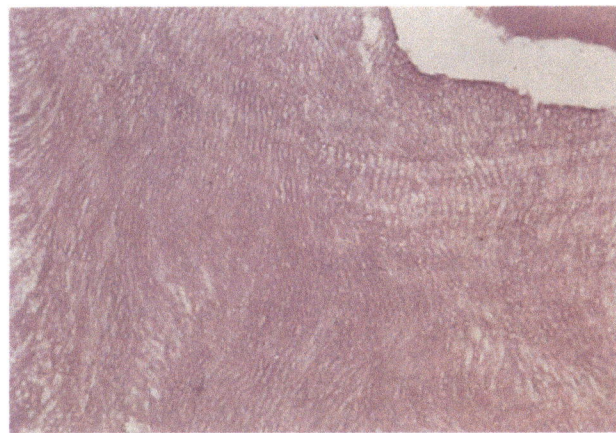

Figure 10.35 A field showing enamel matrix. H & E × 250

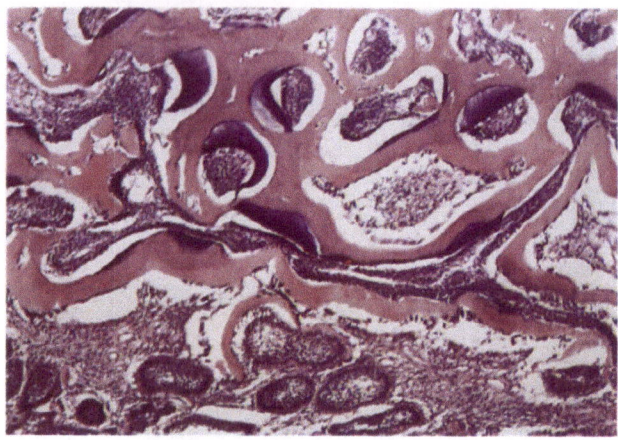

Figure 10.36 In this complex odontome, ameloblastic epithelium is seen at the top of the field. Immature enamel, beginning to calcify, presents as the dark blue areas, close to the eosinophilic dentine, which forms the greater part of the lesion. The general arrangement is rather more organized than that in the lesion shown in Figure 10.34. H & E × 100

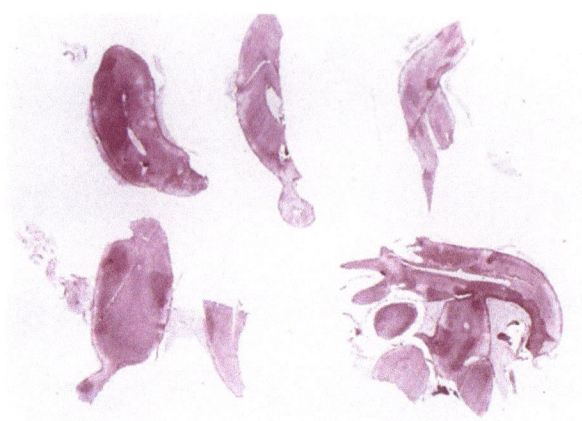

Figure 10.38 Compound odontome. Denticles from a compound odontome. H & E × 4

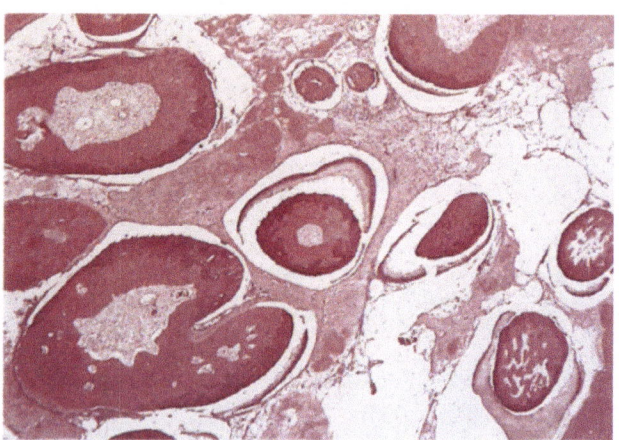

Figure 10.37 A field from a complex odontome in which more recognizably tooth-like structures are present. These are cut in cross-section in this field, and consist of dentine with central pulp and surrounding developing enamel. H & E × 40

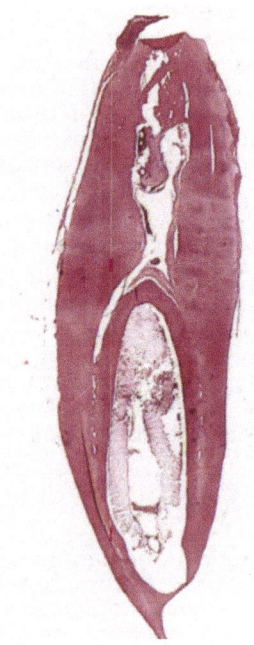

Figure 10.39 Dens invaginatus. In this decalcified section of a maxillary tooth an invagination extends upwards from the crown into the root. The enamel lining the invagination has been lost during the process of decalcification. × 3

fully calcified, it has disappeared from routine decalcified sections and its former presence is indicated by a space. However, enamel matrix that has not yet fully matured may be present. It is haematoxyphilic and the enamel prisms give it a fibrillar or whorled appearance in longitudinal section. Where the section happens to be transverse, it appears to consist of small overlapping hexagons. If the odontome has been removed during its period of active growth ameloblastic epithelium can be seen, but in mature specimens this is absent.

The bulk of the odontome is usually formed by dentine. This is generally normal in appearance, with well developed tubules, but forming irregular masses instead of a normal tooth. Tissue that resembles normal dental pulp and cementum is also present.

Compound odontome. This lesion consists of small separate teeth or denticles enclosed in a fibrous capsule. These denticles may be very numerous, although in most cases they number up to perhaps six or seven. They are recognizably tooth-like, but show many small departures from the normal pattern (Figure 10.38).

Dens invaginatus or *dilated odontome* is a malformation in which an invagination or cavity forms in a tooth during its development. The cavity is lined by enamel. Only the teeth of the permanent dentition are affected by this anomaly, most often the maxillary lateral incisors (Figure 10.39).

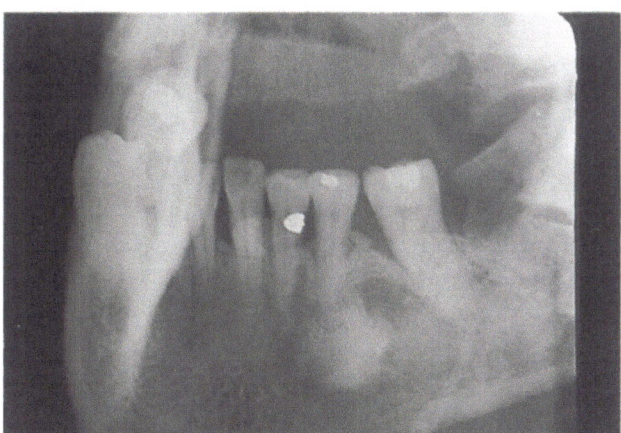

Figure 10.40 Cementoblastoma. The radiograph shows a circumscribed radiopacity at the root of a premolar tooth. There is a surrounding narrow translucent zone.

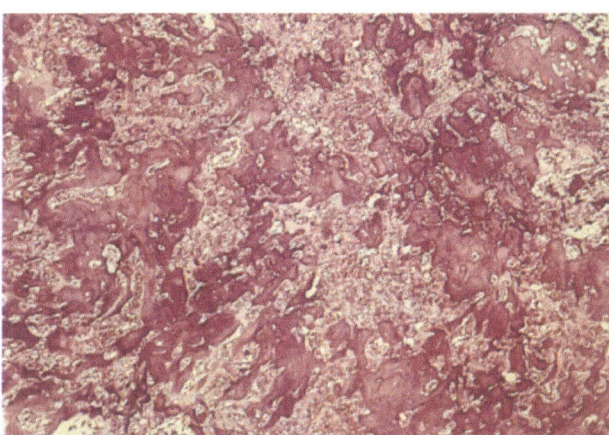

Figure 10.41 Cementoblastoma. The lesion consists of a mass of cementum in a vascular connective tissue matrix. H & E × 100

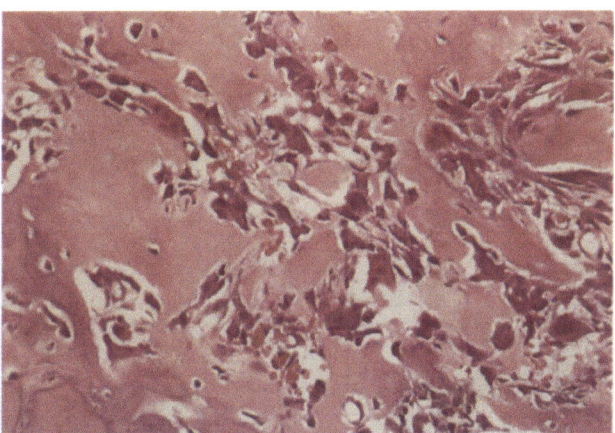

Figure 10.42 Cementoblastoma, showing numerous large osteoblast-type cells. H & E × 250

Differential Diagnosis

The fully mature complex odontome is readily recognized, but when ameloblastic epithelium is present, as in actively growing lesions, other odontogenic tumours have to be differentiated. The essential feature of the ameloblastic epithelium in the odontome is its qualitative normality. Although it is present in abnormal amounts and disposition as compared with a developing tooth, it is reasonably normal in appearance. In the ameloblastic fibro-odontoma, in which dentine and enamel are present as well as the features of ameloblastic fibroma, the epithelium forms islets, as already described, which are more like the follicles of ameloblastoma. The cellular fibroblastic component of ameloblastic fibroma also differs from the much less cellular and less active-appearing fibrous tissue of the odontome. The very rare odontoameloblastoma consists of enamel and dentine as well as epithelium. The epithelium, however, is like the epithelium of ameloblastoma rather than the more normal-looking odontogenic epithelium of the odontome. Dentine may occasionally be seen in other odontogenic tumours, but not usually as such a prominent feature as in odontomes. Moreover, in the other odontogenic tumours such as the adenomatoid odontogenic tumour, calcifying epithelial odontogenic tumour or calcifying odontogenic cyst the epithelium is the predominant tissue, which it very rarely is in odontomes. Rarely, however, one of these other odontogenic tumours may be associated with what appears to be an odontome.

Enameloma

This is the term used for small deposits of enamel that are sometimes found on the roots of teeth. They may be in continuity with the normal enamel of the crown or they may appear as separate small masses. These enamelomas, despite the name, are minor divergences from the normal pattern of enamel formation and are not neoplasms.

Dentinoma

The existence of this tumour as a distinctive entity is doubted by many pathologists. It is said to be a mass or masses of dentine embedded in connective tissue and has usually been described in the mandible, in association with unerupted molar teeth.

Cementoma

The cementomas comprise a group of lesions that are not all neoplasms. In general, they are characterized by overgrowth of calcified tissues at or near the root of a tooth; the radiographic appearances may thus help in giving a clue to the nature of the condition[1].

Cementoblastoma. Most patients are adolescents or young adults, who may or may not complain of pain and swelling of the jaw, more often the mandible than the maxilla. Radiographs show a well defined radiopacity with a surrounding narrow translucent zone involving the root of a tooth, nearly always a premolar or molar (Figure 10.40). The tumour, which forms a globular mass around the root, can often be removed complete with the tooth[1 2] Microscopically, it is seen to consist of a mass of cementum-like tissue, often showing numerous, deeply stained reversal lines. Lacunae scattered throughout this calcified tissue contain osteoblast-like cells. These, together with osteoclast-type giant cells, are seen in the vascular connective tissue that is present here and there throughout the mass of calcified tissue (Figure 10.41). If the tumour is still actively growing there is a zone of uncalcified tissue which lacks reversal lines around the periphery. There and elsewhere there may be many osteoblast-like cells and these are frequently large and deeply staining (Figure 10.42).

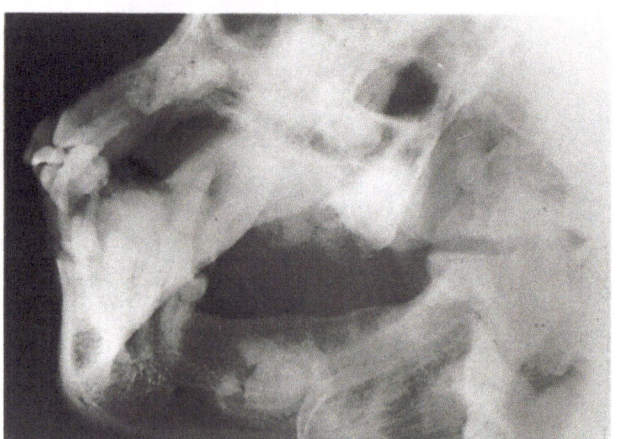

Figure 10.43 Gigantiform cementoma. The radiograph shows a dense irregularly lobulated mass in the mandible

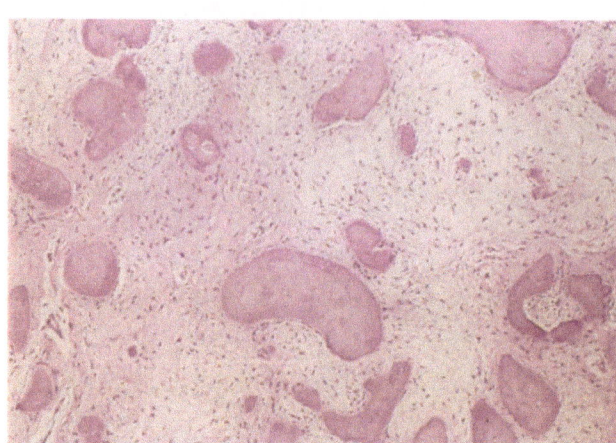

Figure 10.46 Periapical cemental dysplasia. Irreguarly shaped small masses or blunt trabeculae of cementoid tissue form in a connective tissue matrix. H & E × 250

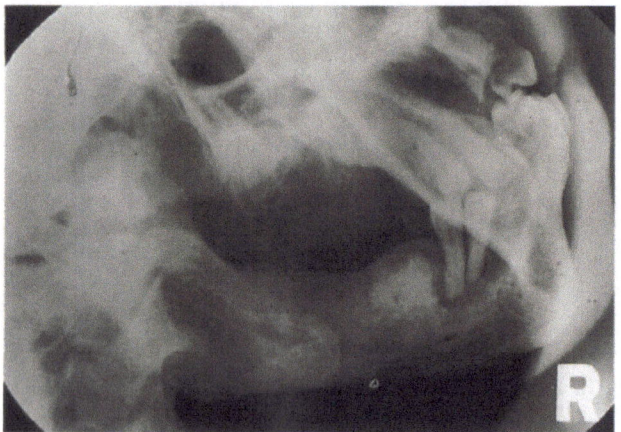

Figure 10.44 The same patient as in Figure 10.43. There is another similar lesion in the mandible on the opposite side

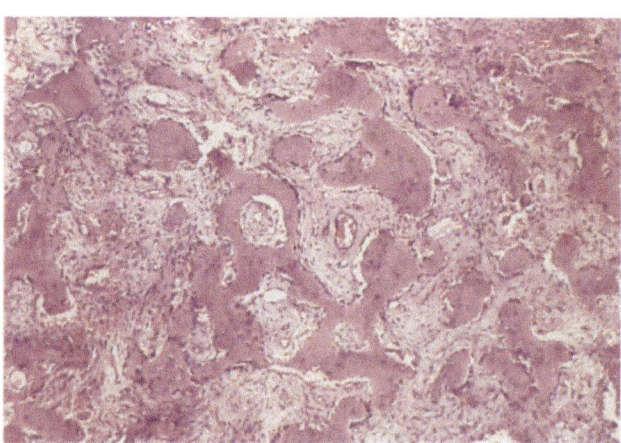

Figure 10.47 Periapical cemental dysplasia. Another field, with appearances very similar to fibrous dysplasia of bone. H & E × 250

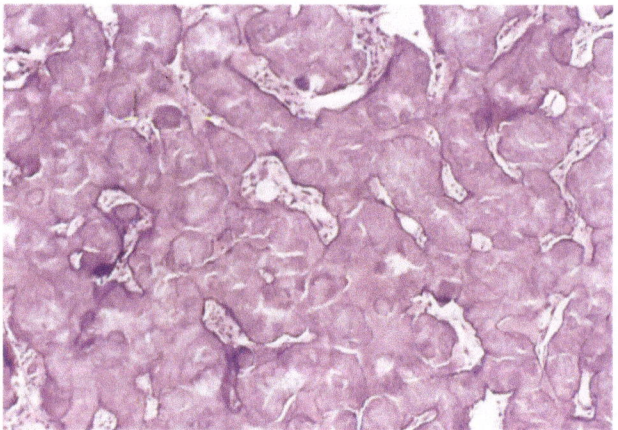

Figure 10.45 Gigantiform cementoma. The lesion consists of a dense mass of acellular cementum. H & E × 100

When the specimen is obtained entire, or even if fragments of hard tissue only are available but the radiograph can also be examined, the correct diagnosis in typical cases is readily made. However, in the absence of adequate clinical or radiographic information the pathologist might think in terms of osteoblastoma, or even of osteosarcoma, because of the cellularity, hyperchromatism and occasional pleomorphism. However, mitoses are absent and the pleomorphism is usually of minor degree only.

Gigantiform cementoma is uncommon. It is usually detected in middle age, in females more than males, and Negroes appear to be especially affected. Although multiple lesions, often symmetrically situated, are characteristic, solitary lesions can also arise. There may be a familial incidence[13]. There is usually painless swelling of the jaw, with a dense lobulated radiopacity (Figures 10.43 and 10.44). Microscopically, the lesion consists of dense, irregular, highly calcified masses of acellular cementum which may be continuous with the normal cementum of the root of a tooth (Figure 10.45). Numerous empty lacunae are often present in some areas.

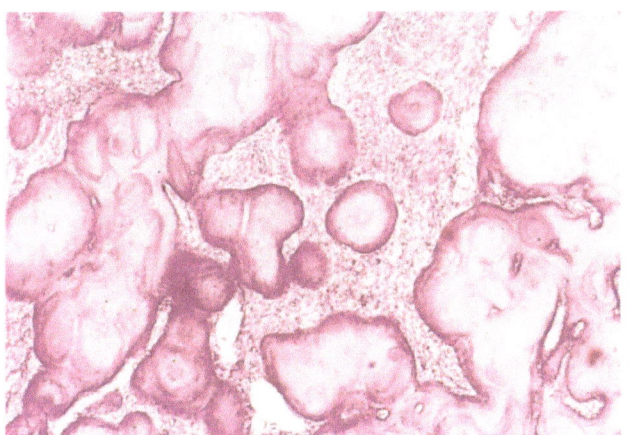

Figure 10.48   Cementifying fibroma. Rounded masses of cementoid tissue form in a cellular fibroblastic matrix.   H & E × 250

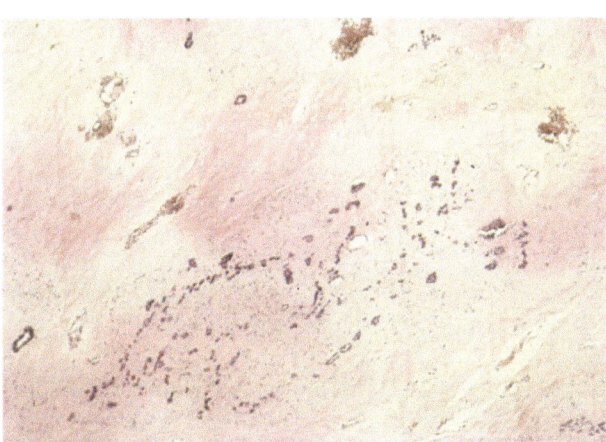

Figure 10.49   Odontogenic fibroma. Strands and groups of odontogenic epithelial cells are present in a fibrous matrix. In this example the fibrous tissue is very largely hyalinized.   H & E × 100

The differential diagnosis includes chronic osteomyelitis and cementifying fibroma. Chronic osteomyelitis is not uncommon and is generally the sequel, ultimately, of dental caries. In such cases there will therefore be a history of caries, possibly pulpitis, and extraction. The chronic sclerosing form of osteomyelitis gives rise to acellular masses of bone so sclerotic that there is no infiltration of inflammatory cells. However, there is no lobulation, as in gigantiform cementoma, and the edges of the lesion where inflammatory infiltration may be detected are less definite.

Periapical cemental dysplasia. This condition is characterized by multiple small symptomless lesions at the apices of the mandibular anterior teeth, usually in women[14]. It is generally detected radiographically. Microscopically, the appearances are very similar to those of fibrous dysplasia. There is a localized area of replacement of bone at the root of a tooth by fibrous tissue. New calcified tissue is laid down, as layers of cementum, cementicles or trabeculae of bone (Figures 10.46 and 10.47). As this gradually increases in amount, the area becomes completely sclerotic.

Cementifying fibroma. This lesion occurs in the mandible, in middle-aged persons. In its earlier stages the appearances are similar to those of periapical cemental dysplasia, but the lesion itself is larger, single rather than multiple and in the premolar or molar region rather than the anterior region. Later, it becomes progressively calcified and islands of cementum tend to fuse to form sclerotic masses of calcified tissue (Figure 10.48).

Odontogenic Fibroma and Myxoma

Odontogenic fibroma. This tumour is usually seen in children and young adults. It is commoner in the mandible than in the maxilla and is often associated with an unerupted or congenitally missing tooth. The tumour forms a well circumscribed mass of fibroblastic tissue of varying degrees of maturity[15]. Some tumours are well collagenized, others are more fibroblastic and look very much like developing dental pulp. Frequently, there are small groups and strands of odontogenic epithelium scattered here and there, but they are not always present (Figures 10.49, 10.50 and 10.51).

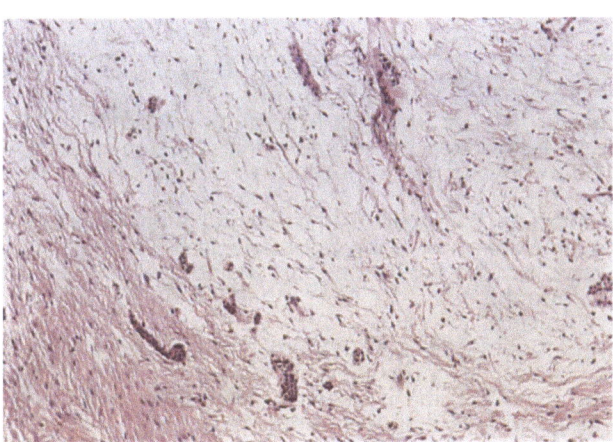

Figure 10.50   Odontogenic fibromyxoma. The tumour consists of fibroblastic and myxomatous tissue. Groups of odontogenic epithelial cells are scattered throughout.   H & E × 100

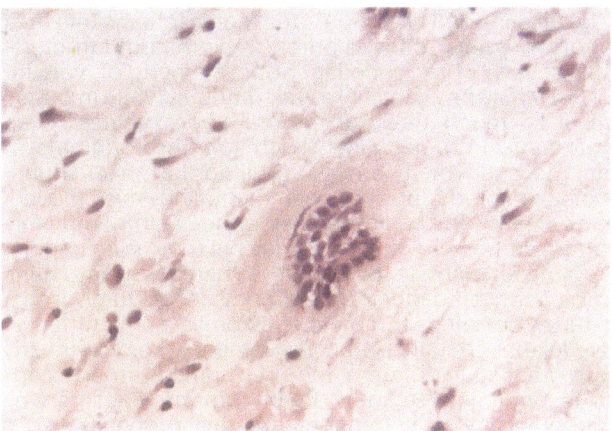

Figure 10.51   Higher magnification from another odontogenic fibromyxoma, showing a myxomatous area with a group of odontogenic epithelial cells. H & E × 625

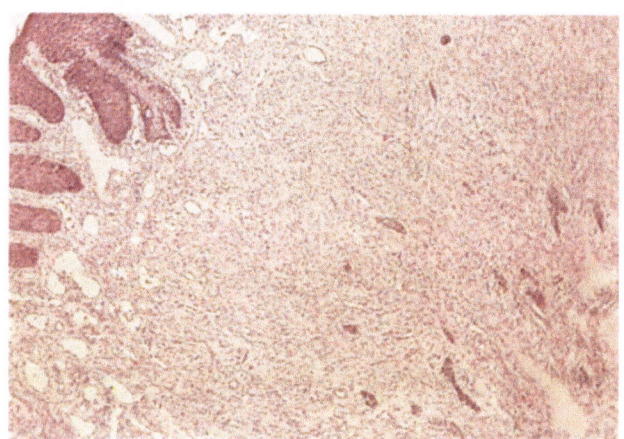

Figure 10.52 Odontogenic fibroma. A peripheral tumour is shown here, situated in the gingiva. The gingival epithelium is seen at top left. The tumour consists of fibroblastic tissue with scattered groups of odontogenic epithelial cells. H & E × 100

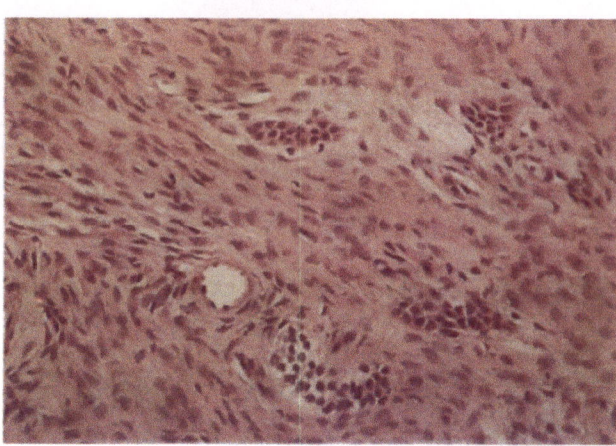

Figure 10.53 Higher magnification showing odontogenic epithelium and richly cellular fibroblastic tissue. H & E × 250

Odontogenic fibroma is essentially a central, intraosseous lesion. A structurally similar lesion, termed peripheral odontogenic fibroma, is seen in the gingiva[16] (Figures 10.52 and 10.53).

Odontogenic myxoma. Although myxomatous tumours elsewhere are often highly debatable lesions, myxoma in the jaws is in a different category, being a lesion peculiar to the odontogenic area. It is probably related to odontogenic fibroma.

Odontogenic myxoma is commoner in the mandible than the maxilla, particularly in the molar region and, like odontogenic fibroma, it is seen more often in children and younger patients than in the older age groups. It is frequently associated with unerupted or congenitally missing teeth[17].

Microscopically, the picture is of typically myxomatous tissue – triangular or stellate cells with long processes set in a matrix of loose mucoid material. The cells have a slightly basophilic cytoplasm and ovoid nuclei. There is no evidence of cellular atypia and practically no mitotic activity. Strands and islets of odontogenic epithelial cells may be present. Not all tumours that come into the myxoma category, however, show a purely myxomatous structure. There is very often a collagenous element of varying amount. It may be scanty in some tumours, while in others there is so much that the tumour approximates to an odontogenic fibroma. Since both tumours originate in dental mesenchyme it is not surprising that there should be a range of gradations between them. They may, indeed, be extremes of the same process rather than completely separate entities. However this may be, there is an important practical point to be noted. Whereas odontogenic fibroma is a well defined and circumscribed tumour that can be enucleated complete, myxomas are infiltrative. Those lesions that are purely myxomatous, or very nearly so, are practically diffluent and they spread through cancellous bone very readily. Even tumours that can be described as fibromyxomas share this propensity to a greater or lesser degree, so that excision for these lesions must be adequate.

Myxomatous tumours also present as peripheral soft tissue lesions. They are in a different category to the intraosseous lesions, being comparable to myxomatous tumours elsewhere in the body.

References

1. Pindborg, J. J. and Kramer, I. R. H. (1971). *International Classification of Tumours. Histological Typing of Odontogenic Tumours, Jaw Cysts and Allied Lesions*. (Geneva: World Health Organization)

2. Lucas, R. B. (1984). *Pathology of Tumours of the Oral Tissues*. 4th Edn. (Edinburgh, London, Melbourne, New York: Churchill Livingstone)

3. Buff, S. J., Chen, J. T. T., Ravin, C. C. and Moore, J. O. (1980). Pulmonary metastasis from ameloblastoma of the mandible: report of case and review of the literature. *J. Oral Surg.*, **38**, 374

4. Gardner, D. G. (1977). Peripheral ameloblastoma. *Cancer*, **39**, 1625

5. Pullon, P. A., Shafer, W. G., Elzay, R. P., Kerr, D. A. and Corio, R. L. (1975). Squamous odontogenic tumor: report of six cases of a previously undescribed lesion. *Oral Surg.*, **40**, 616

6. Robinson, L. and Martinez, M. G. (1977). Unicystic ameloblastoma: a prognostically distinct entity. *Cancer*, **40**, 2278

7. Tsaknis, P. J., Carpenter, W. M. and Shade, N. L. (1977). Odontogenic adenomatoid tumor: report of case and review of the literature. *J. Oral Surg.*, **35**, 146

8. Franklin, C. D. and Pindborg, J. J. (1976). The calcifying epithelial odontogenic tumour: a review and analysis of 113 cases. *Oral Surg.*, **42**, 753

9. Freedman, P. D., Lumerman, H. and Gee, J. K. (1975). Calcifying odontogenic cyst: a review and analysis of seventy cases. *Oral Surg.*, **40**, 93

10. Trodahl, J. N. (1972). Ameloblastic fibroma: a survey of cases from the Armed Forces Institute of Pathology. *Oral Surg.*, **33**, 547

11. Budnick, S. (1976). Compound and complex odontomas. *Oral Surg.*, **42**, 501

12. Abrams, A. M., Kirby, J. W. and Melrose, R. J. (1974). Cementoblastoma: a clinico-pathologic study of seven new cases. *Oral Surg.*, **38**, 394

13. Cannon, J. S., Keller, E. E. and Dahlin, D. C. (1980). Gigantiform cementoma: report of two cases (mother and son). *J. Oral Surg.*, **38**, 65

14. Vegh, T. (1976). Multiple cementomas (periapical cemental dysplasia): report of a case. *Oral Surg.*, **42**, 403

15. Farman, A. G., Nortjé, C. J., Grotepass, F. W., Farman, F. J. and Van Zyl, J. A. (1977). Myxofibroma of the jaws. *Brit. J. Oral Surg.*, **15**, 3

16. Farman, A. G. (1975). The peripheral odontogenic fibroma. *Oral Surg.*, **40**, 82

17. Barros, R. E., Dominguez, F. V. and Cabrini, R. L. (1969). Myxoma of the jaws. *Oral Surg.*, **27**, 225

Tumours of the Oral Tissues
2. Non-odontogenic Tumours

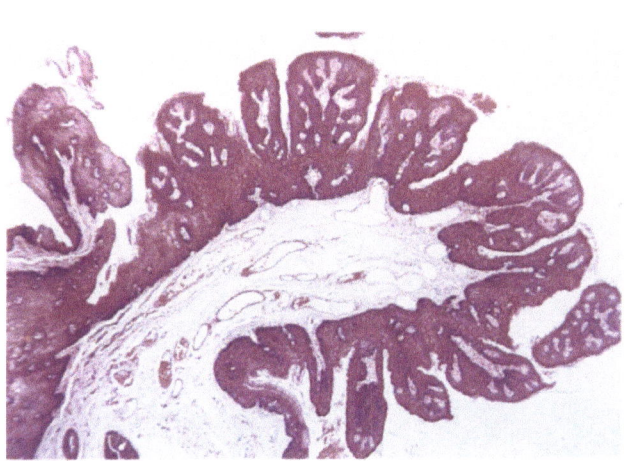

11

Figure 11.1 Squamous cell papilloma of the buccal mucosa.   H & E × 16

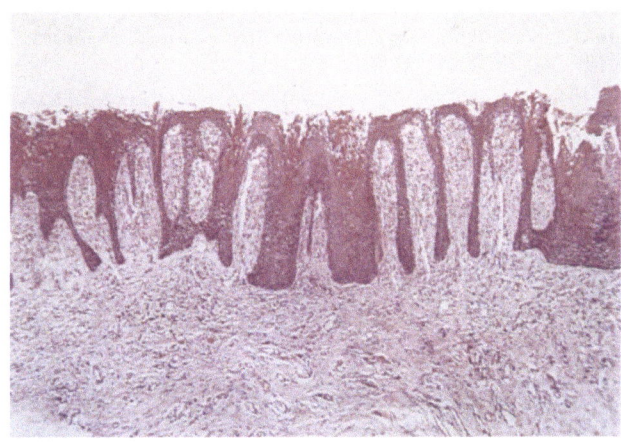

Figure 11.2 Verruciform xanthoma, showing acanthosis and elongation of the rete ridges. Numerous foam cells are present between the ridges.   H & E × 40

Many tumours other than those of the dental tissues appear from time to time in and around the mouth. Salivary gland tumours are illustrated in Chapter 9. Other non-odontogenic tumours are considered here.

Epidermoid Tumours

Squamous Cell Papilloma

Squamous cell papilloma can develop anywhere in the oral mucosa and shows very much the same microscopic features as corresponding tumours of the skin (Figure 11.1). There is usually less keratin formation in oral tumours than in skin tumours, however, and superficial ulceration and infection are commoner, since oral tumours are apt to be traumatized during mastication. Severe dysplastic changes in the epithelium are very rare; there would seem to be very little risk of subsequent malignant change. Although most papillomas are solitary tumours, multiple papillomas can arise, sometimes in association with verruca vulgaris of the skin[1].

Verrucous xanthoma is a verrucous or papilliform lesion of the oral mucosa, in which the rete ridges of the acanthotic epithelium are elongated, with foam cells in the intervening fibrous tissue. These cells do not extend deeper than the level of the tips of the ridges (Figures 11.2 and 11.3). Whether the lesion is essentially an epithelial proliferation with a histiocytic foam cell reaction in the adjacent connective tissue, or whether the foam cells are the primary feature is not yet known[2].

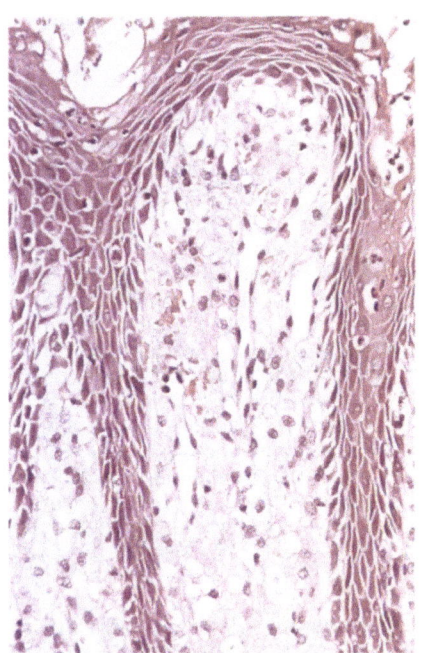

Figure 11.3 Verruciform xanthoma. Higher magnification, showing the foam cells.   H & E × 250

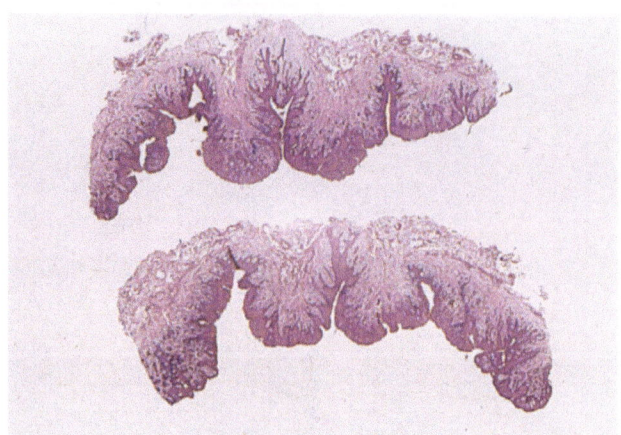

Figure 11.4 Papillary hyperplasia of the palate. The hyperplastic palatal mucosa is thrown into folds and papillary projections. H & E × 5

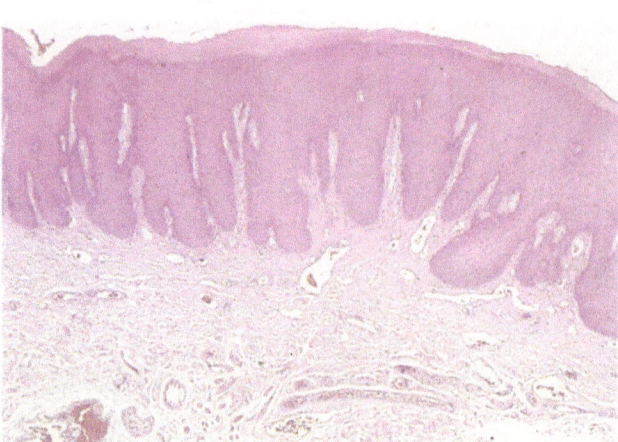

Figure 11.6 Focal epithelial hyperplasia. The epithelium is acanthotic, with elongated and anastomosing rete processes. H & E × 65

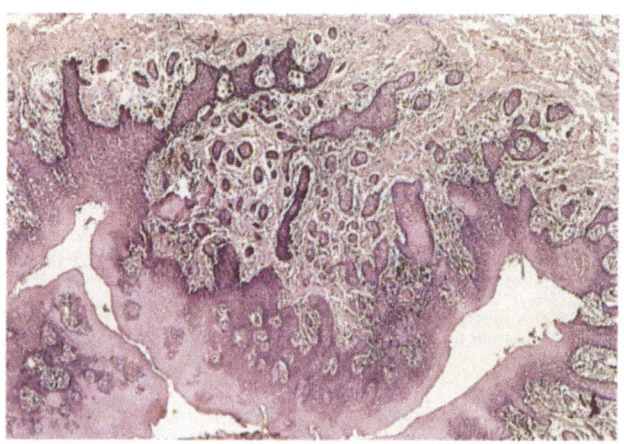

Figure 11.5 Papillary hyperplasia, showing the pseudoepitheliomatous appearance that may be present in some areas. The heavy chronic infalmmatory infiltration is a characteristic feature. H & E × 40

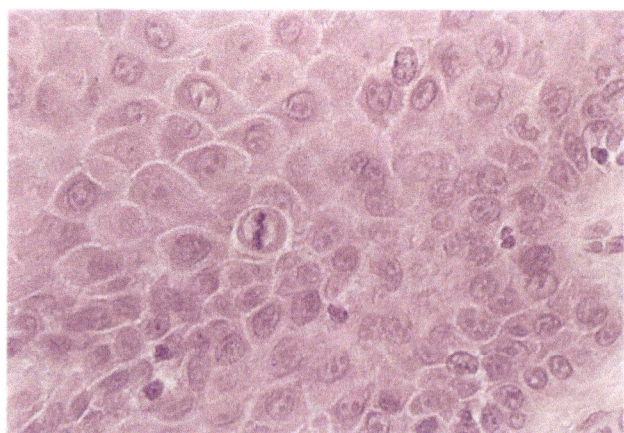

Figure 11.7 Focal epithelial hyperplasia. Higher magnification, showing a cell with mitosis-like nuclear degeneration and several cells with double nuclei. H & E × 400

Papillary Hyperplasia

This condition is seen in persons with a poor standard of oral hygiene and ill-fitting dentures. The palate is the usual site, the mucosa in the denture-bearing area being covered by an extensive warty growth. Microscopically, there are numerous papillary projections of connective tissue covered by acanthotic squamous epithelium (Figure 11.4). There is always heavy chronic inflammatory infiltration of the connective tissue, but there is no ulceration. Although the acanthosis may give rise to a so-called pseudoepitheliomatous appearance in some areas, there is little or no evidence of cellular atypia (Figure 11.5). The condition is reactive and inflammatory and not neoplastic[3].

Focal Epithelial Hyperplasia

This condition is characterized by small, flat, soft nodules in the oral mucosa, particularly of the lower lip. They consist of a connective tissue core covered by acanthotic epithelium in which can be seen cells with large nuclei and also multinucleated cells (Figures 11.6 and 11.7). Chronic inflammatory cells are present in the corium and the ducts of adjacent minor salivary glands may be dilated. The condition is possibly of viral origin[4].

Epithelial Dysplasia

Dysplastic changes may be seen in the oral mucosa in a variety of circumstances[5,6]. The epithelium in such conditions as lichen planus, lupus erythematosus, candidosis and some other mucocutaneous lesions, and the epithelium adjacent to inflammatory or traumatic ulceration, may show dysplasia of varying degree. Other lesions, characterized by patches of white, red or variegated appearance that do not conform to any specific disease entity and may therefore be designated simply as leukoplakia or erythroplasia may also show dysplasia. The epithelium around a frankly invasive carcinoma may be dysplastic.

The histological features of oral epithelial dysplasia are in general similar to those of dysplasia in the skin, the cervix uteri and other mucosae (Figures 11.8–11.12). The problem for the pathologist is therefore not so much the recognition of dysplasia as the evaluation of its significance. The dysplasia that is occasionally present in lichen planus or other mucocutaneous disorders is usually of mild degree and is probably not of great significance. Although squamous cell carcinoma has been reported to follow some of these lesions on occasion, there is practically no available information correlating histological

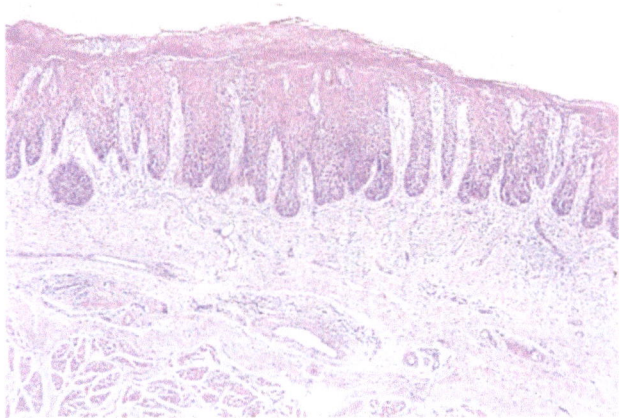

Figure 11.8 Dysplasia. The epithelium shows parakeratosis, acanthosis and elongation of the rete processes. The upper layers of the epithelium are normally stratified, but the cellular arrangement is less orderly in the deeper layers. H & E × 40

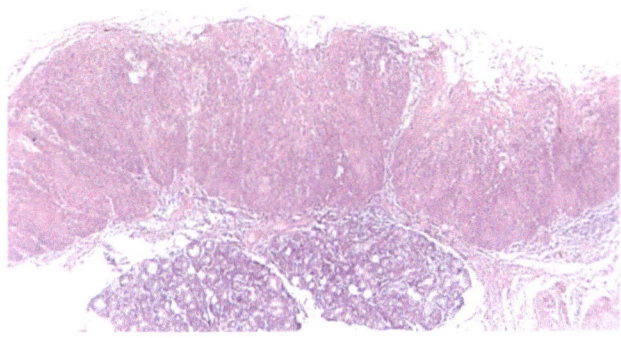

Figure 11.10 Dysplasia adjacent to a carcinoma. The full thickness of the epithelium is dysplastic. H & E × 40

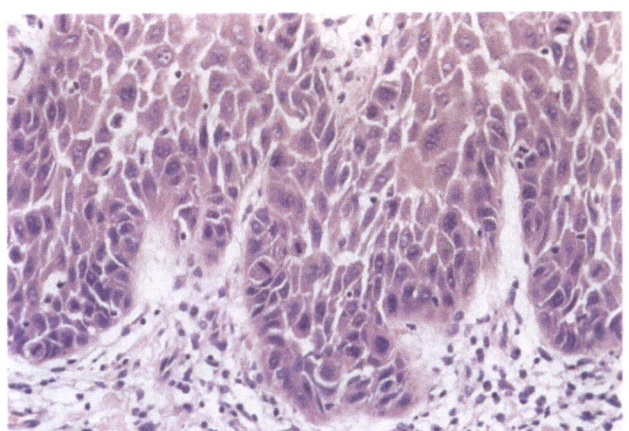

Figure 11.9 Higher magnification, showing the disordered maturation sequence, pleomorphism and hyperchromatism. H & E × 250

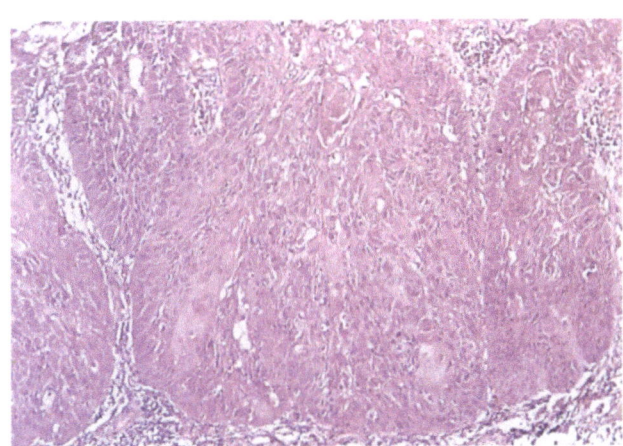

Figure 11.11 Higher magnification, showing severe dysplastic changes in the epithelium, including disorderly or absent stratification, intracellular keratinization pleomorphism and increased mitotic activity. H & E × 100

appearances with the subsequent development of carcinoma. However, should the dysplasia be severe – and this is rare – or even of moderate degree, considerably more caution would be called for.

The degree of dysplasia that may occur in the 'non-specific' mucosal lesions diagnosed clinically as leukoplakia, is more variable in range. The great majority of these lesions show no dysplasia at all. A small number, and especially those that have a variegated appearance with intermingled white and red areas, show significant degrees of dysplasia varying from mild to severe, and a proportion of these will later become invasive. Certain velvety, dusky red lesions – erythroplasias – are especially liable to show severe dysplasia, and to be followed by carcinoma. The term *carcinoma in situ* has sometimes been used when the dysplastic changes extend throughout the whole thickness of·the epithelium.

In the case of an established carcinoma there is often a relatively abrupt transition from apparently normal epithelium to invading neoplastic epithelium. Sometimes, however, there is dysplasia of the epithelium adjoining the area of definite invasion. As this may be the only epithelium present in a small biopsy specimen, the need for thorough sampling and possibly repeat biopsy is clear.

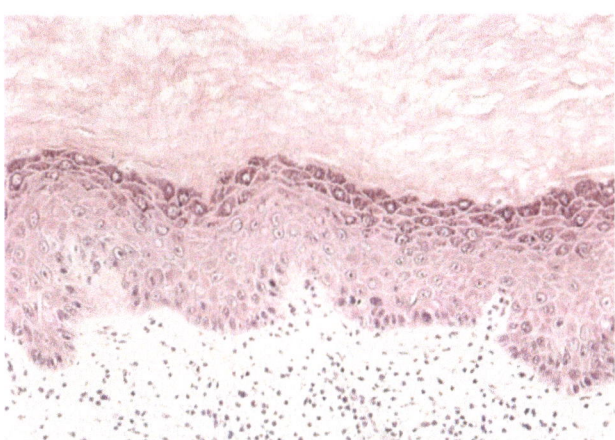

Figure 11.12 Dysplastic epithelium is not infrequently rather atrophic, often with bulbous rete processes. Pronounced hyperkeratinization with a prominent stratum granulosum is seen in this biopsy specimen of a white plaque in the oral mucosa. The deeper layers of the epithelium show cellular atypia. H & E × 200

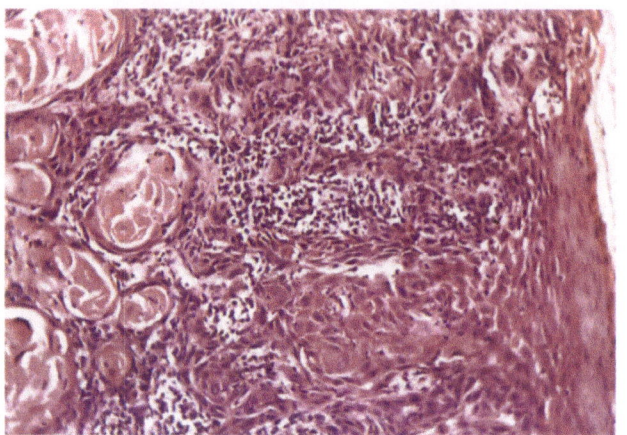

Figure 11.13 Squamous cell carcinoma. A typical well differentiated tumour of the oral mucosa.   H & E × 250

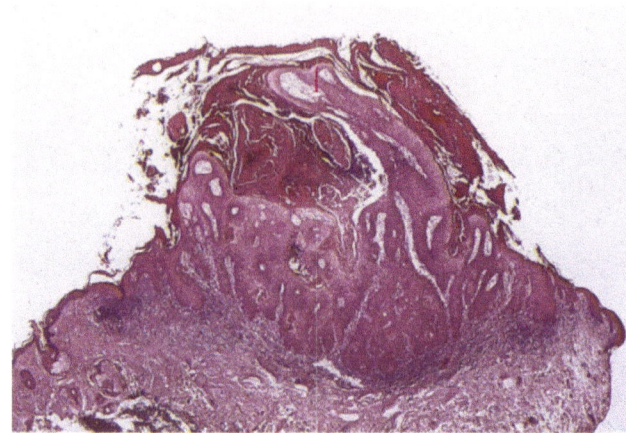

Figure 11.15 Keratoacanthoma. A lip tumour, showing the circumscribed nature of the lesion and the mass of keratin plugging the crateriform depression. H & E × 5·5

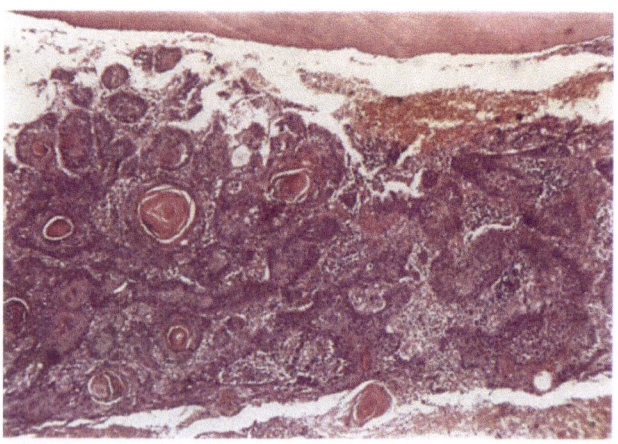

Figure 11.14 Squamous cell carcinoma invading the periodontal ligament (which has torn away from the tooth in the course of preparation).   H & E × 65

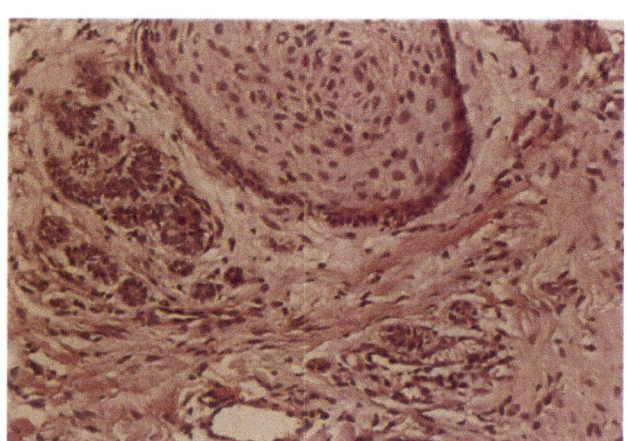

Figure 11.16 Chievitz's organ, consisting of islands of squamous epithelium in the bucco-temporalis fascia.   H & E × 250

The area of the oral mucosa in which a dysplastic lesion is present seems to make little difference to the possible supervention of carcinoma, with one exception. Lesions of the floor of the mouth and ventral surface of the tongue are more likely to become invasive than those elsewhere, so that mild dysplastic changes that would not cause much concern in other areas of the oral mucosa, do so in this situation.

Squamous Cell Carcinoma

Ninety per cent of malignant tumours in the oral tissues are squamous cell carcinomas[6]. About a third of the tumours are in the tongue, a quarter in the lip, and the remainder in the floor of the mouth, gingiva, cheek and palate, in approximately equal proportions.

The large ulcerated growths with rolled edges that figure in the classical descriptions and that immediately suggest malignancy are seen much less frequently nowadays. More often the clinician suspects carcinoma in what might appear to be rather insignificant lesions. These are small ulcers, fissures or cracks in the mucosa of recent onset, but which have not healed after a reasonable trial of local treatment. Three weeks is usually taken as an appro-

priate period, after which biopsy is done. Lesions with a longer history that the patient has probably been harbouring for some time may be biopsied forthwith.

Another type of lesion that comes under suspicion is the white or white-red variegated patch on the mucosa, mentioned in the previous section. Biopsy is done to establish the diagnosis as well as to exclude malignancy.

Microscopically, the great majority of squamous cell carcinomas are well differentiated, presenting no unusual features (Figures 11.13 and 11.14). There is generally little difficulty in making a histological diagnosis in these cases when there is obvious invasion, but early lesions with questionable invasion may be very difficult to distinguish from severe dysplasia. The epithelial hyperplasia that is frequently seen overlying a granular cell myoblastoma can closely resemble well differentiated squamous cell carcinoma, but the adjacent granular cells indicate the correct diagnosis (page 142). The absence of ulceration in a lesion that otherwise looks like squamous cell carcinoma should also indicate caution.

Another non-malignant lesion that may be confused with carcinoma is *keratoacanthoma*. Considerable caution should be employed before making this diagnosis for an oral lesion in any situation other than the lip. Even lip

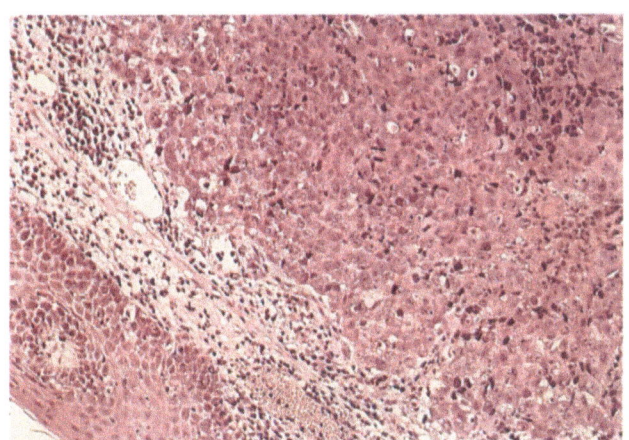

Figure 11.17   Squamous cell carcinoma. A less well differentiated tumour. Intercellular bridges and keratin formation are absent. Relatively normal surface epithelium is seen at bottom left.   H & E × 250

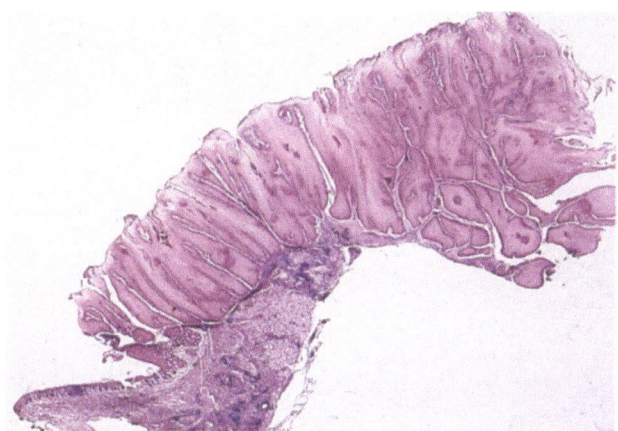

Figure 11.18   Verrucous carcinoma. A tumour of the palate, showing the characteristic exophytic mode of growth.   H & E × 5

lesions are very uncommon and if the tissue submitted is only a portion of the lesion it may be almost impossible to make the distinction from carcinoma. If excision biopsy has provided the entire tumour the diagnosis is much more readily made, since the circumscribed nature of the lesion will be evident, with the characteristic crateriform depression plugged with keratin and surrounded by hyperplastic epithelium (Figure 11.15).

Necrotizing sialometaplasia (page 81) should be borne in mind, especially if minor salivary glands are present in the sections. The metaplastic ducts in this condition have been mistaken for well differentiated squamous cell carcinoma.

The possible presence of Chievitz's organ should be remembered. This structure, which may be the remnants of a vestigial neurosensory organ, is situated in the buccotemporalis fascia on the medial surface of the mandible. It consists of nests of squamous epithelial cells situated close to nerve fibres and may be taken for invasion by squamous cell carcinoma (Figure 11.16).

The term pseudoepitheliomatous hyperplasia has been used for non-neoplastic epithelial overgrowth that might be confused with squamous cell carcinoma. Most of such epithelial hyperplasias are elements of specific conditions that have already been mentioned, but occasionally areas of mucosa that are hyperplastic for no discernible reason may arouse suspicion of malignancy. The acanthosis in these areas can be quite marked, but there is no other evidence of dysplasia and no invasion of the deeper tissues.

The much less common poorly differentiated or anaplastic tumours present the same problems in differential diagnosis in the oral tissues as are encountered with similar growths elsewhere and will therefore not be considered in detail here (Figure 11.17). The tumours that the pathologist would have in mind in this respect would include lymphoma, Ewing's tumour, neuroblastoma, amelanotic melanoma and metastatic tumour from a distant primary growth.

Variants of squamous cell carcinoma seen from time to time in the oral tissues can also give rise to difficulties in diagnosis. They include verrucous carcinoma, spindle cell carcinoma and adenoid squamous cell carcinoma.

Verrucous Carcinoma

The mouth is the commonest site for this tumour. Most tumours arise in the cheek, alveolar or gingival mucosa, followed by the palate and other areas. Characteristically,

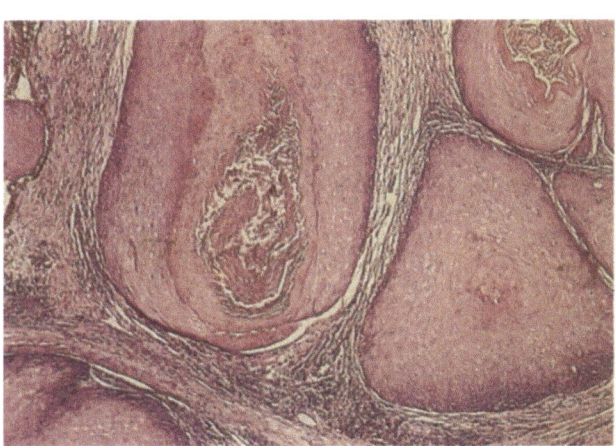

Figure 11.19   Higher magnification, showing the well differentiated epithelium in verrucous carcinoma, invading the connective tissue in rather blunt bulbous processes.   H & E × 100

the tumour has a warty appearance and it grows very slowly, mainly in an outward direction, thus producing the verrucous projection (Figure 11.18). However, in the course of time it invades the underlying tissues, including bone. Microscopically, the tumour epithelium is very well differentiated with little evidence of atypia, so that a small biopsy specimen is easily confused with non-neoplastic epithelial hyperplasia. Adequate samples, however, will show some features that help considerably with the diagnosis. These include the bulbous rete ridge pattern, with the blunt processes all tending to be at the same level (Figure 11.19). In pseudoepitheliomatous hyperplasia the rete ridges are sharp-pointed and elongated rather than bulbous. In addition, the normal epithelium at the edge of a verrucous carcinoma tends to be bent back upon itself because of pressure from the adjacent tumour.

Some areas of a well differentiated squamous cell carcinoma may be very similar to verrucous carcinoma, again particularly if the biopsy specimen is small. However, a greater degree of cellular atypia can nearly always be found in squamous cell carcinoma and the pattern of invasion, with long irregular processes of tumour or discrete islets infiltrating the adjacent tissues, contrasts with the so-called 'pushing edge' of verrucous carcinoma[7].

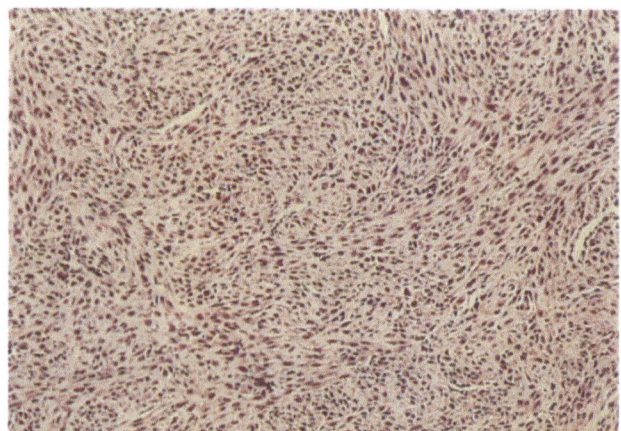

Figure 11.20   Spindle cell carcinoma. A well differentiated tumour consisting of spindle cells of uniform size and shape, arranged in interweaving bundles. H & E × 100

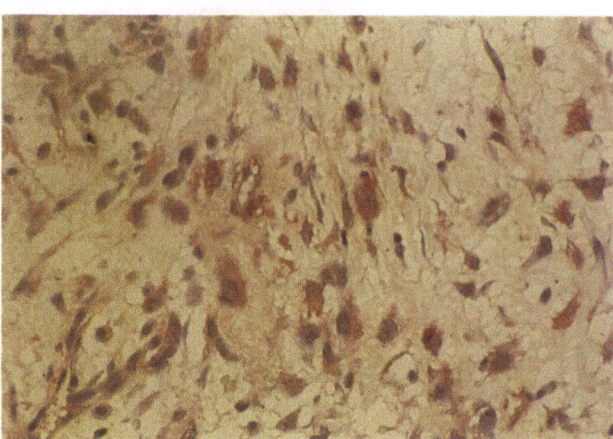

Figure 11.22   Spindle cell carcinoma, showing positive staining for prekeratin. Immunoperoxidase × 400

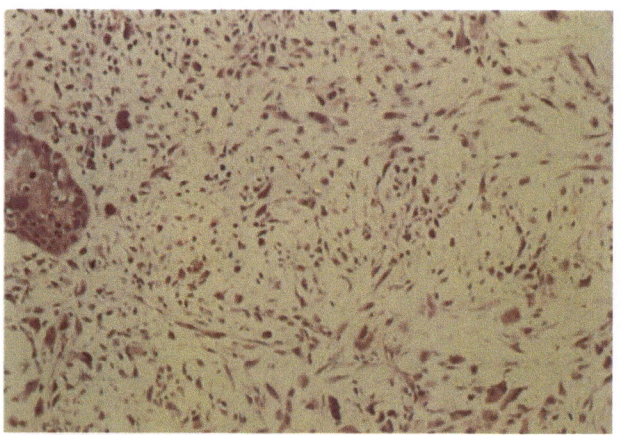

Figure 11.21   A less well differentiated spindle cell carcinoma, with pleomorphic spindle cells and giant cells. An area of more obvious squamous cell growth is present (left edge).   H & E × 250

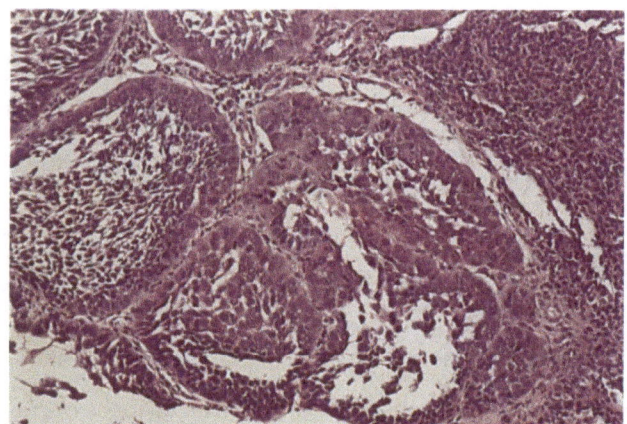

Figure 11.23   Adenoid squamous cell carcinoma. Acantholysis has resulted in the formation of cystic spaces bordered by cubical cells, giving a pseudoglandular appearance.   H & E × 250

Spindle Cell Carcinoma

Although this variant of squamous cell carcinoma may present as a relatively well differentiated tumour composed of spindle cells of fairly uniform size and shape, in some lesions the spindle cells display much variation in size and shape, hyperchromatism, and often numerous abnormal mitoses and tumour giant cells are seen[8]. Areas showing more typical squamous cell carcinoma may be found, which gives the clue to the diagnosis (Figures 11.20 and 11.21). In the absence of such areas the possibility of a mesenchymal tumour must be considered. Electron microscopy can be of help here by demonstrating the characteristics of epithelial cells such as desmosomes and tonofibrils, as can also the immunocytochemical demonstration of prekeratin in epithelial cells (Figure 11.22).

Adenoid Squamous Cell Carcinoma

Although the head and neck are the common sites for this tumour it is rare in the oral tissues. The tumour has been reported in the lip where, like many of those of the skin, it appears to be related to solar damage[9]. Microscopically, a process of acantholysis appears to be taking place in a squamous cell carcinoma. This results in the formation of spaces containing desquamated cells, while the remaining cells that line the spaces tend to be cubical. Hence there is a pseudoglandular appearance (Figure 11.23).

Carcinoma in the Jaws

Rarely, carcinoma may arise as a purely intraosseous growth. The possible sources of origin for tumours of this type are the epithelium of odontogenic cysts, the epithelial rests that normally remain in the jaws after the teeth have developed and intraosseous inclusions of salivary tissue.

Radicular, dentigerous and keratocysts have all been reported as giving rise to squamous cell carcinoma but, although the pathologist may be satisfied as to the histological identity of the tumour, its assignment to a cystic origin is a matter for detailed clinical and radiographic as well as pathological investigation. Tumours considered to have originated within bone and subsequently perforated the cortex may in fact have commenced in the soft tissues and then invaded the bone. Similarly, tumours that look as if they have originated in cysts may in reality be neoplasms in which cystic change has taken place as a secondary phenomenon. Metastasis from a distant primary growth is a possibility that should always be kept in mind.

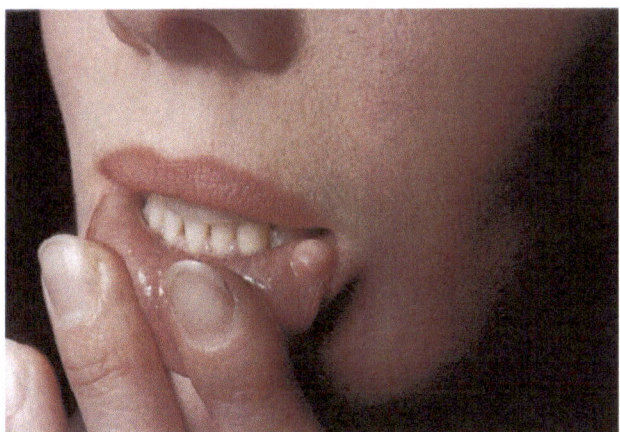

Figure 11.24 Fibroepithelial polyp of the lip

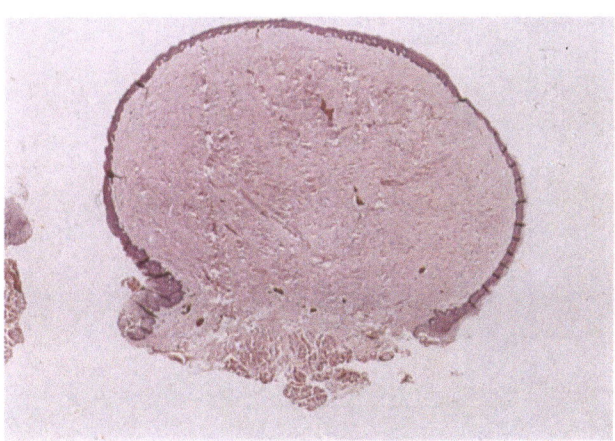

Figure 11.26 Fibroepithelial polyp. The lesion consists of hyperplastic fibrous tissue covered by squamous epithelium. H & E × 4·5

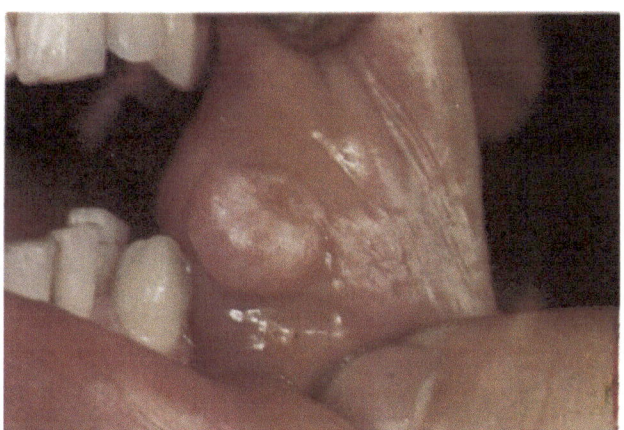

Figure 11.25 Fibroepithelial polyp of the cheek

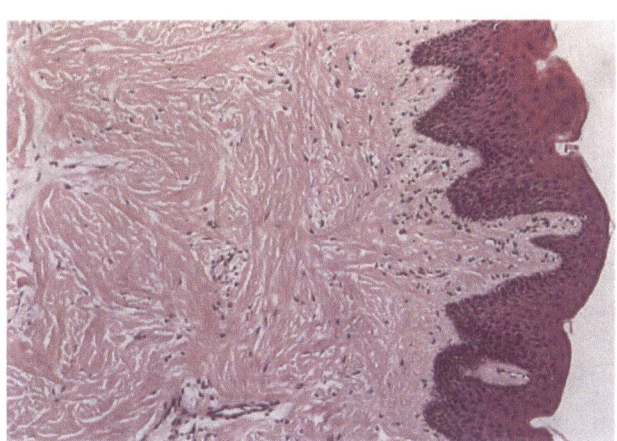

Figure 11.27 Higher magnification from Figure 11.26, showing the well formed collagen bundles that constitute the lesion. H & E × 250

Primary intraosseous tumours, other than those arising from cysts and which are thought to originate in remnants of odontogenic epithelium, may have a pattern suggesting this odontogenic origin. They may thus have an alveolar or plexiform arrangement, with palisading of the peripheral cells. However, these are rare tumours and the possibility of some other, extraosseous, origin should be excluded.

Salivary tumours may rarely arise within the jaws. The majority of such growths are mucoepidermoid tumours.

Basal Cell Carcinoma

Basal cell carcinomas in the oral region are seen mainly in the skin of the lip, especially the upper, from where they may spread to involve the mucocutaneous areas. Tumours that would be accepted histologically as basal cell carcinomas if they had occurred in skin have been reported, rarely, in the oral mucosa. Their precise nature is problematical.

Multiple basal cell carcinomas of the skin are seen in the multiple naevoid basal cell carcinoma and jaw cyst syndrome (page 104).

Tumours of Fibrous Tissue

Proliferative lesions of fibrous tissue are the commonest of all tumour-like lumps or overgrowths in the oral tissues, but only a small minority are true neoplasms. Most of them are reactive hyperplasias. They are conveniently considered as 'peripheral' lesions affecting the soft tissues and 'central' lesions originating in the jawbones. The peripheral soft tissue lesions comprise a number of entities which have had many indiscriminately applied synonyms, the commonest and the least accurate being 'fibroma'. Very few indeed are neoplastic[10].

Reactive and Inflammatory Hyperplasias

Fibrous hyperplasia. Circumscribed tumour-like nodules of fibrous tissue are common in the cheek, lip, tongue, palate and gingiva (Figures 11.24–11.27). They are due to mild trauma or other irritation and often this may be obvious. For example, cheek lesions are frequently situated opposite the line of occlusion of the upper and lower teeth and the patient may know that he keeps biting his cheek in this area. Similarly, nodules often arise at the border of the tongue for the same reason. In other cases

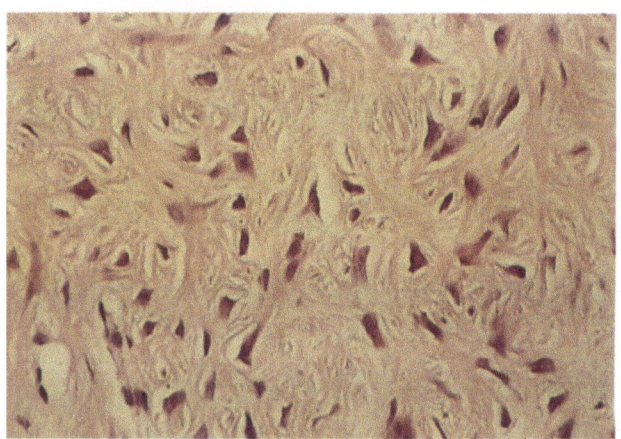

Figure 11.28 Spindle and stellate cells are seen in some fibrous lesions. H & E × 320

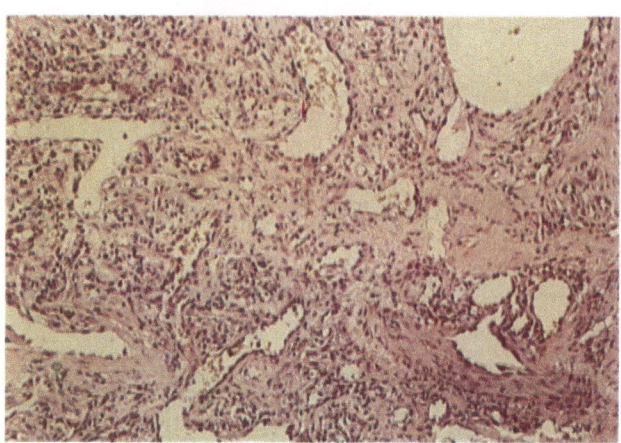

Figure 11.31 Higher magnification, showing the prominent vascularity that is characteristic of pyogenic granuloma. H & E × 100

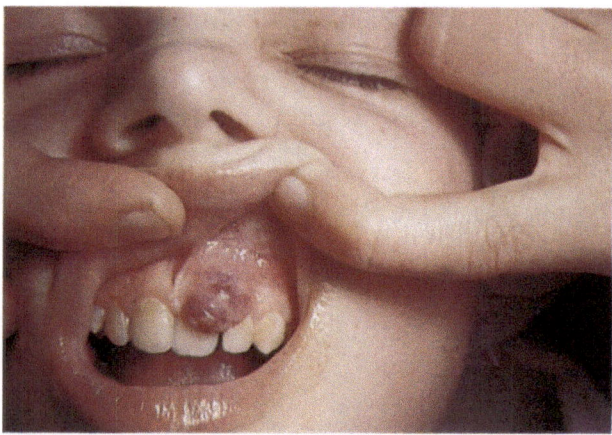

Figure 11.29 Pyogenic granuloma. A gingival lesion

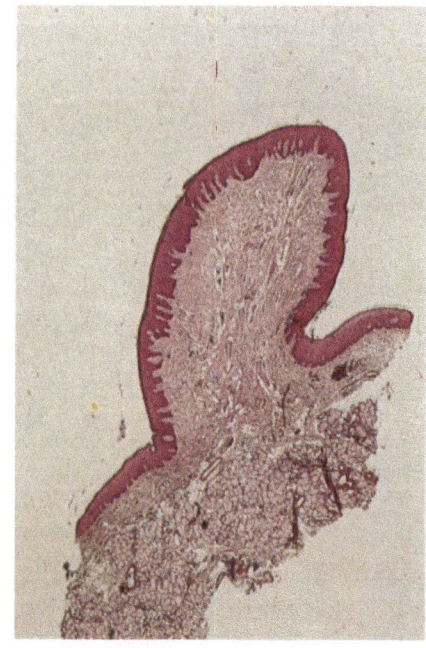

Figure 11.32 Denture-induced hyperplasia. The edge of the denture has produced a groove in the tissues, with concomitant overgrowth of fibrous tissue. H & E × 4

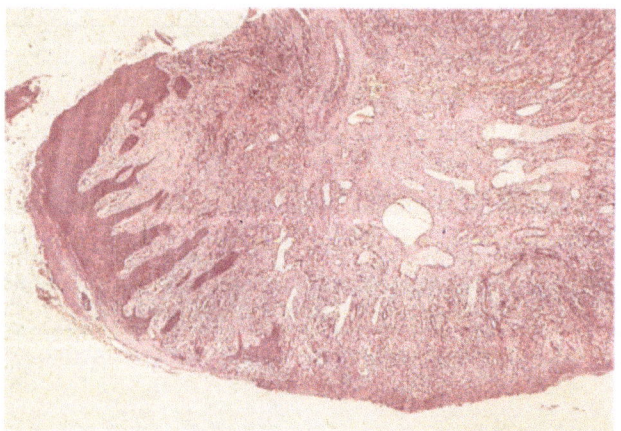

Figure 11.30 Pyogenic granuloma. The lesion consists of vascular fibrous and granulation tissue covered by squamous epithelium. There is superficial ulceration over the convexity of the lesion. H & E × 40

the causal factor may not be readily apparent. Microscopically, lesions of this type consist of bundles of well collagenized fibrous tissue running in all directions, but rarely forming a capsule. There may be areas of inflammatory infiltration, but frequently these fibrous nodules remain uninflamed. The overlying epithelium may be stretched and slightly atrophic, or it may show variable acanthosis (Figures 11.26 and 11.27). The designation *fibroepithelial polyp* is frequently used for lesions of this type. Gingival lesions (*fibrous epulis*) are often much more fibroblastic than those in other sites (page 44).

In an uncommon variant that has been termed giant cell fibroma there are numerous spindle and stellate cells, together with multinucleated cells (Figure 11.28)[11].

Pyogenic granuloma. Although usually seen in the gingiva between two teeth, this lesion can also occur in the lip, tongue and elsewhere (Figure 11.29). As in the

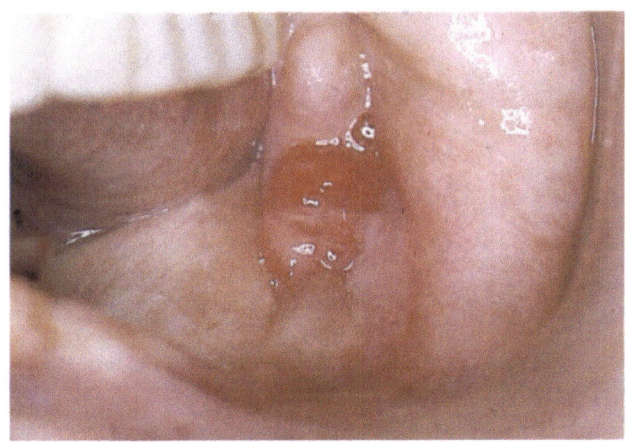

Figure 11.33 Fasciitis. This lesion presented as a fleshy swelling of the edentulous alveolus

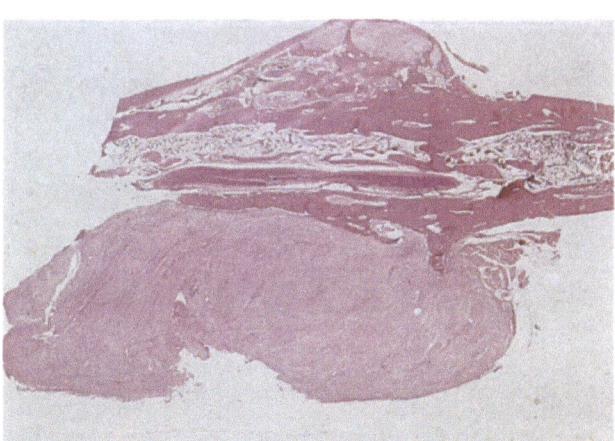

Figure 11.35 Fibromatosis. A lesion in the submandibular area in a child 3 years, extending to infiltrate the mandible. H & E × 8

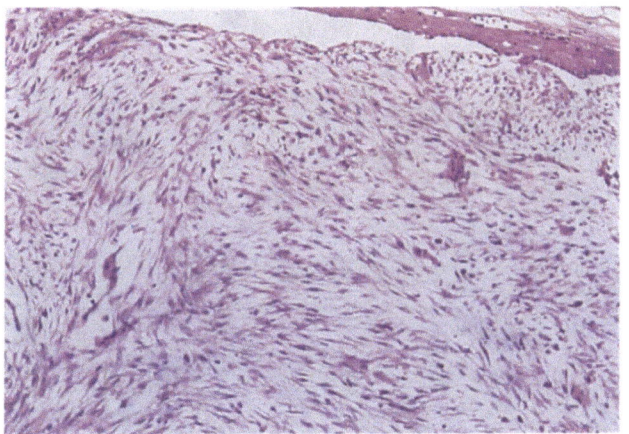

Figure 11.34 The lesion shown in Figure 11.33. There is fibroblastic proliferation, with a loose textured feathery appearance.

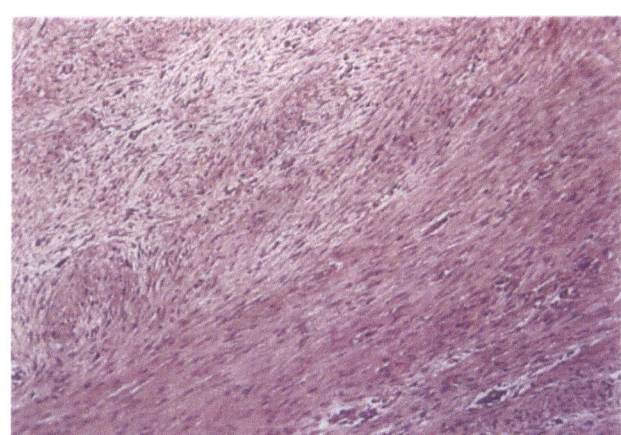

Figure 11.36 Higher magnification, showing the lesion to consist of fibroblastic proliferation and collagen bundles. H & E × 70

corresponding lesion of the skin, the dominating microscopic features are vascularity and inflammation[12]. The lesion consists of granulation tissue with heavy inflammatory infiltration, often with a prominent acute element. There are many dilated capillaries and the overlying epithelium is frequently ulcerated (Figures 11.30 and 11.31).

Hyperplasia related to dentures. When the flange of a denture bears unduly into the tissues a groove is formed, with overgrowth of the surrounding fibrous tissue which comes to form a leaf or lobelike protuberance (Figure 11.32). The lesion is sometimes referred to as denture-induced fibrosis, fibroma or hyperplasia. Treatment is excision of the redundant tissue, which is seen on microscopic examination to consist of collagenous fibrous tissue covered by squamous epithelium which may be of variable thickness, slightly atrophic or slightly hyperplastic, or a combination of these changes. There is usually some chronic inflammatory infiltration in the subepithelial zone and there may be superficial ulceration[13].

Fasciitis. Fasciitis is uncommon in the oral tissues and usually presents as a soft tissue swelling in the mandibular region (Figure 11.33). As in similar lesions elsewhere, oral lesions have a short history, generally less than a month. Microscopically, they show areas of fibroblastic proliferation intermingled with patchy chronic inflammatory infil-

tration. The fibroblasts are haphazardly arranged in a myxoid matrix which results in a rather loose textured, feathery appearance (Figure 11.34). They vary in size and shape and are usually larger than normal with plump nuclei and prominent nucleoli. Some have a rather triangular appearance. The fibroblastic proliferation involves adjacent muscle bundles, which tend to be broken up by the infiltrating cells[14].

Fibromatosis

Congenital and juvenile fibromatosis. The head and neck are the commonest areas for the proliferative and locally infiltrative fibrous lesions that are seen in infants and children. In the oral region lesions usually involve the soft tissues, but they may also extend into the mandible or maxilla[15]. Identical lesions are seen in adults, but they are much rarer. Microscopically, the prominent feature of these lesions is fibroblastic proliferation with the formation of interweaving bundles of spindle cells, in some areas infiltrating muscle or bone (Figures 11.35 and 11.36). Prominent, thin-walled vessels are a notable feature of some lesions. Although the fibroblasts vary to some extent in size and shape, hyperchromatic or abnormal nuclei are

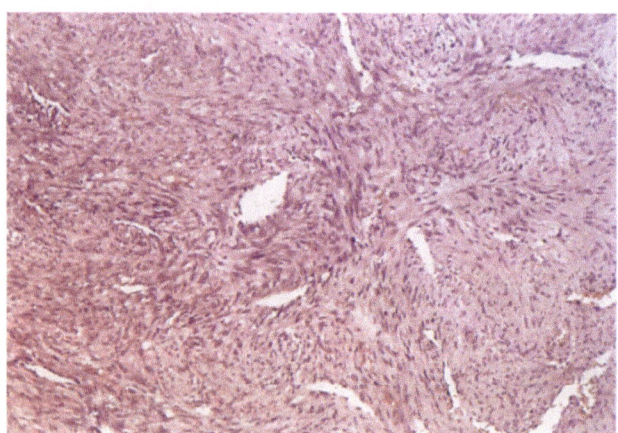

Figure 11.37   Fibromatosis. A lesion in the submandibular area and neck in a woman of 38 years, consisting of interweaving bundles of spindle cells and collagen. Thin-walled vessels are prominent.   H & E × 100

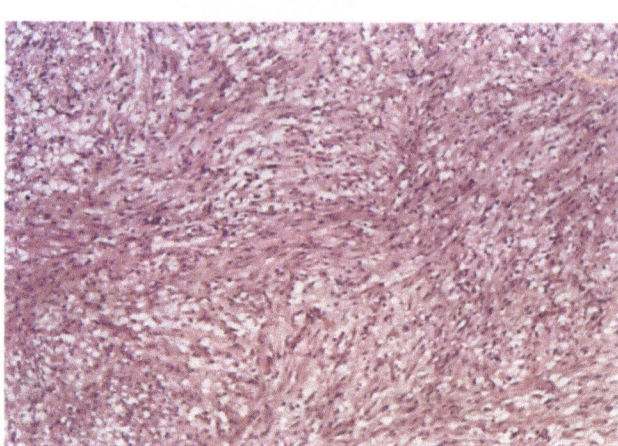

Figure 11.39   Desmoplastic fibroma. A mandibular tumour, consisting of spindle-shaped fibroblasts and bundles of collagen.   H & E × 100

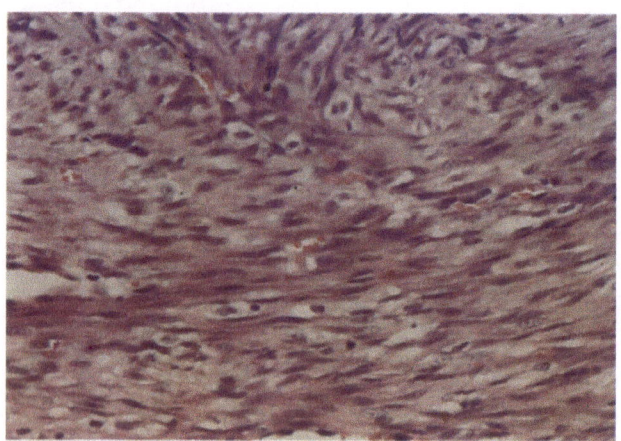

Figure 11.38   Higher magnification, showing the regularity of the fibromatous tissue, and absence of significant atypia.   H & E × 250

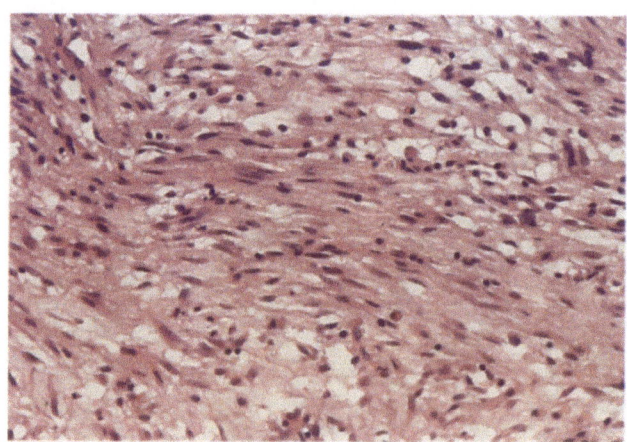

Figure 11.40   Higher magnification, showing the small, evenly staining and regular nuclei of the fibroblasts.   H & E × 250

not observed nor is there any significant mitotic activity (Figures 11.37 and 11.38).

Gingival fibromatosis. This hereditary condition, which may be associated with other developmental defects, is characterized by overgrowth of the gingivae. A condition that clinically resembles gingival fibromatosis is caused by phenytoin, used in the control of epilepsy (page 38).

Neoplasms

Fibroma. This is a rare tumour in the oral tissues. The soft tissue lesions that form tumour-like protuberances and nodules in the mouth are practically all reactive hyperplasias or neoplasms of various other types, as already mentioned. Intraosseous lesions are uncommon and comprise a number of different entities.

Desmoplastic fibroma. This tumour is seen especially in young people, below the age of 20, and much more often in the mandible than in the maxilla[16]. It presents as a painless, gradual enlargement of the jaw with a variable radiographic appearance, usually as a radiolucency which is well defined and uni- or multilocular. The tumour is not associated with embedded teeth. Microscopically, it is a cellular fibroblastic lesion producing mature collagen fibres. The fibroblasts are spindle-shaped and have relatively small and evenly staining nuclei. There is no pleomorphism and no mitotic activity. Metaplastic bone formation is absent and there is no odontogenic epithelium present (Figures 11.39 and 11.40).

Odontogenic fibroma. This tumour is described in Chapter 10 (page 123).

Fibrosarcoma. In the jaws, fibrosarcoma occurs mainly as a mandibular tumour[17]. It is very rare in the maxilla. It can develop at any age and the jaw swelling is often accompanied by pain and loosening of teeth. Radiographs show an ill defined radiolucency. In the soft tissues the tumour presents as a localized swelling, resembling at first the common fibrous hyperplasias but growing more rapidly and frequently ulcerating. Histologically, the features are those of fibrosarcoma elsewhere (Figures 11.41 and 11.42).

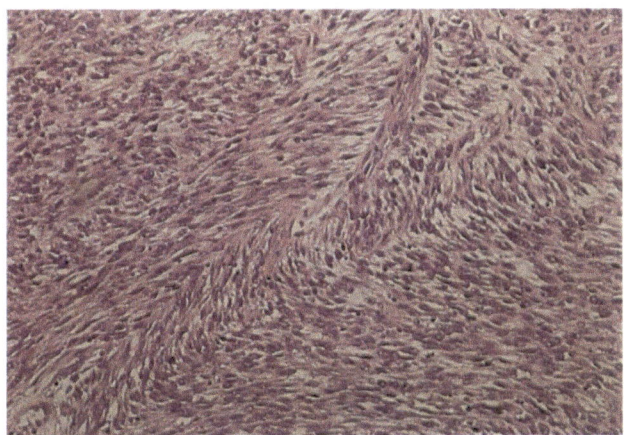

Figure 11.41 Fibrosarcoma of the mandible, showing the typical herring-bone pattern formed by the bundles of collagen. H & E × 100

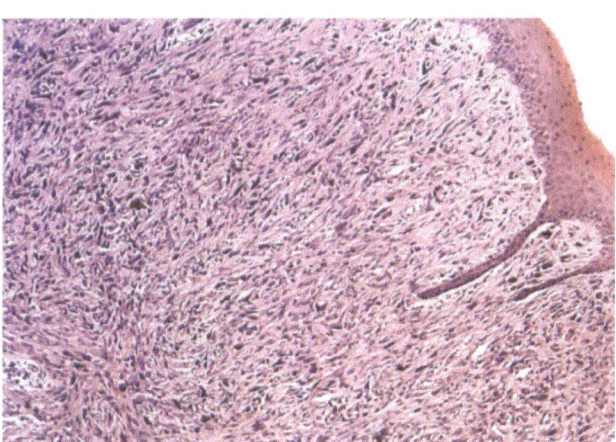

Figure 11.43 Malignant fibrous histiocytoma. A maxillary lesion, in the sub-epithelial connective tissue. H & E × 100

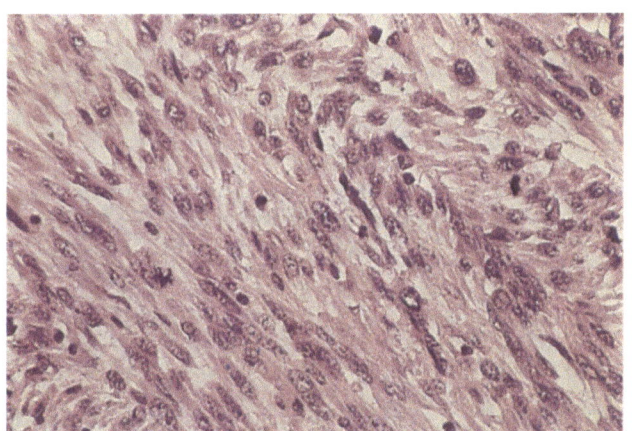

Figure 11.42 Fibrosarcoma. Higher magnification, showing pleomorphism and other features of atypia of the fibroblasts, contrasting with the small, regular fibroblasts in fibromatosis. H & E × 250

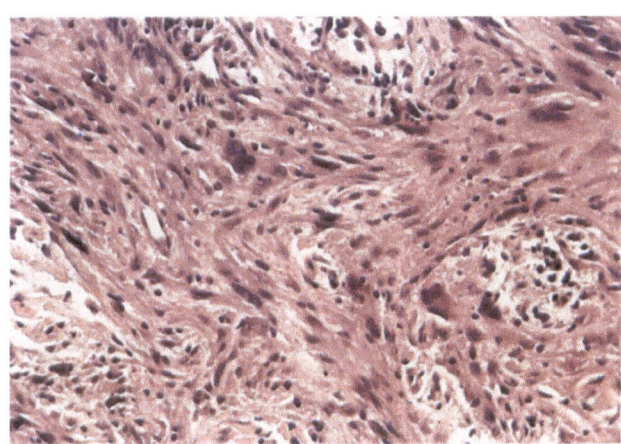

Figure 11.44 Higher magnification, showing the characteristic storiform pattern formed by the fibrous tissue, and the pleomorphism of the fibroblastic–histiocytic cells. H & E × 250

Fibrous histiocytoma. Benign fibrous histiocytoma is very rare in the oral tissues, malignant fibrous histiocytoma a little less so. Most of the reported cases have originated in the soft tissues and subsequently invaded bone, usually the mandible[18]. The histological appearances are as seen in these tumours in other parts of the body (Figures 11.43 and 11.44).

Differential diagnosis of fibrous tumours. Although at least 95% of fibrous lesions in the oral tissues are benign, any of the malignant fibrous tumours may appear on occasion. These are much more likely to involve bone than to be solely soft tissue lesions. When bone is involved, this may be due to a tumour that has originated centrally and may remain within the bone, although most central malignant tumours will in time perforate the cortex and invade adjacent soft tissues. Alternatively, the bony involvement may be due to a soft tissue tumour spreading to involve adjacent bone.

The problems of histological diagnosis are those that apply to fibrous tumours in any other situation and are therefore not dealt with here in detail. They include the differentiation of the fibrous hyperplasias and fibromatoses from well differentiated fibrosarcoma and malignant fibrous histiocytoma. Other spindle cell tumours such as neural tumours have to be considered, as well as salivary tumours. Submandibular gland tumours are those likely to invade the mandible and very occasionally they may be of undifferentiated spindle cell type. Another epithelial spindle cell tumour is the spindle cell variant of squamous cell carcinoma. Although it is uncommon, the mouth is one of its more frequent sites. Bone-forming tumours may on occasion produce very little bone and, unless thoroughly sampled, may appear to consist entirely of fusocellular tissue. The benign ossifying fibroma can come into this category since, especially in young children, it may form very little calcified tissue while at the same time growing very rapidly and causing anxiety on clinical grounds alone (page 72). Fibrosarcomatous varieties of osteosarcoma must also be kept in mind. They may form very little tumour bone, but alkaline phosphatase activity can be demonstrated. This is absent from fibrosarcoma.

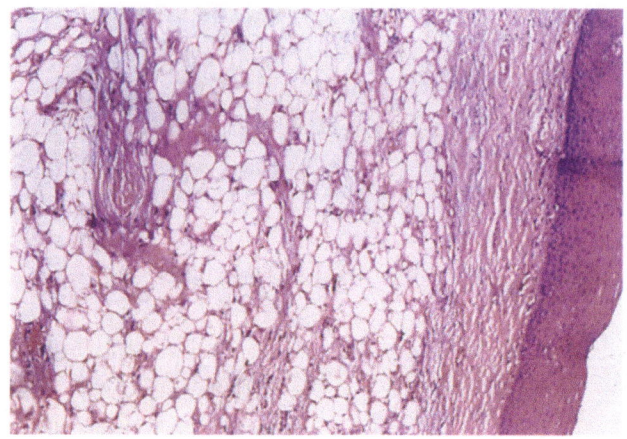

Figure 11.45 Lipoma of cheek. The tumour consists of fat cells with intermingled fibrous tissue, situated in the subepithelial connective tissue.   H & E × 100

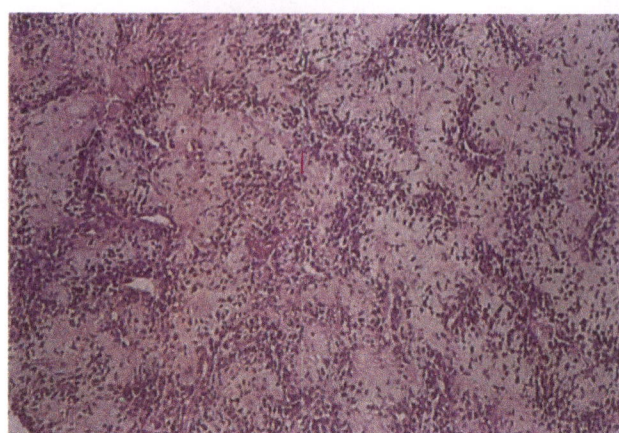

Figure 11.47   Mesenchymal chondrosarcoma of maxilla. The tumour consists of small round and oval cells in a fibrocartilagenous matrix.   H & E × 100

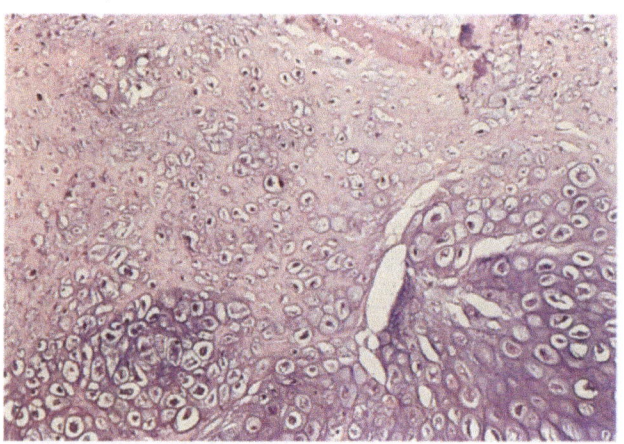

Figure 11.46   Chondrosarcoma of maxilla, showing irregular and cellular cartilage, with pleomorphic cells.   H & E × 250

Tumours of Adipose Tissue

Oral lipomas usually appear as round or ovoid, occasionally lobulated, masses that originate in the submucous fat. Histologically, they show the usual features of these growths (Figure 11.45). Intraosseous lipoma is very rare; most reported tumours have been in the mandible. Liposarcoma in the oral tissues is likewise very rare[19].

Tumours of Cartilage

Chondroma and Chondrosarcoma

Cartilage tumours occur in the jaws at any age, although the maximum incidence is in adults in the fifth or sixth decades. Unlike many other jaw tumours, the maxilla is more often affected than the mandible[20]. In the maxilla the anterior region is the usual site, whereas in the mandible the molar-premolar region or the symphysis are most commonly affected. The tumours are often painless, at least in the earlier stages, and the rate of growth is variable. The roots of teeth may be involved, which leads to their loosening and exfoliation. This may be an early symptom. Radiologically, there is evidence of bone destruction. The

radiolucency may or may not have well defined margins and sometimes it may contain areas of patchy calcification.

Histologically, the usual features of cartilage tumours are seen and, as in other bones, there is often the problem of differentiating between benign and malignant lesions (Figure 11.46). Malignancy is indicated by an increased number of cells with plump nuclei, more than the occasional binucleate cell and the presence of giant cartilage cells. If these features are pronounced there is little doubt that the tumour is a chondrosarcoma. However, even a very well differentiated tumour may still be a low grade chondrosarcoma, as will become evident in due course. It is probable that most oral intraosseous cartilage tumours are malignant, although some have a low growth potential. Rarely, a cartilage tumour in the jaws will be a secondary chondrosarcoma from a primary growth elsewhere.

Apart from the areas of the maxilla and mandible already mentioned, the other sites for cartilage tumours in the jaws are the mandibular condyle and the coronoid process. The lesions here have been referred to under a variety of designations – chondroma, osteochondroma, hypertrophy, hyperplasia – and their exact nature is not always clear.

Soft tissue chondromatous tumours are seen occasionally in the oral region, the tongue being the commonest site, where they are sometimes called lingual choristomas. Islands of ectopic cartilage may be found in the palate and gingivae, especially behind the upper incisor teeth. Occasionally islands of metaplastic cartilage related to irritation from ill-fitting dentures may be seen.

Mesenchymal Chondrosarcoma

The skull and jaws are relatively common sites for this rare tumour[21]. Unlike the usual type of chondrosarcoma, it affects younger persons in the second to fourth decades. It involves soft tissue as well as bone and consists of masses of small round or oval cells together with cartilage (Figure 11.47). There is very little pleomorphism of the small round cells and the cartilage is very well differentiated. This helps to distinguish the tumour from the usual type of chondrosarcoma which, if cellular to a comparable degree, would show considerable pleomorphism of its cartilaginous element. Alternatively, a well differentiated chondrosarcoma would not be as cellular as a mesenchymal chondrosarcoma.

Chondroblastoma and *chondromyxoid fibroma* have been reported in the jaws but are very rare.

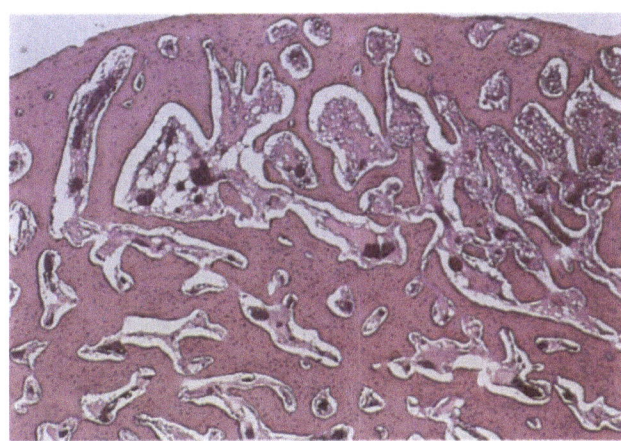

Figure 11.48 Osteoma of maxilla. The tumour, which presented as a circumscribed outgrowth, consists of mature cancellous lamellar bone. H & E × 70

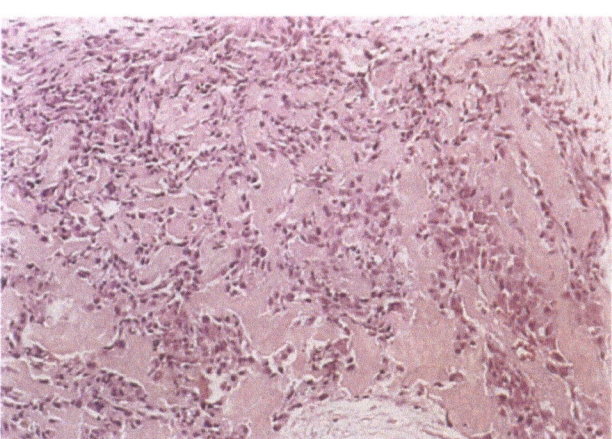

Figure 11.50 Osteosarcoma of the mandible, showing pleomorphic osteoblasts and osteoid tissue. H & E × 200

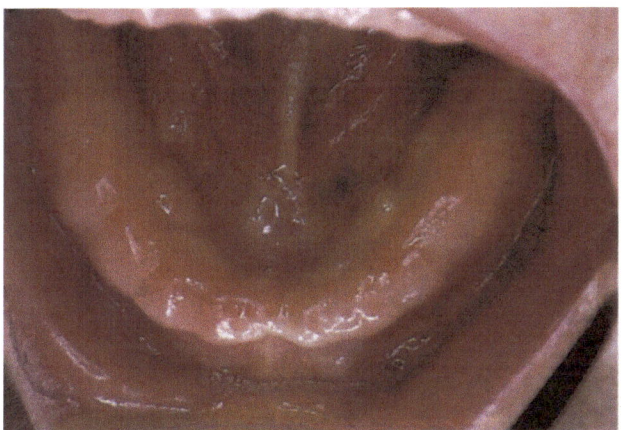

Figure 11.49 Torus mandibularis. This bony growth from the mandible consists of compact lamellar bone. H & E × 70

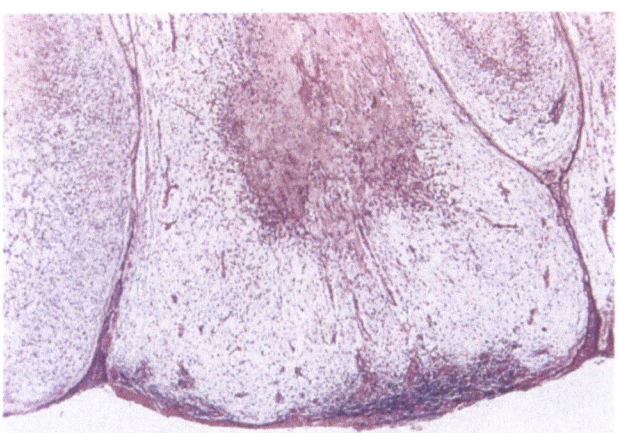

Figure 11.51 Parosteal osteosarcoma. This mandibular tumour presented as a localized outgrowth and was at first thought to be a fibrous epulis. The lesion consists of osteoid and bone in a fibrocellular matrix. H & E × 100

Tumours of Bone

Osteoma

This tumour arises almost exclusively in membrane bones in the skull and in the jaws. The two histological varieties, cancellous and compact, form dense radiopaque lumps that protrude from the bone, more often the mandible than the maxilla. The cancellous tumour consists of trabeculae of mature lamellar bone with the intervening spaces containing fibrous or fatty marrow (Figure 11.48). The compact osteoma is a dense mass of lamellar bone with very few marrow spaces.

Cancellous or compact bone similar to that constituting the osteomas can be seen in a variety of conditions. Diagnosis therefore depends not only on the histology but also on the clinical and radiological findings. This is not difficult in those tumours that arise subperiostally and grow out from the bone to form the characteristic dense masses. It is much more difficult to decide whether a lesion that forms a tumour-like mass centrally within bone is an osteoma, since certain types of ossifying fibroma and some varieties of cementoma or of fibrous dysplasia may have similar histological appearances. It is in fact problematic as to whether a true central osteoma does indeed exist[22].

Soft tissue osteomas, or lesions that are conveniently described as such, are rare in the oral tissues. Most of the reported lesions, which consist of dense lamellar bone, have presented in the posterior third of the tongue. Metaplastic bone formation is common in fibrous epulides (page 44).

Torus palatinus and *torus mandibularis* are developmental lesions that form bony outgrowths from the palate and the mandible respectively. They consist of compact bone of normal structure (Figure 11.49).

Osteoid osteoma and osteoblastoma are seen occasionally in the jaws.

Osteosarcoma

Osteosarcoma is less common in the jaws than in many other bones. When it does occur the mandible is more often affected than the maxilla. In the usual type of central growth there is generally a painful swelling of the jaw that increases in size fairly rapidly and is often accompanied by such symptoms as loosening of teeth and numbness of the lip and chin. Parosteal tumours are also encountered and these may present as alveolar lumps that look very like the common fibrous nodules or epulides[23].

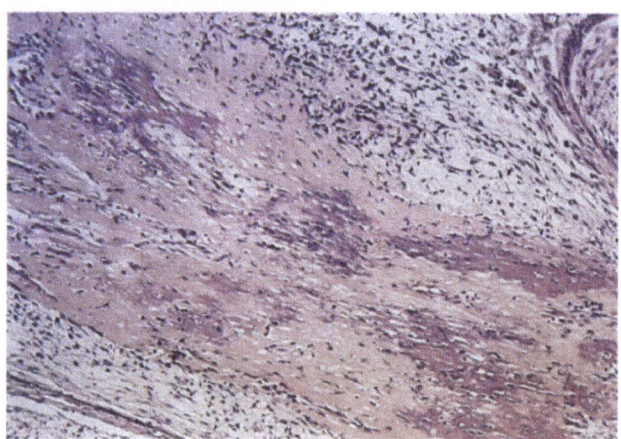

Figure 11.52 Higher magnification from Figure 11.51, showing the irregular tumour bone and osteoblasts. H & E × 250

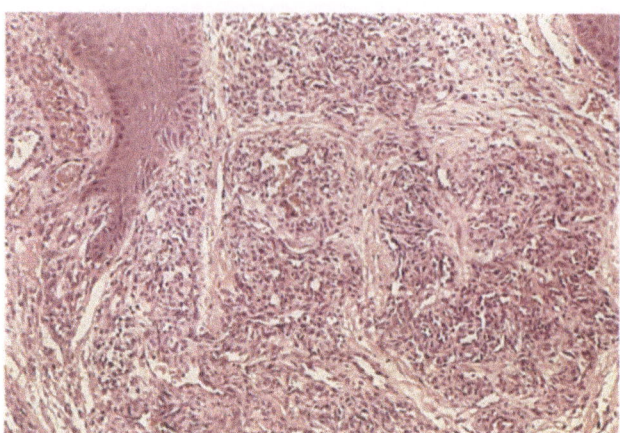

Figure 11.54 Higher magnification, showing the proliferating endothelium and capillaries. H & E × 200

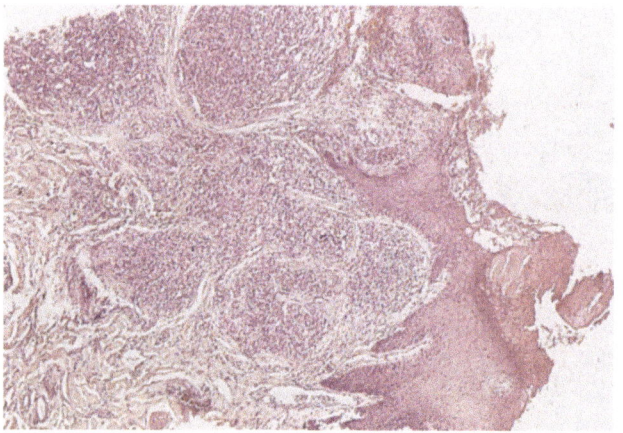

Figure 11.53 Haemangioma of the gingiva. The lesion consists of masses of endothelial cells and small capillaries, situated in the subepithelial fibrous tissue. H & E × 100

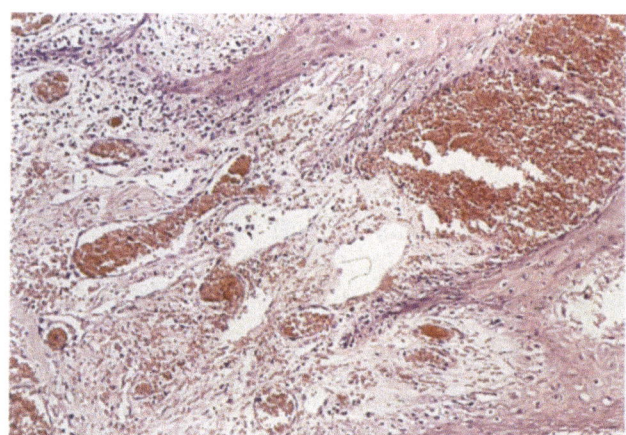

Figure 11.55 A gingival haemangioma with larger capillaries and vascular spaces. H & E × 250

Histologically, central tumours show the usual features of osteosarcoma and the diagnostic problems are essentially the same as those elsewhere in the skeleton (Figures 11.50–11.52). In the jaws, cementoblastoma must be kept in mind (page 121). The bone-forming lesions like fibrous dysplasia, ossifying fibroma and the cementomas are not likely to cause confusion since the bone is usually formed metaplastically. Even when numerous osteoblasts are present, these cells remain of normal appearance and do not show the pleomorphism, hyperchromatism and mitotic activity of malignant osteoblasts.

Vascular Tumours

Haemangioma

The oral and perioral tissues are a relatively common site for haemangiomas, using the term in its broad sense to include, as well as localized swellings, lesions such as portwine stains and cirsoid and arteriovenous aneurysms. In the oral mucosa these lesions usually appear as solitary, small reddish or purple swellings. Rarely, there may be multiple lesions or more extensive ones comparable to the portwine lesions of the skin. Although these unusual types of lesion may be seen in an otherwise normal indi-

vidual, their presence always suggests the possibility of an angiomatous syndrome (Sturge–Weber syndrome and others). Histologically, these angiomas are of the usual capillary or cavernous type, or very often a mixture of the two patterns (Figures 11.53–11.57). In infants the lesions are often more cellular and solid.

Muscle is a not uncommon site for haemangioma and in the oral region this is usually the masseter[24].

Haemangiomas of bone are found most often in the vertebrae and skull; in the jaws the mandible is much more often affected than the maxilla. There are some suggestive clinical signs that may be present in jaw tumours, such as bleeding around teeth that have become unaccountably loose, compressibility or pulsation of the tumour or the presence of a bruit. These signs usually make the surgeon very chary about extracting teeth or doing a biopsy, as such manoeuvres can result in massive haemorrhage. If surgical treatment is required, this will probably be complete excision, so the pathologist's specimen is likely to be a segment of jaw[25].

Microscopically, the lesion is usually of the cavernous type. There are often appreciable amounts of fibrous tissue between the cavernous spaces, in which osteoid and bone may be formed (Figure 11.58). The possibility of the lesion being an aneurysmal bone cyst arising either alone or in association with some other bone lesion such as

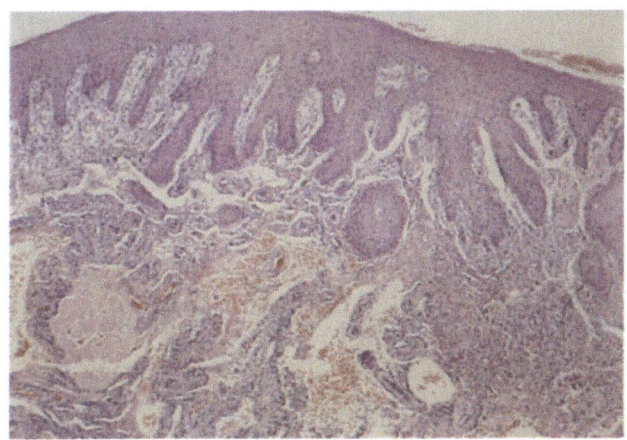

Figure 11.56 A gingival lesion in the Sturge–Weber syndrome. Numerous capillaries and larger vascular spaces are seen in the subepithelial tissue, together with chronic inflammatory infiltration. H & E × 100

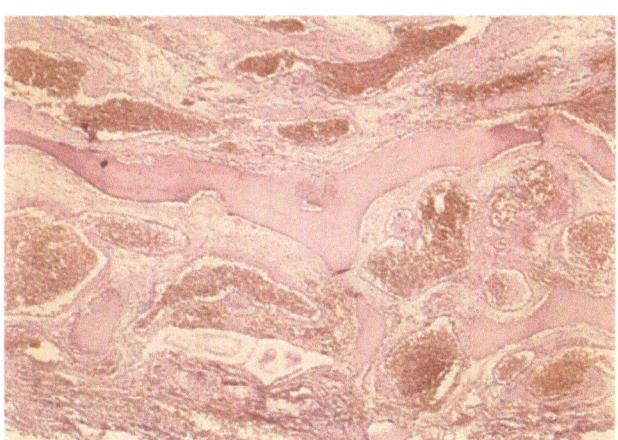

Figure 11.58 Haemangioma of mandible. This intraosseous lesion consists of cavernous vascular spaces in the mandibular bone. H & E × 100

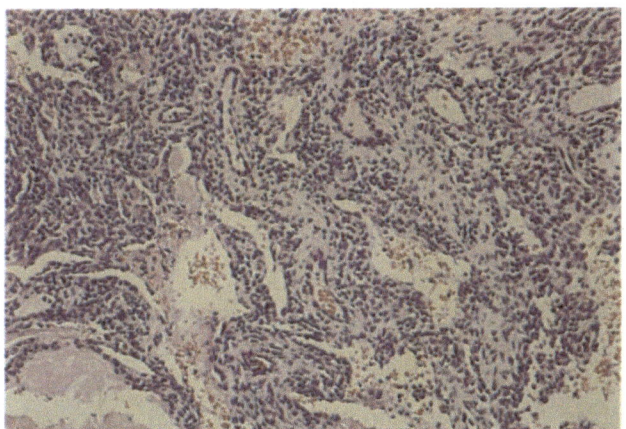

Figure 11.57 Higher magnification from Figure 11.56, showing the capillaries and proliferated endothelial cells. H & E × 250

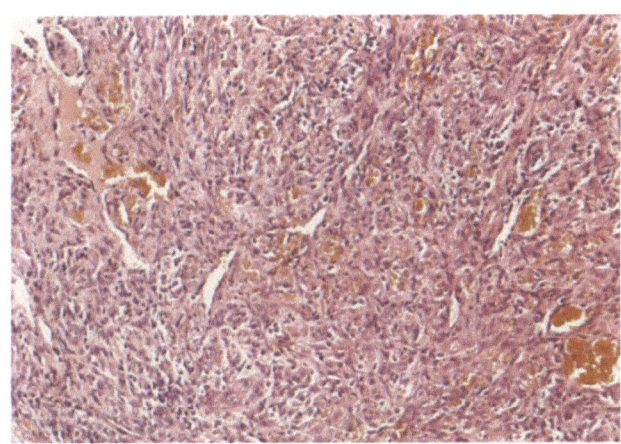

Figure 11.59 Kaposi's sarcoma. This oral lesion presented as a dark blue raised area in the cheek mucosa of a patient who had numerous skin and other lesions. It consists of endothelial cells lining numerous vascular channels, intermingled with spindle cells. H & E × 250

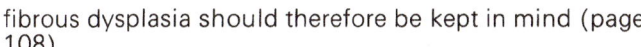

fibrous dysplasia should therefore be kept in mind (page 108).

Haemangiopericytoma is occasionally seen in the oral tissues, where it displays no unusual features.

Angiosarcoma

Angiosarcoma is rare in the oral region, where it occurs in both the soft tissues and the jaws. The usual histological features are seen. Kaposi's sarcoma is also rare, but oral lesions, which appear in some 10% of cases, are becoming increasingly evident with the rising incidence of the acquired immune deficiency syndrome (Figure 11.59).

Lymphangioma

The mouth, especially the tongue, is the commonest site for lymphangioma[26]. Lesions may also arise in the lip, cheek, palate or, less often, elsewhere in the oral mucosa (Figure 11.60). The ramifying, dilated lymph channels that constitute the lesion are separated by a fine connective tissue stroma, but where there have been repeated attacks of inflammation there is likely to be a considerable degree of fibrosis and sometimes calcification. These inflammatory episodes are not uncommon in oral tumours because of their liability to trauma.

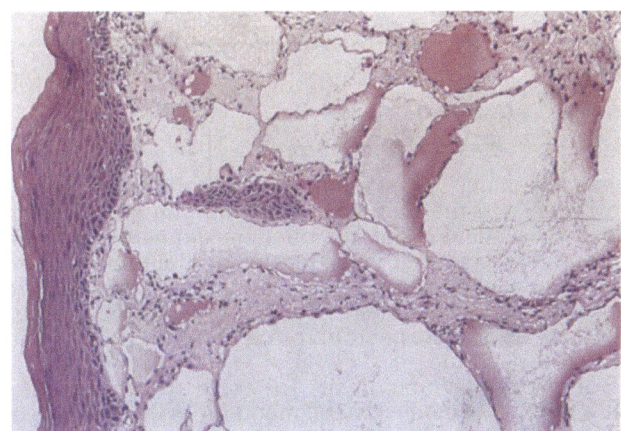

Figure 11.60 Lymphangioma. A lip lesion, consisting of ramifying dilated lymph channels in the subepithelial connective tissue. H & E × 100

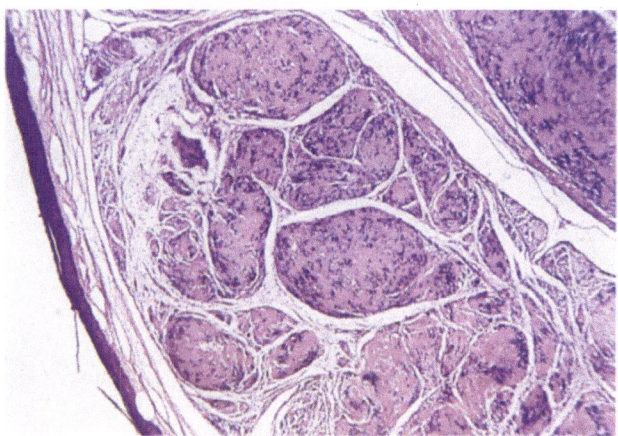

Figure 11.61   Neurilemmoma of mandibular gingiva.   H & E × 100

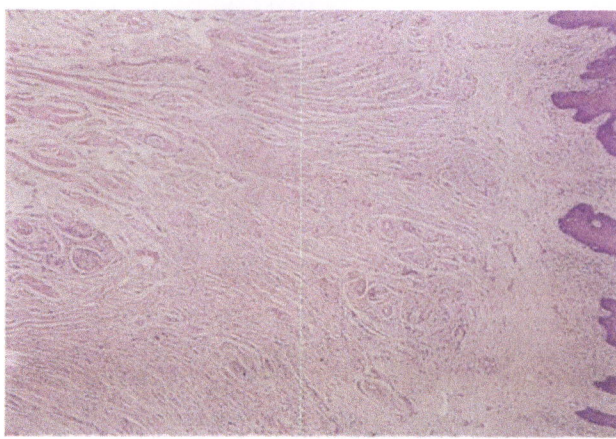

Figure 11.63   Traumatic neuroma, showing numerous nerve fibres intermingled with connective tissue in the oral mucosa.   H & E × 70

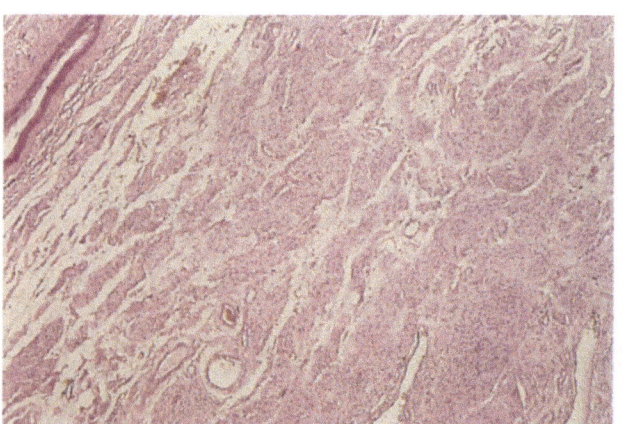

Figure 11.62   Plexiform neuroma. The lesion consists of a mass of thickened and convoluted nerves. A mucous gland duct is seen at top left.   H & E × 100

Neural Tumours

Neurilemmoma and Neurofibroma

These tumours occur both in the oral soft tissues and in the jaws[27]. In the soft tissues the tongue is much the commonest site. Solitary tumours present very much like the commoner fibrous hyperplasias and epulides; these are the usual clinical diagnoses. Multiple lesions are almost certain to be manifestations of neurofibromatosis. They may be discrete neurofibromas or the more ramifying plexiform neuroma.

Bone is not a common site for nerve sheath tumours, but when they do develop the mandible is the bone most commonly affected (Figure 11.61). Most of the tumours are neurofibromas. There is swelling of the jaw, often accompanied by pain or paraesthesia and radiographs show a variable defect. This tends to be unilocular and well defined when the tumour is a neurilemmoma. Neurofibromas are usually associated with a less constant appearance, the radiolucency being unilocular or multilocular and well or poorly defined. When the radiolucency is due to a tumour of the mandibular nerve within the mandibular canal, which it expands, the canal may sometimes still be seen on either side of the radiolucent area and continuous with it.

Neurofibromatosis

Oral lesions are present in some 7% of cases of neurofibromatosis, varying from one or two isolated tumours to widespread involvement of the soft tissues. Rarely, there may be an intraosseous tumour. Macroglossia, usually unilateral and appearing in infants or children, is caused by a plexiform neuroma type of lesion (Figure 11.62). Multiple plexiform neuromas are also seen in the oral mucosa as well as in other mucous membranes in the multiple endocrine neoplasia syndrome.

Malignant Nerve Sheath Tumours

These are very rare and when seen are usually due to malignant change in pre-existing neurofibromas, especially in cases of neurofibromatosis.

Traumatic Neuroma

Traumatic neuromas in the oral tissues are not very common. They may appear following extraction of teeth, or resection or fracture of the jaws (Figure 11.63).

Melanotic Neuroectodermal Tumour of Infancy

This tumour is seen in infants under the age of 12 months, most frequently in the maxilla[28]. Mandibular tumours are much less common and extraoral tumours, mainly in the skull, are rarer still.

The tumour may or may not be well circumscribed and in some cases it has appeared to be multicentric. The cut surface is typically slate blue to grey-black in appearance. Microscopically, two types of cell in a collagenous stroma are seen. Some cells are cubical or slightly flattened with large pale nuclei and they contain small rod-shaped particles of melanin which are often present in large numbers. These pigmented cells are frequently arranged around small cleft-like spaces, or they may form solid masses. The second type of cell is small and round with a well stained nucleus that occupies most of the cell body. These cells,

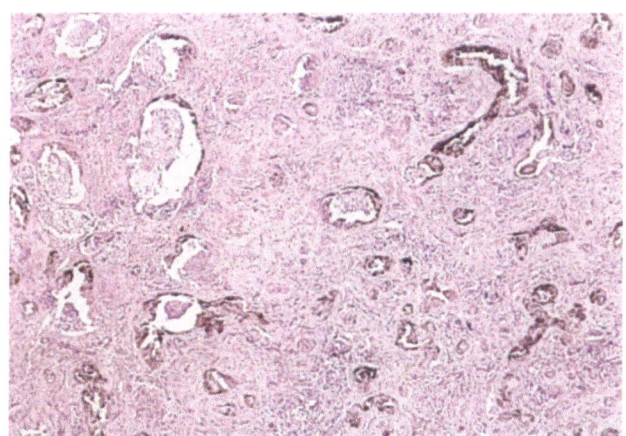

Figure 11.64 Melanotic neuroectodermal tumour. Pigmented cells line spaces in a fibrous stroma. Smaller nonpigmented cells are also present, often within the spaces.   H & E × 100

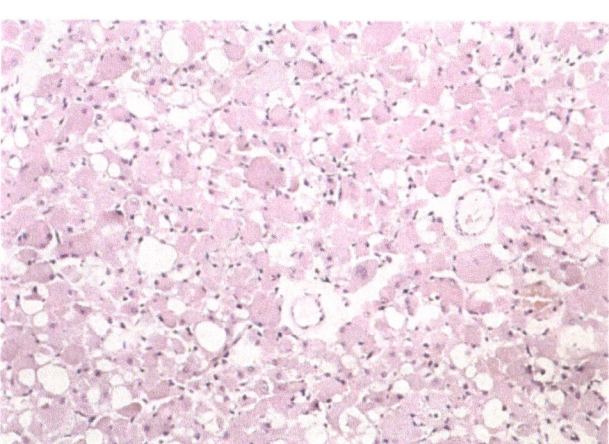

Figure 11.66 Rhabdomyoma. A tumour of the floor of the mouth, consisting of large round cells with eosinophilic granular cytoplasm, which is frequently vacuolated.   H & E × 100

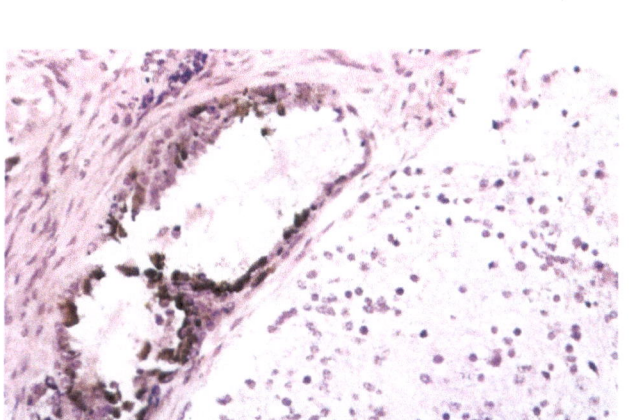

Figure 11.65 Higher magnification, showing a space lined by cells containing the granules of melanin, and smaller nonpigmented cells in a fibrillar matrix. H & E × 250

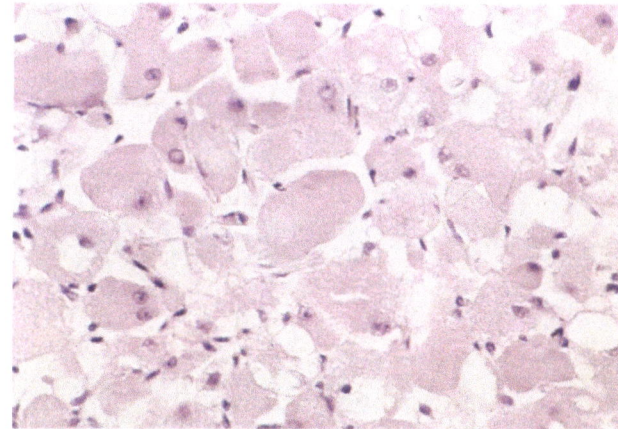

Figure 11.67 Higher magnification from Figure 11.66.   Cross-striations are seen.   H & E × 250

which are nonpigmented, are arranged in groups, often within the spaces lined by the pigmented cells. There may be a fine fibrillar matrix between the cells (Figures 11.64 and 11.65).

The microscopic features of this tumour, combined with its characteristic clinical presentation, which includes increased urinary vanilmandelic acid excretion levels in some cases, will ensure the correct diagnosis. It was only in the earlier cases, before the tumour had become well recognized, that melanoma was considered as a possible diagnosis.

Tumours of Muscle

Rhabdomyoma

The floor of the mouth and the tongue are the commonest sites for this tumour, which is very rare elsewhere in the body, as indeed it is in the mouth[29]. The large granular cells give the tumour a characteristic microscopic appearance; they are not likely to be confused with the granular cells of other tumours such as myoblastoma, since they are much larger, and particularly because cross-striations can readily be demonstrated (Figures 11.66–11.68).

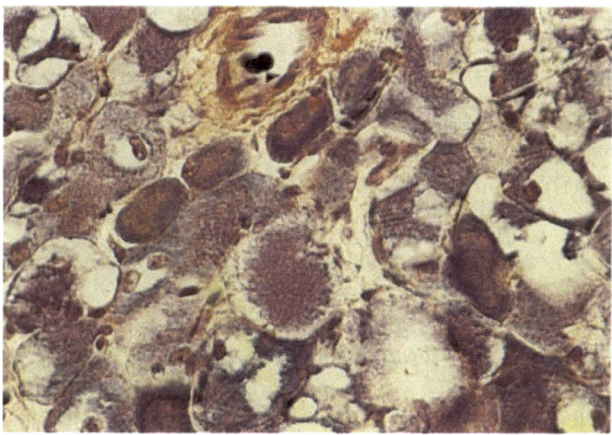

Figure 11.68 The cross-striations are well demonstrated in this PTAH preparation.   × 250

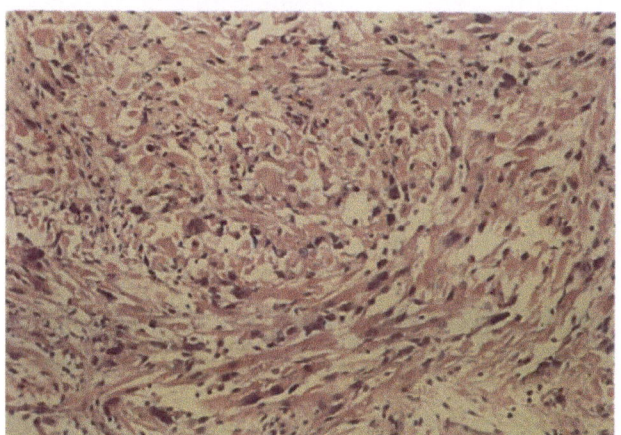

Figure 11.69 Rhabdomyosarcoma. A tumour of the palate, showing the pleomorphic tumour muscle cells.   H & E × 200

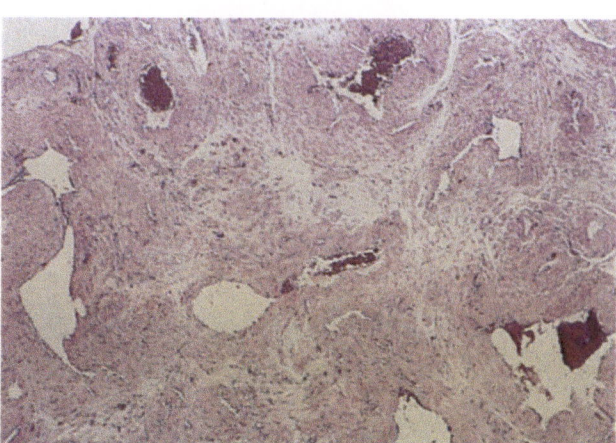

Figure 11.71 Angiomyoma. A tumour of the cheek, consisting of blood vessels with thick muscular walls and surrounding muscle fibres.   H & E × 100

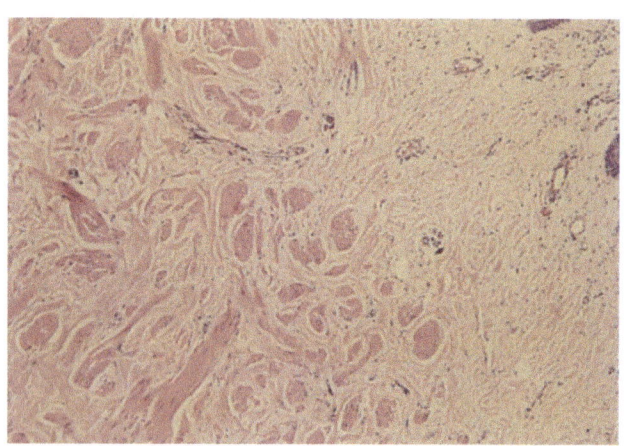

Figure 11.70 Leiomyoma. A tumour of the buccal mucosa, consisting o bundles of smooth muscle fibres.   H & E × 100

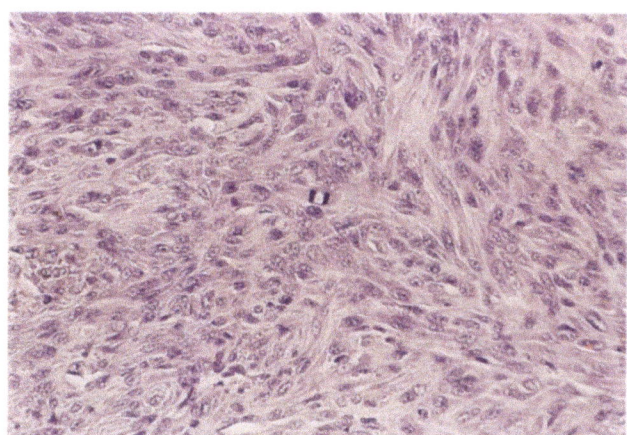

Figure 11.72 Leiomyosarcoma of the cheek, showing pleomorphic smooth muscle cells.   H & E × 400

Rhabdomyosarcoma

When rhabdomyosarcoma arises in the oral tissues, where the tongue, palate, lip and floor of the mouth are the likely sites, it tends to do so as a rather fleshy and polypoid growth, with the usual microscopic features (Figure 11.69)[30].

Leiomyoma and Leiomyosarcoma

These tumours are rare in the mouth, where they present the same microscopic features as elsewhere[31]. Many of the oral lesions are of the angiomyoma type (Figures 11.70–11.72).

Myoblastoma

This tumour is mentioned here for convenience rather than for its questionable origin from muscle cells. The tongue is the commonest site and lesions are occasionally multiple. Differential histological diagnosis centres around two features: the granular cells and the overlying epi-

thelium (Figures 11.73 and 11.74). Granular cells not dissimilar to those of myoblastoma form an occasional component of some odontogenic tumours, notably ameloblastoma, but the odontogenic epithelium is unmistakable and no confusion arises. Rarely, odontogenic fibromas may have a large granular cell element, but again some odontogenic epithelium is likely to be present, even though in small amounts. The congenital epulis, which is seen in the gingiva of newborn infants, is very similar to myoblastoma, but the absence of hyperplasia of the overlying epithelium, the age of the patient and the provenance of the lesion are distinctive features[32].

The epithelium overlying a myoblastoma is frequently the site of striking pseudoepitheliomatous hyperplasia which may closely simulate squamous cell carcinoma. A mistaken diagnosis of carcinoma due to failure to note the underlying granular cells is by no means unknown. As the dorsum of the tongue is a common site for myoblastoma and a rare site for squamous cell carcinoma, a careful examination of the underlying muscle should never be omitted in lesions from this site which appear to be early carcinomas.

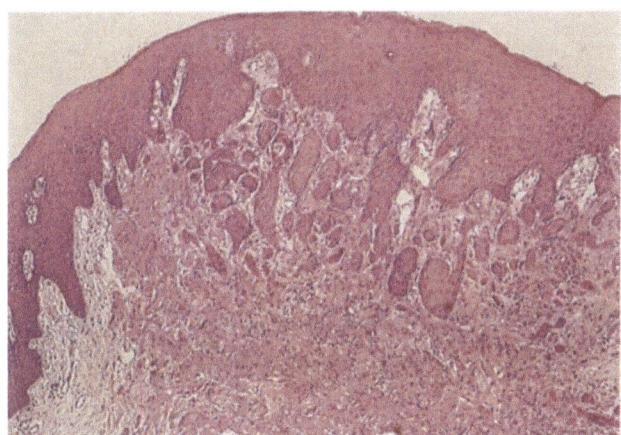

Figure 11.73　Myoblastoma of the cheek. A mass of granular cells occupies the subepithelial area. The overlying epithelium shows pseudoepitheliomatous hyperplasia.　H & E × 70

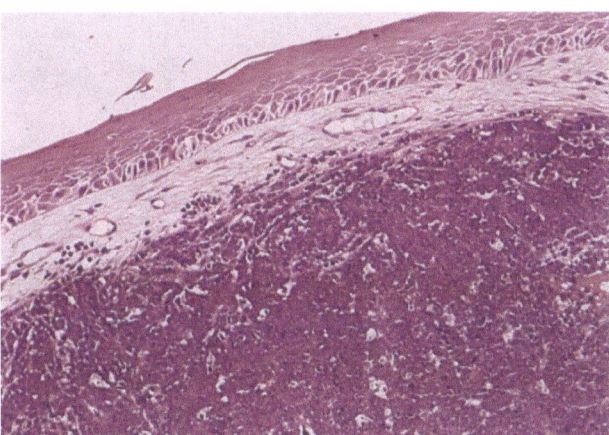

Figure 11.75　Lymphoma. A palatal lesion, showing a clear zone between the lymphomatous tissue and the oral epithelium.　H & E × 100

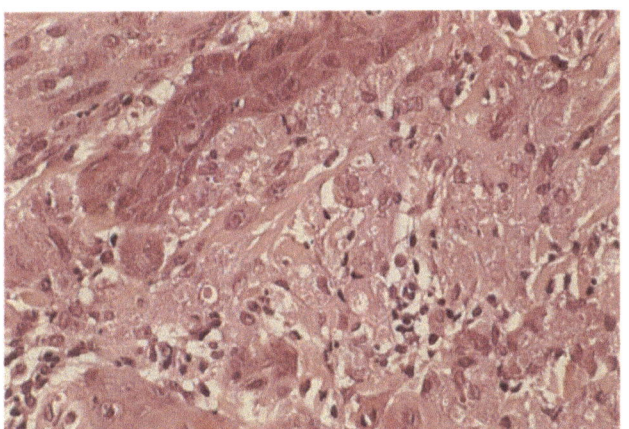

Figure 11.74　Myoblastoma. Higher magnification, showing the granular cells. A strand of squamous epithelium is seen (top), and isolated atypical epithelial cells (bottom).　H & E × 250

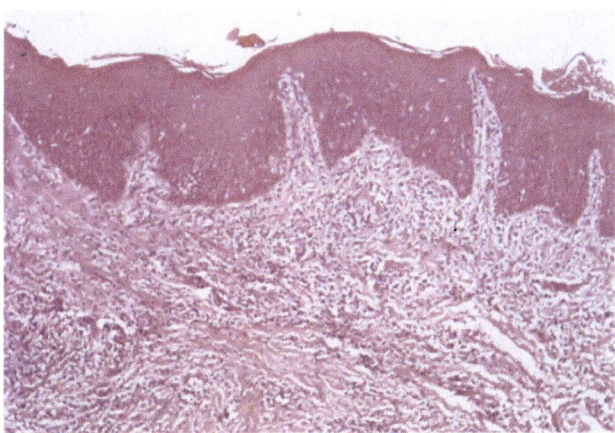

Figure 11.76　Lymphoma. A gingival lesion, with diffuse infiltration of the subepithelial tissues.　H & E × 100

Tumours of Lymphoid Tissue

A detailed account of the histopathology of the lymphomas is given in another volume in this series[33]. Only those features directly concerned with lesions in the oral tissues are noted here.

Oral lesions may be the presenting sign of lymphoma and the presence of a rapidly growing, fleshy, ulcerated tumour would lead the clinician to suspect malignancy. On the other hand, the lesion may be less characteristic and the clinician may suggest acute necrotizing ulcerative gingivitis (Vincent's infection) or some other diagnosis. The pathologist should therefore be prepared to encounter lymphomas in a variety of clinical circumstances[34].

Most lymphomas in the oral tissues are non-Hodgkin lymphomas[35]. Hodgkin's lymphoma is relatively uncommon and the less usual types of lymphoma are rare in the mouth apart from Burkitt's tumour in endemic areas. Microscopically, the important differential diagnosis is from chronic inflammation, which is so common in the oral tissues that neither the clinician nor the pathologist may have the possibility of lymphoma in mind in the same

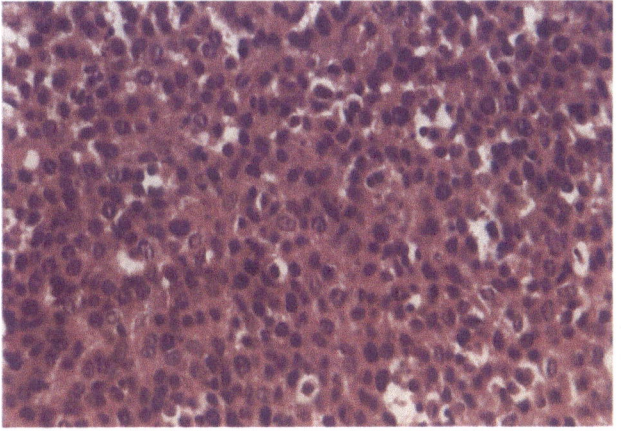

Figure 11.77　Higher magnification, showing the lymphoma cells.　H & E × 250

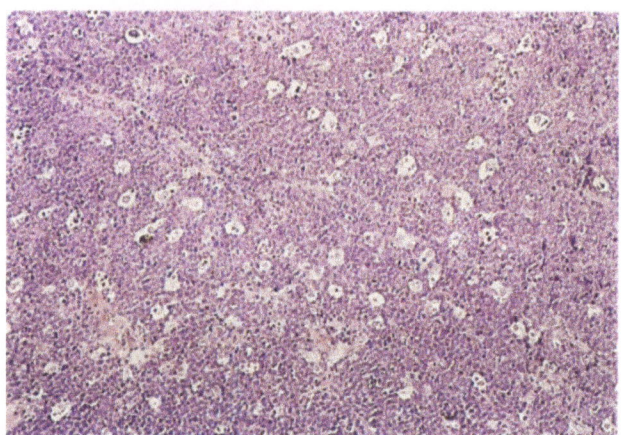

Figure 11.78 Burkitt's lymphoma. A mandibular tumour, showing the 'starry sky' appearance produced by the fat-containing and degenerating histiocytes scattered among the lymphoid cells. H & E × 100

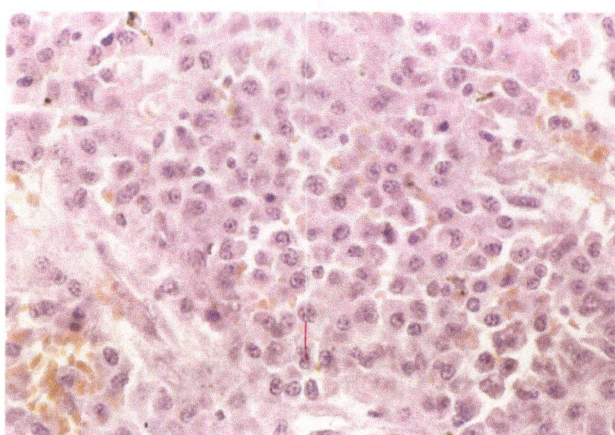

Figure 11.81 Myeloma. A mandibular lesion, consisting of a uniform mass of plasma cells. H & E × 320

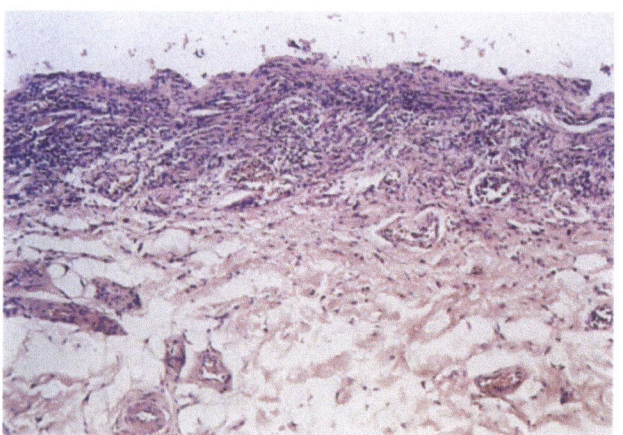

Figure 11.79 An ulcer of the gingiva in chronic myeloid leukaemia. H & E × 100

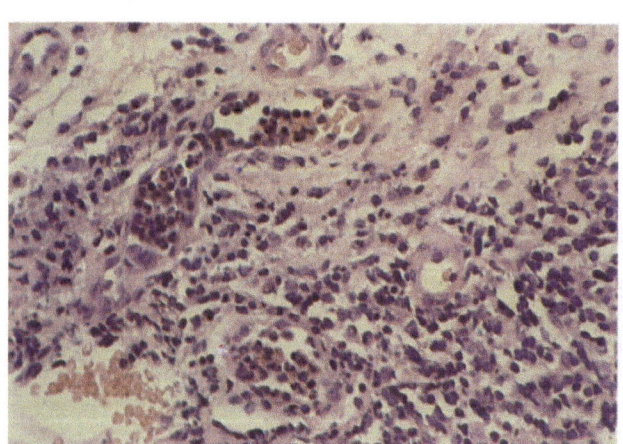

Figure 11.80 Higher magnification from Figure 11.79, showing infiltration by mature and immature myeloid cells. H & E × 250

way that they would if dealing with, say, an enlarged lymph node. A lymphomatous infiltration in the gingivae or other oral tissues presents the same features as elsewhere, but whereas a purely inflammatory infiltration generally extends throughout the corium up to the epithelium, there is often a cell-free zone between a lymphomatous infiltrate and the epithelium. However, if there has been ulceration or infection, this feature may be obscured (Figures 11.75–11.77).

Burkitt's lymphoma is particularly associated with oral lesions, one or more tumours of the jaw frequently being the presenting symptom. These tumours, and the others in the abdominal viscera and elsewhere that are also present, consist of masses of lymphoblasts with interspersed large phagocytic histiocytes (Figure 11.78).

Oral lesions appear in about half the cases of acute leukaemia and are characterized by much swelling, bleeding and ulceration of the mucosa, usually in the gingivae. Other areas of the oral mucosa may sometimes be affected. Biopsy is usually avoided in these cases because of the risk of haemorrhage, the diagnosis being confirmed by haematological examination. However, if biopsy is done the microscopic appearances are the usual ones of a leukaemic infiltration.

Oral lesions are much less common in the chronic leukaemias but, when present, the usual microscopic appearances are seen (Figures 11.79 and 11.80).

Myeloma

Both the multiple and the solitary lesions of myeloma are seen in the oral tissues. Lesions in the jaws appear in 30% or more of cases and there are nearly always multiple lesions in other bones. Occasionally, however, jaw lesions are the first to be noted. Pain, which may be severe, is a common symptom and radiographs generally show the punched-out radiolucencies that are typical of myeloma, although sometimes the appearances are less characteristic. As the lesions expand the bone is destroyed and ultimately the cortex is perforated with the tumour appearing as a fleshy submucosal mass. The microscopic appearances of these lesions, intrabony or in the soft tissues, are the same as those of lesions elsewhere (Figure 11.81).

Amyloidosis is present in up to 10% of patients and it may affect the tongue, causing macroglossia. This can be an early manifestation of the disease, even preceding bone lesions. Amyloid may also be present in the gingivae and buccal mucosa[36].

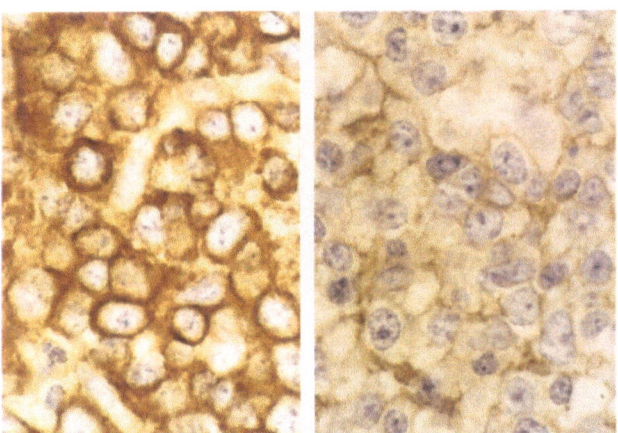

Figure 11.82 Plasmacytoma. This tumour presented clinically as an epulis. Immunoperoxidase staining gives, left, a strong reaction for κ chains, showing the lesion to be monoclonal. Staining for λ chains, right, is essentially negative, as most of the staining seen here is background. ×1000

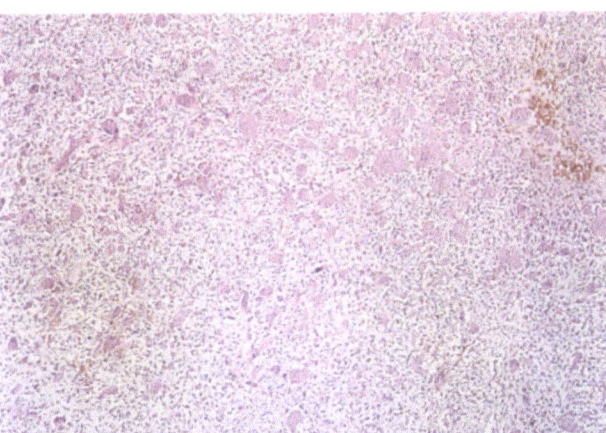

Figure 11.84 Giant cell granuloma of the mandible, showing osteoclast-like giant cells in a spindle cell and fibrous matrix, Small scattered foci of haemorrhage are present, a common feature in these lesions. H & E × 100

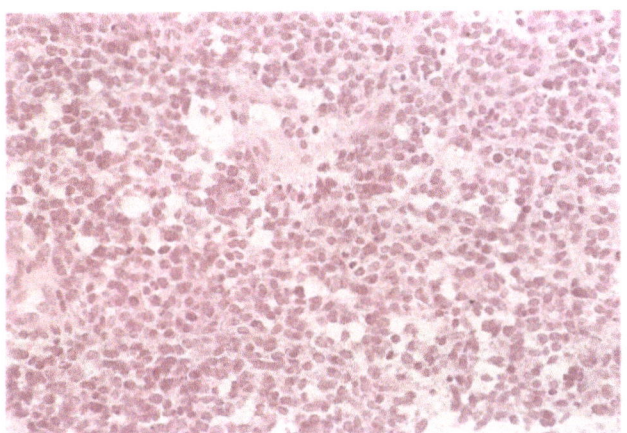

Figure 11.83 Ewing's tumour. A mandibular tumour, consisting of small round cells with rather indistinct outlines. H & E × 250

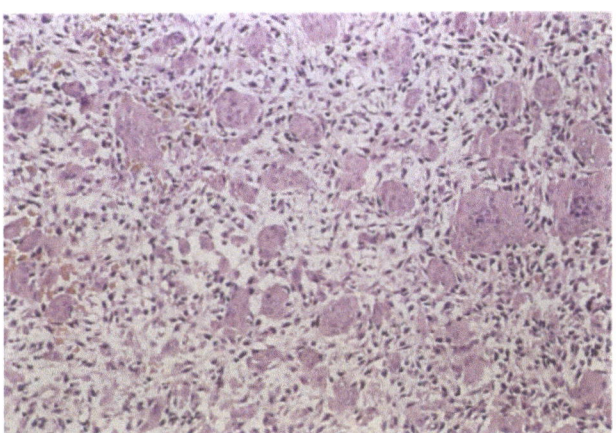

Figure 11.85 Higher magnification from Figure 11.84. Neither the giant cells nor the intervening spindle cells show significant atypia. H & E × 250

Plasmacytoma may develop in the oral soft tissues, usually as a polypoid or pedunculated swelling. Sessile or diffuse lesions are seen less commonly. Plasmacytoma has to be differentiated from non-neoplastic plasma cell infiltration. Inflammatory lesions tend to be more vascular than plasmacytoma and invariably show other types of inflammatory cells. However, as dense plasma cell infiltration is common in many oral inflammatory lesions, especially those of the gingivae, a diagnosis of plasmacytoma should be made with caution. Immunohistochemical demonstration of monoclonality of the plasma cells is the most useful method of confirming the diagnosis (Figure 11.82).

Ewing's Tumour

This tumour is rarely seen in the oral region and when present the mandible is much more often affected than the maxilla[37]. Bone destruction is rapid and the cortex is perforated so that the lesion frequently presents as an ulcerating mass in the soft tissues. Histological diagnosis raises the same difficulties and problems as in other sites (Figure 11.83).

Giant Cell Lesions

Central Giant Cell Granuloma

This tumour-like lesion appears to be practically specific to the jaws. It arises in adolescents and young adults, more often in the mandible than the maxilla, and is characterized by swelling and occasionally pain. The radiographic appearances of a unilocular or multilocular and generally well defined defect are not diagnostic.

Microscopically the lesion is composed of osteoclast-like giant cells in a fibrous matrix that contains many spindle cells (Figure 11.84). To this extent it resembles the giant cell tumour of long and other bones, but the giant cells are usually more patchily distributed than they are in the tumour. However, the nuclear hyperchromatism and pleomorphism that are sometimes seen in the tumour are practically never seen in the granuloma (Figure 11.85). Occasionally a jaw lesion can resemble a long bone tumour very closely, numerous giant cells being evenly distributed throughout the lesion rather than in the usual patchy manner. Sometimes there is moderate mitotic activity in the plump stromal cells[38]. However, the principal distinction between the two lesions is the one with the

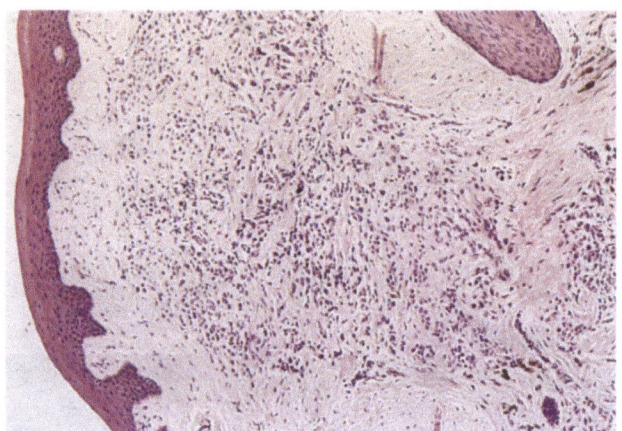

Figure 11.86   Naevus of gingiva. Nests of naevus cells are present in the corium. H & E × 100

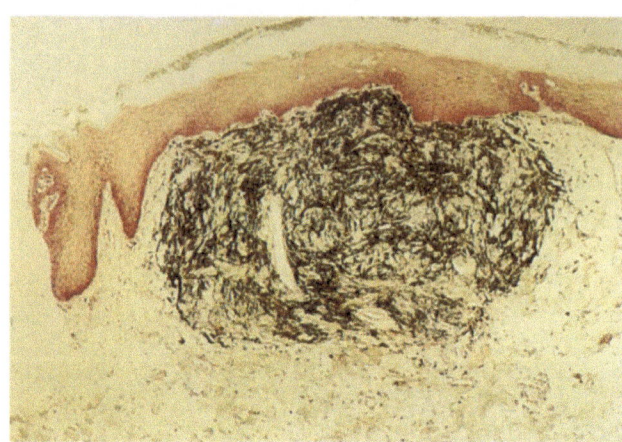

Figure 11.88   Blue naevus. The same lesion as shown in Figure 11.87.   Fontana × 100

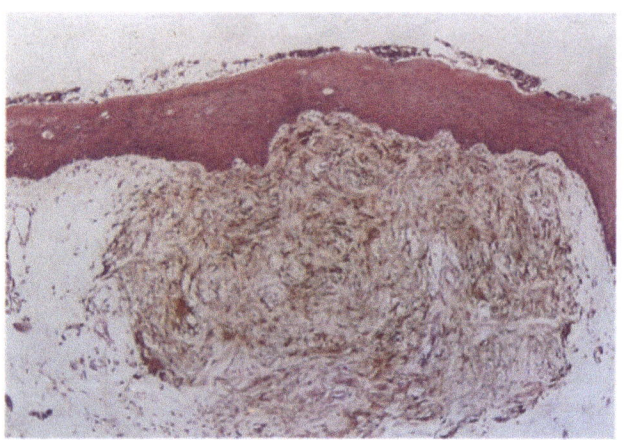

Figure 11.87   Blue naevus. A palatal lesion, consisting of fusiform cells and melanophages.   H & E × 100

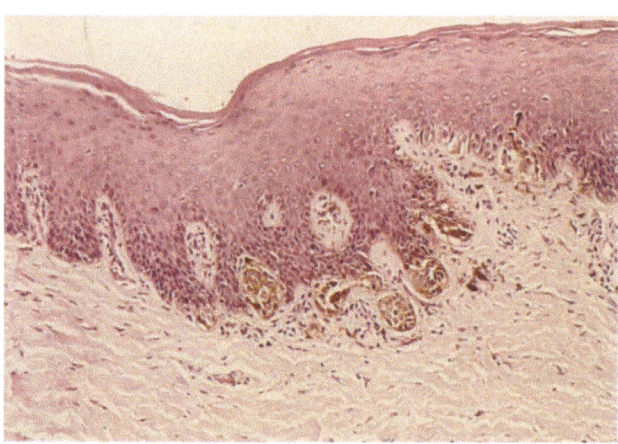

Figure 11.89   Junctional naevus. A palatal lesion. There are focal aggregates of highly pigmented melanocytes at the epitheliomesenchymal junction.   H & E × 250

greatest validity: the difference in behaviour. Although jaw lesions can on occasion prove to be rather aggressive locally, apart from a few exceptional cases they virtually never metastasize, whereas the long bone tumour may occasionally do so. Thus, whatever the histological details of a jaw lesion (provided, of course, that it really is a giant cell granuloma and not some other lesion containing giant cells), there need be no fears of malignancy. Recurrence, however, is not rare. This is mainly due to the desire of the surgeon not to resect the lesion but to curette it, wherever feasible, since this is usually a satisfactory treatment. However, it may occasionally leave small portions of lesional tissue, for example between roots of teeth, so that recurrence is then likely.

Osteoclast-like giant cells may be seen in a number of jaw lesions. Aneurysmal bone cyst can closely resemble giant cell granuloma and these lesions may indeed be related. However, the large blood spaces of the cyst are not seen in a typical granuloma (page 108). Small numbers of giant cells may be seen in fibrous dysplasia and ossifying fibroma (page 71), but a lesion that can be identical to giant cell granuloma and to giant cell tumour is the giant cell lesion of hyperparathyroidism (brown tumour). The lesions in cherubism are also practically identical to those of giant cell granuloma (page 72).

Giant Cell Lesions in Hyperparathyroidism

The focal bone lesions of hyperparathyroidism have a predilection for the jaws and a solitary jaw lesion may be the presenting manifestation. Commencing as an intrabony lesion it is likely, in time, to perforate the cortex and may then be taken for a lesion of the gingiva or giant cell epulis. Since this lesion can be virtually identical to giant cell granuloma and to the 'brown tumour' of hyperparathyroidism, all patients with either intrabony or soft tissue lesions of the giant cell granuloma type should be screened for parathyroid disease.

Naevus and Melanoma

Although the usual varieties of pigmented naevi are seen in the oral mucosa, they are much less common there than in the skin. The usual histological features are observed[39]. Like the benign naevi, malignant melanoma is much rarer in the oral mucosa than it is in the skin, and again the clinicopathological features and varieties are virtually the same for mucosal as for dermal tumours (Figures 11.86–11.90)[40].

Non-neoplastic pigmented lesions are discussed on page 61.

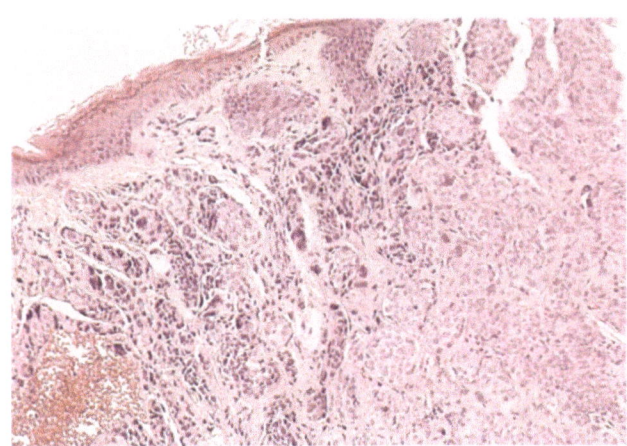

Figure 11.90 Melanoma. A tumour of the palate showing nests and sheets of malignant melanocytes invading the corium.　× 250

References

1. Abbey, L. M., Page, D. G. and Sawyer, D. R. (1980). The clinical and histopathologic features of a series of 464 oral squamous cell papillomas. *Oral Surg.*, **49**, 419

2. Nowparat, B., Howell, F. V. and Rick, G. M. (1981). Verruciform xanthoma. A clinicopathologic review and report of 54 cases. *Oral Surg.*, **51**, 619

3. Bhaskar, S. N., Beasley, J. D. and Cutright, D. E. (1970). Inflammatory papillary hyperplasia of the oral mucosa: report of 341 cases. *J. Amer. Dent. Ass.*, **81**, 949

4. Clausen, F. P. (1969). Histopathology of focal epithelial hyperplasia. *Tandlaegebl.*, **73**, 1013

5. World Health Organization Collaborating Centre for Oral Precancerous Lesions (1978). Definition of leukoplakia and related lesions: an aid to studies on oral precancer. *Oral Surg.*, **46**, 518

6. Pindborg, J. J. (1980). *Oral Cancer and Precancer.* (Bristol: J. Wright & Sons Ltd)

7. Fonts, E. A., Greenlaw, R. H., Rush, B. F. and Rovin, S. (1969). Verrucous squamous cell carcinoma of the oral cavity. *Cancer*, **23**, 152

8. Ellis, G. L. and Corio, R. L. (1980). Spindle cell carcinoma of the oral cavity. A clinicopathologic assessment of fifty-nine cases. *Oral Surg.*, **50**, 523

9. Tomich, C. E. and Hutton, C. E. (1972). Adenoid squamous cell carcinoma of the lip: report of cases. *J. Oral Surg.*, **30**, 592

10. Barker, D. S. and Lucas, R. B. (1967). Localized fibrous overgrowths of the oral mucosa. *Brit. J. Oral Surg.*, **5**, 86

11. Regezi, J. A., Courtney, R. M. and Kerr, D. A. (1975). Fibrous lesions of the skin and mucous membranes which contain stellate and multinucleated giant cells. *Oral Surg.*, **39**, 605

12. Lee, K. W. (1968). The fibrous epulis and related lesions. Granuloma pyogenicum, 'pregnancy tumour', fibro-epithelial polyp and calcifying fibroblastic granuloma. A clinicopathological study. *Periodontics*, **6**, 277

13. Cutright, D. E. (1974). The histopathologic findings in 583 cases of epulis fissuratum. *Oral Surg.*, **37**, 401

14. Werning, J. T. (1979). Nodular fasciitis of the orofacial region. *Oral Surg.*, **48**, 441

15. Melrose, R. J. and Abrams, A. M. (1980). Juvenile fibromatosis affecting the jaws. Report of three cases. *Oral Surg.*, **49**, 317

16. Freedman, P. D., Cardo, V. A., Kerpel, S. M. and Lumerman, H. (1978). Desmoplastic fibroma (fibromatosis) of the jawbones. Report of a case and review of the literature. *Oral Surg.*, **46**, 386

17. Van Blarcom, C. W., Masson, J. K. and Dahlin, D. C. (1971). Fibrosarcoma of the mandible. A clinicopathologic study. *Oral Surg.*, **32**, 428

18. Van Hale, H. McM., Handlers, J. P., Abrams, A. M. and Strahs, G. (1981). Malignant fibrous histiocytoma, myxoid variant metastatic to the oral cavity. Report of a case and review of the literature. *Oral Surg.*, **51**, 156

19. Cannell, H., Langdon, J. D., Patel, M. F. and Rapidis, A. D. (1976). Lipomata in oral tissues. *J. Max-Fac. Surg.*, **4**, 116

20. Huvos, A. G. (1979). *Bone Tumors. Diagnosis, Treatment and Prognosis.* (Philadelphia, London, Toronto: W. B. Saunders Company)

21. Caravolas, J. J., Pierce, J. M., Andrews, J. E. and Nazif, M. M. (1981). Mesenchymal chondrosarcoma of the mandible. *Oral Surg.*, **52**, 478

22. Schneider, L. C., Dolinsky, H. B. and Grodjesk, J. E. (1980). Solitary peripheral osteoma of the jaws: report of case and review of literature. *J. Oral Surg.*, **38**, 452

23. Roca, A. N., Smith, L. J. and Jing, B.-S. (1970). Osteosarcoma and parosteal osteogenic sarcoma of the maxilla and mandible. Study of 20 cases. *Amer. J. Clin. Pathol.*, **54**, 625

24. Ivey, D. M., Delfino, J. J., Sclaroff, A. and Pritchard, L. J. (1980). Intramuscular hemangioma. Report of a case. *Oral Surg.*, **50**, 295

25. Eveson, J. W. and Campbell, H. D. (1977). Central haemangioma of an edentulous mandible. *Brit. J. Oral Surg.*, **14**, 240

26. Dingman, R. O. and Grabb, W. C. (1977). Lymphangioma of the tongue. *Plast. Reconstr. Surg.*, **27**, 714

27. Wright, B. A. and Jackson, D. (1980). Neural tumors of the oral cavity. A review of the spectrum of benign and malignant oral tumors of the oral cavity and jaws. *Oral Surg.*, **49**, 509

28. Cutler, L. S., Chaudhry, A. P. and Topazian, R. (1981). Melanotic neuroectodermal tumor of infancy. An ultrastructural study, literature review and re-evaluation. *Cancer*, **48**, 257

29. Eveson, J. W. and Merchant, N. E. (1978). Sublingual rhabdomyoma. *Int. J. Oral Surg.*, **7**, 27

30. Sada, V. M. (1978). Rhabdomyosarcomas. *Int. J. Oral Surg.*, **7**, 316

31. Farman, A. G. and Kay, S. (1977). Oral leiomyosarcoma. Report of a case and review of the literature pertaining to smooth muscle tumors of the oral cavity. *Oral Surg.*, **43**, 402

32. Regezi, J. A., Batsakis, J. G. and Courtney, R. M. (1979). Granular cell tumors of the head and neck. *J. Oral Surg.*, **37**, 402

33. Arno, J. (1980). *Atlas of Lymph Node Pathology.* (Lancaster: MTP Press Limited)

34. Lehrer, S., Roswit, B. and Federman, Q. (1976). The presentation of malignant lymphoma in the oral cavity and pharynx. *Oral Surg.*, **41**, 441

35. Hashimoto, N. and Kurihara, K. (1982). Pathological characteristics of oral lymphomas. *J. Oral Pathol.*, **11**, 214

36. Flick, W. G. and Lawrence, F. R. (1980). Oral amyloidosis as initial symptom of multiple myeloma. A case report. *Oral Surg.*, **49**, 18

37. Rapoport, A., Sobrinho, J. de A., de Carvalho, M. B., Magrin, J., Costa, F. de Q. and Quadros, J. V. (1977). Ewing's sarcoma of the mandible. *Oral Surg.*, **44**, 89

38. Franklin, C. D., Craig, G. T. and Smith, C. J. (1979). Quantitative analysis of histological parameters in giant cell lesions of the jaws and long bones. *Histopathol.*, **3**, 511

39. Buchner, A. and Hansen, L. S. (1979). Pigmented nevi of the oral mucosa: a clinicopathologic study of 32 new cases and review of 75 cases from the literature. Part I. A clinicopathologic study of 32 new cases. *Oral Surg.*, **48**, 131. Part II. Analysis of 107 cases. *Oral Surg.*, **49**, 55

40. Regezi, J. A., Hayward, J. R. and Pickens, T. N. (1978). Superficial melanomas of oral mucous membranes. *Oral Surg.*, **45**, 730

Index